Asia's Role in Governing Global Health

Asia is rising. The West is not. Similarly, Asian health standards and practices are improving significantly: from the discovery of a new virus in Malaysia to a cost-innovative approach to head surgery in India or to an innovative universal health insurance scheme in Thailand. In short, the world can learn a lot from Asia in this area. And it can also pay more attention to Asian ideas for improving global health governance. This is why this book is both timely and valuable: it provides new and unique insights into new thinking and developments in Asia. Both academics and practitioners will profit by studying this volume in depth.

Kishore Mahbubani, Dean
Lee Kuan Yew School of Public Policy
National University of Singapore

The first of its kind, this informative and insightful volume assembles some of the world's leading global health scholars to examine Asian countries' participation in global health governance. It not only addresses some critical issues of global health governance, but also explores the "distinctiveness" of Asia's conceptions of and contributions to global health governance. It should be of strong interest to students, scholars, practitioners, even laypeople who are keen to learn more about the rise of Asia and its global governance implications.

Yanzhong Huang, Editor
Global Health Governance

With its stellar list of authors from around the world, this book should be required reading for anyone who wants to be sure that global health is not left behind in the changing world order.

David L. Heymann
Head and Senior Fellow, Centre on Global Health Security,
Chatham House, London

This publication is a stellar example of the convergence of technical deliberations and research outputs as policy relevant-normative input – beyond that it is also an important contribution in global health from a region that is fast emerging as an epicenter.

Sania Nishtar, Founder and President
Heartfile

Global geopolitics and health are undergoing unprecedented transitions. How is Asia's growing influence linked to the governance of global health? This book reveals surprising and compelling answers.

Richard Horton, Editor,
The Lancet

The distinguished editors, all with close connections to Asia, have put together a significant contribution to the field of global health politics. The book covers a major gap in the academic literature, Asian countries' approach to global health governance. It is essential reading for those working at the interface of global health and international relations.

Devi Sridhar
Department of Public Health, University of Oxford

Health is occupying an increasingly central role in the global agenda, and Asia has become one of the leading regions in the world. The message of the book edited by Lee, Pang and Tan is that the overlap of these two processes is one of the key developments of our times. This book addresses with clarity, vision and ambition a topic of enormous relevance for everyone working at the intersection of health and globalization.

Julio Frenk
Dean of the Harvard School of Public Health

In an era of rapid and extensive globalisation, the world faces a wide range of transboundary problems that require effective collective action. Key among these are threats to human health that do not recognise national borders, and include emerging and re-emerging infections, rising rates of chronic diseases, inadequate access to affordable and safe medicines, spreading anti-microbial resistance and the health effects of climate change. These threats require a transnational response and thus pose significant challenges to global health governance, as well as to long established notions of national sovereignty.

This book investigates the neglected question of the impact of a rising Asia on the management of transboundary health problems. The chapters examine the role played by Asia in the governance of a range of global health issues, from development assistance in health, to global health instruments dealing with tobacco control and disease outbreaks, to health research and knowledge products, and the book concludes by examining the broad themes of a rising Asia's role in the complexity of global health governance. The various analyses are tied together by a common focus on Asian countries' use of the sovereignty principle, and seek to understand how traditional notions of national sovereignty can both clash with, and enhance, governance objectives in global health. In addition, the contributors examine the interaction between global, regional and domestic institutions, and present current ideas in Asia on the challenge of governing global health.

With an inter-disciplinary approach that combines international relations, public policy and public health, this book will be invaluable to both scholars and policy makers working in these fields, as well as Asian politics, social policy and governance more generally.

Kelley Lee is a Professor in the Faculty of Health Sciences, Simon Fraser University, Canada and the London School of Hygiene and Tropical Medicine, UK.

Tikki Pang is a Visiting Professor at the LKY School of Public Policy, National University of Singapore and was previously Director of Research Policy & Cooperation, World Health Organization, Geneva, Switzerland.

Yeling Tan is a PhD candidate at the John F Kennedy School of Government, Harvard University, USA.

Routledge Contemporary Asia Series

1. Taiwan and Post-Communist Europe
Shopping for Allies
Czeslaw Tubilewicz

2. The Asia-Europe Meeting
The Theory and Practice of Interregionalism
Alfredo C. Robles, Jr

3. Islamic Legitimacy in a Plural Asia
Edited by Anthony Reid and Michael Gilsenan

4 .Asian-European Relations
Building Blocks for Global Governance?
Edited by Jürgen Rüland, Gunter Schubert, Günter Schucher and Cornelia Storz

5. Taiwan's Environmental Struggle
Toward a Green Silicon Island
Jack F. Williams and Ch'ang-yi David Chang

6. Taiwan's Relations with Mainland China
A Tail Wagging Two Dogs
Su Chi

7. The Politics of Civic Space in Asia
Building Urban Communities
Edited by Amrita Daniere and Mike Douglass

8. Trade and Contemporary Society Along the Silk Road
An Ethno-History of Ladakh
Jacqueline Fewkes

9. Lessons from the Asian Financial Crisis
Edited by Richard Carney

10. Kim Jong Il's Leadership of North Korea
Jae-Cheon Lim

11. Education as a Political Tool in Asia
Edited by Marie Lall and Edward Vickers

12. Human Genetic Biobanks in Asia
Politics of Trust and Scientific Advancement
Edited by Margaret Sleeboom-Faulkner

13. East Asian Regionalism from a Legal Perspective
Current features and a vision for the future
Edited by Tamio Nakamura

14. Dissent and Cultural Resistance in Asia's Cities
Edited by Melissa Butcher and Selvaraj Velayutham

15. Preventing Corruption in Asia
Institutional Design and Policy Capacity
Edited by Ting Gong and Stephen Ma

16. Expansion of Trade and FDI in Asia
Strategic and Policy challenges
Edited by Julien Chaisse and Philippe Gugler

17. Business Innovation in Asia
Knowledge and technology networks from Japan
Dennis McNamara

18. Regional Minorities and Development in Asia
Edited by Huhua Cao and Elizabeth Morrell

19. Regionalism in China-Vietnam Relations
Institution-Building in the Greater Mekong Subregion
Oliver Hensengerth

20. From Orientalism to Postcolonialism
Asia-Europe and the Lineages of Difference
Edited by Sucheta Mazumdar, Kaiwar Vasant and Thierry Labica

21. Politics and Change in Singapore and Hong Kong
Containing Contention
Stephan Ortmann

22. Inter-Ethnic Dynamics in Asia
Considering the Other through Ethnonyms, Territories and Rituals
Edited by Christian Culas and François Robinne

23. Asia and Latin America
Political, Economic and Multilateral Relations
Edited by Jörn Dosch and Olaf Jacob

24. Japan and Africa
Globalization and Foreign Aid in the 21st Century
Edited by Howard P. Lehman

25. De-Westernizing Communication Research
Altering Questions and Changing Frameworks
Edited by Georgette Wang

26. Asian Cities, Migrant Labor and Contested Spaces
Edited by Tai-Chee Wong and Jonathan Rigg

27. Diaspora Literature and Visual Culture: Asia in Flight
Sheng-mei Ma

28. Alterities in Asia
Reflections on Identity and Regionalism
Edited by Leong Yew

29. Soft Power in Japan-China Relations:
State, Sub-state and Non-state Relations
Utpal Vyas

30. Enhancing Asia-Europe Co-operation through Educational Exchange
Georg Wiessala

31. History Textbooks and the Wars in Asia
Divided Memories
Edited by Gi-Wook Shin and Daniel C. Sneider

32. The Politics of Religion in South and Southeast Asia
Edited by Ishtiaq Ahmed

33. The Chinese/Vietnamese Diaspora
Revisiting the Boatpeople
Edited by Yuk Wah Chan

34. The Dynamics of Social Capital and Civic Engagement in Asia
Vibrant Societies
Edited by Amrita Daniere and Hy Van Luong

35. Eurasia's Ascent in Energy and Geopolitics
Rivalry or Partnership for China, Russia and Central Asia?
Edited by Robert E. Bedeski & Niklas Swanström

36. Asian Popular Culture in Transition
Edited by John A. Lent and Lorna Fitzsimmons

37. Sexual Diversity in Asia, c. 600 – 1950
Edited by Raquel Reyes and William G. Clarence Smith

38. Asia's Role in Governing Global Health
Edited by Kelley Lee, Tikki Pang and Yeling Tan

Asia's Role in Governing Global Health

Edited by
Kelley Lee, Tikki Pang
and Yeling Tan

Routledge
Taylor & Francis Group
LONDON AND NEW YORK

First published 2013
by Routledge
2 Park Square, Milton Park, Abingdon, Oxon OX14 4RN

Simultaneously published in the USA and Canada
by Routledge
711 Third Avenue, New York, NY 10017

Routledge is an imprint of the Taylor & Francis Group, an informa business

British Library Cataloguing in Publication Data
A catalogue record for this book is available from the British Library

Library of Congress Cataloging in Publication Data
Asia's role in governing global health / edited by Kelley Lee, Tikki Pang, and Yeling Tan.
p. ; cm. — (Routledge contemporary Asia series ; 38)
Includes bibliographical references and index.
I. Lee, Kelley, 1962- II. Pang, T. (Tikki) III. Tan, Yeling. IV. Series: Routledge contemporary Asia series ; 38.
[DNLM: 1. World Health—Asia. 2. Health Policy—Asia. 3. Health Services Administration—Asia. 4. International Cooperation—Asia. 5. Politics—Asia. WA 530 JA1]
362.1095—dc23

2012042915

ISBN: 978-0-415-50343-3 (hbk)
ISBN: 978-0-203-08121-1 (ebk)

Typeset in Times New Roman
by RefineCatch Limited, Bungay, Suffolk

Contents

Illustrations

Figures

Tables

Boxes

Contributors

Sara Bennett Ph.D. is Associate Professor at the Johns Hopkins Bloomberg School of Public Health. Her research seeks to understand and address institutional and capacity challenges in promoting stronger governance for health in low- and middle-income countries. Dr Bennett was previously the Executive Director of the WHO's Alliance for Health Policy and Systems Research of which she is now a board member, She is also editor of the journal *Health Policy and Planning*. Dr Bennett has authored over 35 peer-reviewed papers, 4 books and multiple policy and briefing notes.

Somsak Chunharas is Secretary General of the National Health Foundation, a non-governmental agency in Thailand promoting evidence-based health systems and policy development. He is a medical doctor, founding Director of the Health System Research Institute (HSRI) and Director of the Bureau of Policy and Planning in the Thai Ministry of Public Health. He served as a member of various international boards and committees dealing with health research including the WHO Global Advisory Committee on Health Research and Global Alliances for Health Policy and System Research. Two key areas of work are the development of national health research systems and equal research partnerships between developing and developed country partners, and health system strengthening.

David P. Fidler, BA, MPhil, JD, BCL, is the James Louis Calamaras Professor of Law at the Indiana University Maurer School of Law and Associate Fellow of the Centre on Global Health Security at Chatham House. He is a leading expert on international law and global health.

Lawrence O. Gostin is Professor in Global Health Law at Georgetown, Faculty Director of the O'Neill Institute for National and Global Health Law, and Director of the WHO Collaborating Centre on Public Health Law and Human Rights. He has chaired numerous National Academy of Sciences committees, proposed a Framework Convention on Global Health endorsed by the UN Secretary General, served on the WHO Director's Ad Hoc Advisory Committee on Reforming the WHO, drafted a Model Public Health Law for WHO and the CDC, directed the National Council of Civil Liberties and the National

Association for Mental Health in the United Kingdom, where he wrote the Mental Health Act and brought landmark cases before the European Court of Human Rights. In the United Kingdom, he was awarded the Rosemary Delbridge Prize for a person 'who has most influenced Parliament and government to act for the welfare of society'.

Aravinda Meera Guntupalli, BSc, MA, MPS, Ph.D., is a lecturer in the Faculty of Social and Human Sciences at the University of Southampton. Her research interests are well-being and health, and her recent work is concerned with life-course epidemiology, gender differentials, nutritional transition and reproductive health. Since 2001, she has worked on inequality, welfare and health issues using large-scale surveys and historical datasets. Dr Guntupalli applies both qualitative and quantitative methods and her interdisciplinary background is reflected in her published work.

Adam Kamradt-Scott is Senior Lecturer in International Security Studies, Centre for International Security Studies, Department of Government and International Relations at the University of Sydney; and Honorary Lecturer in the Department of Global Health and Development, London School of Hygiene and Tropical Medicine. His research and teaching interests include global health security, health diplomacy and pandemic preparedness (with a particular regional focus on the Asia-Pacific region). Dr. Kamradt-Scott has published numerous journal articles and book chapters on these themes, and has two forthcoming books entitled *Disease diplomacy* (Johns Hopkins University Press with Sara Davies and Simon Rushton) and *Managing global health security* (Palgrave Macmillan).

Wayne Kao, BA, MA, is a Ph.D. candidate in health and leisure studies at New York University. His current work focuses on tobacco-control programs, including monitoring Taiwan's progress in the implementation of the Framework Convention on Tobacco Control.

Mathias Koenig-Archibugi is Senior Lecturer in Global Politics at the London School of Economics and Political Science. His research focuses on global governance, especially in the domain of health and labour, and on the possibility of democratising global politics. His articles have been published in the *European Journal of International Relations*, *Governance*, *International Organization*, *Philosophy and Public Affairs*, and other journals, and he has co-edited five books on various aspects of global politics.

Kelley Lee, BA, MPA, MA, DPhil, FFPH, is Associate Dean, Research, Director of Global Health and Professor in the Faculty of Health Sciences, Simon Fraser University; and Professor of Global Health Policy at the London School of Hygiene and Tropical Medicine. Her research and teaching focuses on the impacts of globalisation on communicable and non-communicable diseases, and the implications for emerging forms of global governance. She has authored over 75 scholarly papers, 40 book chapters and 9 books including

The World Health Organization (Routledge, 2008) and *Global health and international relations* (Polity Press, 2012 with Colin McInnes).

Hang Li is Director of the International Training Project in the Center for Human and Economic Development at Peking University. His academic interests include the application of management in the area of human development. He is the co-translator of the Chinese version of Amartya Sen's monumental work, *The idea of justice* (Penguin, 2010). He is also experienced in project management and international training programmes.

Aming Liu, Ph.D., is Associate Professor in the Institute of International Relations at the Shanghai Academy of Social Sciences. Her research and teaching focuses on international relations in East Asia and China's foreign policy. She has authored over 20 scholarly papers and one book.

Minquan Liu, MPhil, DPhil, is Professor and Chair of the Department of Development Economics, and the Founding Director of the Center for Human and Economic Development Studies at Peking University. His research has focused on human development in China and other Asian economies. He has contributed to high-level consultations by the UN Department of Economic and Social Affairs on poverty eradication and the post-2015 agenda. He has also led major research projects on rural development, rural finance, health, education, environment and poverty in China. His publications have appeared in leading Chinese and international journals.

Suerie Moon, BA, MPA, Ph.D., is Research Director and Co-Chair of the Forum on Global Governance for Health, Harvard Global Health Institute, and Project Co-Director, Innovation and Access to Technologies for Sustainable Development, Sustainability Science Program, Harvard Kennedy School of Government. Her work focuses on global governance, the evolution of international regimes, the political economy of global health (particularly innovation, access to medicines, intellectual property and equity), and innovative policies for addressing global problems. She has authored numerous articles, papers and other scholarly works including *Informal norms in global governance: negotiating global intellectual property rules, human rights and access to medicines* (Ashgate 2012 with Wolfgang Hein).

Karthik Nachiappan is a Research Associate at the Centre on Asia and Globalisation, Lee Kuan Yew School of Public Policy at the National University of Singapore. His current research investigates Asia's evolving relationship with global governance, with a specific focus on health and energy governance.

Tikki Pang (Pangestu), BSc(Hons), Ph.D., FRCPath, is Visiting Professor, Lee Kuan Yew School of Public Policy, National University of Singapore and former Director of Research Policy and Cooperation at the World Health Organization in Geneva, Switzerland. His research, work experience and teaching focuses on global health and global health research governance, the use of evidence in policy formulation, knowledge translation, national health research systems and emerging/re-emerging infectious diseases. He has authored over 200 scholarly papers, 20 book chapters and authored/edited 10 books including *Genomics and world health* (WHO, 2002 with David Weatherall) and the *World report on knowledge for better health* (WHO, 2004).

Christine Pilcavage, BA, MIA, MPH, is the Director and a founding partner of Innovative Development Expertise and Advisory Services, an international consultancy group based in Boston dedicated to strengthening health systems in resource-constrained countries. For nearly 20 years, Ms Pilcavage has advised government, non-governmental and grass roots organisations on business processes, cultural competence, governance, leadership and the application of best practices in public health. She has extensive field experience in Asia and Africa while working with USAID and JICA. She was raised in Japan and is a graduate of the University of California, San Diego and Columbia University.

Thaworn Sakunphanit, MD, BA, MSc, FRCP, is Deputy Director of the Health Insurance System Research Office, Health System Research Institute, Thailand. He serves on many subcommittees of the Social Security Office, Civil Servant Medical Benefits Scheme, the National Health Security Office and Ministry of Public Health. His research focuses on health care financing, health care management, health system research and social protection policy. He has authored around 30 publications and book chapters in Thai and English.

Nicole Szlezák, MPA, MD, DrMed, Ph.D., was born in Zürich and grew up in Switzerland, Germany, and the United States. Trained in medicine and public policy, her main interests are in the interconnections of science, health policy and society. She was a Research Rellow at the Center for International Development at Harvard University from 2003–2008. Since 2009, she has worked for McKinsey & Company where she advises clients in the health care domain on topics of strategic management and organizational development. Dr Szlezák has also worked as a clinical researcher on malaria and other tropical diseases. She has published in *PLoS Medicine,* the *Bulletin of the World Health Organization, Nature Medicine* and the *Proceedings of the National Academies of Science.*

Yeling Tan, BA, MPA, is a Ph.D. candidate at the John F. Kennedy School of Government, Harvard University. Her research interests are on China and global governance. As a Research Fellow at the National University of Singapore, she analysed governance innovations at local and global levels. In the Policy Office of the Singapore Ministry of Defence, she covered Singapore's defence relations with Indonesia and the United States. She has also worked for The Asia Foundation in Singapore, Bangladesh and Indonesia. She is co-author (with Ann Florini and Hairong Lai) of *China experiments: from local innovations to national reform* (Brookings Institution Press, 2012).

Jenny Qu Wang is a Ph.D. candidate in political science at the University of Vienna. She is a Research Fellow in the Center for Human and Economic

Development Studies at Peking University, and Vienna University of Economics and Business. She has studied and published extensively on China's health care and health care-system reforms, especially on maternal and child health. Her recent research has focused on governance issue of health care, including local and global governance issues.

Tao Wei, BM, MPH, is Associate Research Librarian in the Library of the Kunming Medical University, a Ph.D candidate at the Public Health School of the Kunming Medical University a Member of Yunnan Participatory Research Association, and a Member of the Yunnan Health and Development Research Association. His research and teaching focuses on information literacy, evidence-based medicine and social medicine. He has authored over twenty scholarly papers, three book chapters and one book entitled *Community health and development* (Han, 2006).

Jingying Xu, BSc, PgDip, MSc, is a Ph.D. candidate in the Department of Global Health and Development at the London School of Hygiene and Tropical Medicine. Her doctoral research examines China's policy on counterfeit medicines and its implications for global health governance. She holds a Masters in management and economics and a Postgraduate Diploma in econometrics and mathematical economics from the London School of Economics and Political Science. She has worked previously as a research assistant in the Centre on Global Change and Health, LSHTM and the Institute for Global Health, Peking University.

Sungwon Yoon, B.Soc.Sc, MPH, Ph.D., is a postdoctoral fellow in the Department of Community Medicine, Li Ka Shing Faculty of Medicine and the School of Public Health of the University of Hong Kong. Her research interest lies in global health governance, primarily with regard to the role of state and non-state actors in global health policy-making as well as health and development issues in East Asia. More recently, she has expanded the scope of her research interests to include public health issues related to alcohol policy.

Foreword

Global health has grown in prominence on the international agenda over the past decade. This is a logical development, considering that health is at the core of every individual's existence, regardless of where they live. But the discourse on global health remains fragmented. Even discussions about health systems, which by definition should take a comprehensive perspective, tend to splinter into analyses of individual building blocks rather than focusing on complex, integrated systems.

Of the six building blocks of health systems identified by the World Health Organization – service delivery, health workforce, information, medical products, financing and governance – it is the last element, governance, that is the key to integrating all of the components of health systems. But this is also the area that has suffered from a dearth of in-depth analysis and consideration.

There have been many attempts in global health policy making to create more synergy between efforts to deal with specific diseases and broader efforts to strengthen health systems, with both approaches aiming for the ultimate goal of improving health outcomes. However, in practice, there simply is not a sufficient body of policy research to promote a real merger of these two approaches. On top of that, even in the area of health-system strengthening, priority has been put on three components of health systems – financing, human resources and information – and policies regarding each tend to be limited to the individual component.

So even while policy-oriented research on specific aspects of health system strengthening and policy research on individual topics within the global health field have progressed, there has been little strategic and practical research that promotes health-system strengthening by looking at the whole system in each country and developing a plan for a comprehensive health system. In addition, there are more than 150 global health initiatives around the world, which can be confusing to partner countries and communities. So one policy question that we must ask ourselves is how can we reform and strengthen the governance system in the global health field so that it can more effectively address the real challenges that we face in the field?

In that sense, research on health system governance needs to look at the big picture and explore the various aspects of health systems in a comprehensive manner. To do that, policies need to be designed in a way that brings the different areas together, and one might say that this question of governance is the most important research topic today.

The 23 young authors whose work is presented in this volume have made an important contribution to the field of global health through their examination of various topics of global health governance. By focusing their study on Asian perspectives, they also bring a significant voice to the table that is not always heard in the global health governance discourse.

I have no doubt that this publication will go a long way in furthering debate about how to create and maintain health systems that can achieve their ultimate goal – improving the health status and lives of the people they serve and helping us create a global system of governance that will enhance human security. I hope that it is only one of many such studies to come on this crucial topic of global health governance.

Keizo Takemi
Senior Fellow, Japan Center for International Exchange
Tokyo, April 2012

Acknowledgements

This book is the product of many hands and many minds. The editors wish to thank Dr Seng Tee Lee, above all, for his support for strengthening global health governance research in Asia through his generous core funding of this project. Additional financial support for specific case studies was provided through the National Cancer Institute, US National Institutes of Health (Grant Number CA91021), and the European Research Council under the European Community's Seventh Framework Programme – Ideas Grant 230489 GHG. The project also received support from the Rockefeller Foundation Bellagio Centre which served as the venue for one of the project's key workshops.

We are very grateful to the Dean of the Lee Kuan Yew School of Public Policy, Professor Kishore Mahbubani and Professor Ann Florini, former Director of the Centre on Asia and Globalization at the School, for their initial conceptualisation of the project, steering the overall development of the S. T. Lee Project on Global Governance, and securing the major sources of financial support.

For providing essential administrative support for this project, including the production of this book, we acknowledge the important role of Sung Lee, National University of Singapore. Additional key support was received from Jasmin Kaur, Juliana Wilson, Claire Leow, Sandra Ng and Michele von Rautenkranz at the Lee Kuan Yew School of Public Policy, National University of Singapore. At the London School of Hygiene and Tropical Medicine, we would like to thank Ela Gohil and, at Simon Fraser University, Jennifer Fang was invaluable in assembling the final manuscript.

Finally, we express our appreciation for the valued inputs of the following individuals who contributed to our intellectual journey either through their participation in workshops, commenting on draft chapters or facilitating the conduct of the case studies: Laurie Garrett, Steve Stedman (Stanford University), Fatima Alvarez Castillo (University of the Philippines), Lucy Chen (Beijing University), Abdul Ghaffar (Alliance for Health Policy and Systems Research), Pak K. Lee (University of Kent), Sanir Nishtar (Heartfile, Pakistan), Phua Kai Hong (National University of Singapore), Devi Sridhar (Oxford University) and Keizo Takemi (Tokai University).

Abbreviations

ADB	Asian Development Bank
AfDB	African Development Bank
AIDS	acquired immune deficiency syndrome
APACT	Asian Pacific Conference on Tobacco or Health
APEC	Asia-Pacific Economic Cooperation
APEIR	Asian Partnership on Emerging Infectious Diseases Research
APHIS	animal and plant health inspection service
APSED	Asia-Pacific Strategy for Emerging Diseases
ART	antiretroviral therapy
ARV	antiretroviral
ASEAN	Association of Southeast Asian Nations
ASH	Action on Smoking and Health
BAT	British American Tobacco
BIEC	Bureau of International Economic Cooperation
BMGF	Bill and Melinda Gates Foundation
BMS	Bristol Myers Squibb
BRICS	Brazil, Russia, India, China and South Africa
CAP	Country Assistance Programme
CBD	Convention on Biological Diversity
CDC	Center for Disease Control
CESCR	UN Committee on Economic, Social and Cultural Rights
CHAFC	China's health aid to foreign countries
CIDA	Canadian International Development Agency
CIPIH	WHO Commission on Intellectual Property, Innovation and Public Health
CL	compulsory licensing
CMTs	Chinese Medical Teams
CNDR	Commission of National Development and Reform
CNTC	China National Tobacco Corporation
COHRED	Council on Health Research for Development
COP	Conference of the Parties
CSO	civil society organization
CWF	China Women's Federation

DAC	Development Assistance Committee
DAFC	Department of Aid to Foreign Countries (China)
DAH	development assistance for health
ddI	didanosine
DEA	Department of Economic Affairs (India)
DIC	Department of International Cooperation (China)
DITEA	Department of International Trade and Economic Affairs (China)
DNDi	Drugs for Neglected Diseases
DPJ	Democratic Party of Japan
ECO	Economic Counselor's Office
EHF	ebola haemorrhagic fever
EIBC	Export–Import Bank of China
EINet	Emerging Infectious Network
EMRO	Eastern Mediterranean Regional Office of the World Health Organization
ETS	environmental tobacco smoke
FAO	Food and Agriculture Organization
FCA	Framework Convention Alliance
FCGH	Framework Convention on Global Health
FCTC	Framework Convention on Tobacco Control
FOCAC	Forum of China and Africa Cooperation
G7	Group of Seven
G8	Group of Eight
GA	grant assistance
GATT	Generalized Agreement on Tariffs and Trade
GAVI	Global Alliance for Vaccines and Immunisation
GDP	gross domestic product
GFATM	Global Fund to Fight HIV/AIDS, Tuberculosis and Malaria
GGH	global governance for health
GHG	global health governance
GHRG	global health research governance
GII	Global Issues Initiative
GISN	Global Influenza Surveillance Network
GNI	gross national income
GOARN	Global Outbreak Alert and Response Network
GSK	GlaxoSmithKline
HBV	hepatitis B vaccine
HDI	Human Development Index
HIPCs	highly indebted poor countries
HRP	Special Program on Human and Reproductive Health Research
HSRI	Health Systems Research Institute (Thailand)
HTF	Health Task Force (ASEAN)
IAVI	International AIDS Vaccine Initiative
IBSA	India–Brazil–South Africa

ICO	International Communication Office of the CPC (China)
IDB	Inter-American Development Bank
IDI	Infectious Diseases Initiative
IDRC	International Development Research Centre (Canada)
IGO	intergovernmental organisation
IGWG	intergovernmental working group
IHP	International Health Partnership
IHR	International Health Regulations
IMCJ	International Medical Center of Japan
IMF	International Monetary Fund
INB	Intergovernmental Negotiating Body
INGO	international non-governmental organizations
IP	intellectual property
IPAB	Intellectual Property Appellate Board
IPRs	intellectual property rights
ISR	International Sanitary Regulations
ITEC	Indian Technical and Cooperation Programme
JALI	Joint Action and Learning Initiative on National and Global Responsibilities for Health
JCIE	Japan Center for International Exchange
JICA	Japan International Cooperation Agency
JICE	Japan International Cooperation Center
JOCS	Japan Overseas Christian Medical Cooperative Services
JOCV	Japan Overseas Cooperation Volunteers
JOICFP	Japanese Organization for International Cooperation in Family Planning
JTI	Japan Tobacco International
KEI	Knowledge Ecology International
LDCs	Least Developed Countries
LDP	Liberal Democratic Party
LMICs	low- and middle-income countries
LoC	letters of credit
LTDL	Legacy Tobacco Document Library
MBDS	Mekong Basin Disease Surveillance
MDG	Millennium Development Goals
MEA	Ministry of External Affairs (India)
METI	Ministry of Economy, Trade and Industry
MHLW	Ministry of Health, Labour and Welfare
MMV	Medicines for Malaria Venture
MOA	Ministry of Agriculture
MOC	Ministry of Commerce (China)
MOE	Ministry of Education
MOF	Ministry of Finance
MOFA	Ministry of Foreign Affairs
MOFTEC	Ministry of Foreign Trade and Economic Cooperation

MOH	Ministry of Health
MoPH	Ministry of Public Health (Thailand)
MoU	Memorandum of Understanding (on the Protection of Intellectual Property)
MSF	Médecins Sans Frontières
NACO	National AIDS Control Organisation
NCDs	non-communicable diseases
NEPAD	New Partnership for Africa's Development
NGO	non-governmental organisation
NHSO	National Health Security Office (Thailand)
NIC	National Influenza Centre
ODA	Official Development Assistance
OECD	Organisation for Economic Cooperation and Development
OIE	Organization for Animal Health
PBC	People's Bank of China
PEPFAR	US President's Emergency Plan for AIDS Relief
PHEIC	public health emergencies of international concern
PIPF	Pandemic Influenza Preparedness Framework
PLRC	Party Literature Research Center of the CPC (China)
PLWHA	People Living with HIV/AIDS
PMA	Pharmaceutical Manufacturers' Association (USA)
PMI	Philip Morris International
PPE	personal protective equipment
ppy	per patient/year
R2P	responsibility to protect
R&D	research and development
RRT	rapid response team
SARS	severe acute respiratory syndrome
SCAAP	Special Commonwealth Assistance for Africa Programme
SEA IRCN	Southeast Asian Influenza Research Network
SEAMEC	Southeast Asian Ministers of Education Organization Council
SEAMEO-TROPMED	Southeast Asian Ministers of Education Organization Regional Tropical Medicine and Public Health Network
SEARO	Southeast Asia Regional Office
STMA	State Tobacco Monopoly Administration
SWAp	Sector-Wide Approach
TC	technical cooperation
TDR	Special Program for Research and Training in Tropical Diseases
TFI	Tobacco Free Initiative
TNP+	Thai Network of Positive People
TTC	transnational tobacco company
TICAD	Tokyo International Conference on African Development
TRIPS	Agreement on Trade-Related Intellectual Property Rights
TTC	transnational tobacco companies

TWG	Takemi Working Group
UN	United Nations
UNDP	United Nations Development Program
UNFPA	United Nations Population Fund
UNICEF	United Nations Children's Fund
UNSIC	United Nations System Influenza Coordination
USTR	US Trade Representative
WHA	World Health Assembly
WHO	World Health Organisation
WHO CC	WHO Collaborating Centres
WIC	World Influenza Centre
WIPO	World Intellectual Property Organization
WPRO	Western Pacific Regional Office
WTO	World Trade Organisation
XHNA	Xinhua News Agency

1 Introduction

Kelley Lee, Tikki Pang and Yeling Tan

In an era of accelerated and extensive globalisation, the world faces a number of challenges to tackle a wide range of transboundary problems that require effective collective action. These challenges come at a time of major shifts in world order, characterised by the emergence of multi-polarity, contestation over the meaning and interpretation of sovereignty, and reassessment of the contributions of state and non-state actors. In this context, transboundary threats to human health, including emerging and re-emerging infections, rising rates of chronic diseases, inadequate access to affordable and safe medicines, spreading antimicrobial resistance and the health effects of climate change, serve as exemplars of these global governance challenges.

Since the mid-1990s recognition of the need for effective collective action, for what has become known as 'global health', has led to the creation of numerous new initiatives and the mobilisation of unprecedented resources. For the most part, however, the institutional arrangements for enabling collective action, known as global health governance (GHG), have been formed in an ad hoc, rather than systematic or strategic, manner. Significantly, the global health landscape has been characterised by a large number of diverse state and non-state actors, engaged in wide-ranging and generally uncoordinated activities, unstructured in terms of a clear distribution of authority and responsibility, and informed by different and often competing normative frameworks. In addition to traditional governmental and intergovernmental (IGO) action, non-state actors ranging from charitable foundations to pharmaceutical companies to non-governmental organisations (NGOs) have sought to tackle health challenges. However, many of these initiatives have been defined by diverse, and often competing, interests and values, resulting in actions that have been uncoordinated at best, and mutually undermining at worst. The result has been a cacophony of institutional actors, largely unregulated, rarely transparent, and too often acting at cross purposes.

The desire to support and strengthen collective action in order to tackle pressing global health needs, has generated substantial attention within the policy and scholarly communities, with research on GHG having the potential to contribute to a fuller understanding of how to respond effectively to contemporary challenges. However, there is recognition that analysis to date has been narrowly focused on selected institutional actors and arrangements. Despite being home to more than half of the world's population (3.8 billion people), Asia has been particularly neglected, cast as the source of global health risks (e.g. antimicrobial resistance, pandemic influenza, counterfeiting, climate change), or as protecting narrow national interests (e.g. Indonesia's refusal to share influenza virus samples), rather than as a potential contributor to collective action. This neglect is increasingly anachronistic, given the region's substantial progress in improving basic socioeconomic indicators. For example, China's Human Development Index (HDI) score rose from 0.43 to 0.72, and Indonesia's score rose from 0.47 to 0.69, between 1980 and 2010 (United Nations Development Program, 2011). Asia's share of global gross domestic product (GDP) has tripled over the past three decades, growing from 8 per cent in 1980 to 24 per cent in 2010. The share held by the Group of Seven (G7) countries, in contrast, has fallen from 56 to 40 per cent over the same period (International Monetary Fund, 2011). As Asia achieves greater prosperity, and becomes more integrated with the world economy, there are growing expectations for the region to make a fuller contribution to governing transboundary problems such as economic crises, disease pandemics, climate change and transnational crime. There is indeed growing evidence that a rising Asia is beginning to bring forth a new set of increasingly influential players with their own values, worldviews and histories and strategic considerations (Gu and Humphrey, 2008; Kawai *et al.*, 2009). It is thus recognised that the region will be called upon to contribute future economic, political and intellectual inputs and leadership to improving global health, as part of its increasing role in global governance as a whole.

The S. T. Lee project on global governance and study group on global health governance

In January 2008 the Lee Kuan Yew School of Public Policy, and its Centre on Asia and Globalisation, launched the three-year S. T. Lee Project on Global Governance. The project brought together leading thinkers and practitioners from Asia and the West to develop insights and recommendations on how to govern a world that includes a rising Asia. Focusing on the global governance of energy (Dubash and Florini, 2011) and health, the project addressed two key sets of questions:

1. How can states, the private sector and civil society better organise to address the deficiencies in global governance? In a world of emerging multipolarity and deepening globalisation, how can the global community take effective collective action?
2. What is Asia's role in dealing with these issues? How can, and should, Asia translate its emerging economic clout into positive political influence that will strengthen global governance?

The Study Group on Global Health Governance (GHG) was convened in 2009 (chaired by Tikki Pang and Kelley Lee) with the recognition that while health has risen rapidly on the global agenda, GHG has increasingly suffered from a dysfunctional mélange of institutional arrangements. Thus, despite new resources and political will, institutional gaps and lack of strategic coherence reflected important tensions driving GHG efforts. To explore the state of GHG within an Asian context, the Study Group brought together an array of scholars of Asian origin, as well as senior experts and practitioners, for the purpose of understanding Asian contributions to GHG. The Study Group produced a series of discussion papers focused on three analytical lenses: (i) sovereignty; (ii) institutional diversity; and (iii) conceptions of GHG within Asia. The papers were developed and improved through workshops held in Bellagio, Italy (September 2009), Singapore (June 2010) and Beijing (December 2010).

Sovereignty and global health governance in Asia

The project was interested in how well traditional concepts of sovereignty function as a principle for managing global issues amid growing requirements for collective action to address transboundary health problems. By looking closer at Asian countries and their use of the sovereignty principle in managing different global health issues, we attempted to understand when, why and how sovereignty is used as a governing principle. The chapters reveal several ways in which the sovereignty principle relaxes, clashes, converges and even evolves with governance objectives in global health. While there is evidence that national interests are sometimes pursued on the basis of sovereignty, and at the expense of global health outcomes, there are other instances where sovereignty concerns have been downplayed in favour of other goals. Asian states have also challenged global rules and regimes that have undermined health outcomes by contravening existing norms and pushing for greater national policy space. In other cases, sovereignty turns out to be a principle of last resort in ordering relations in an ethnically and historically fractious region where trust remains thin. The multifaceted ways in which sovereignty and globalisation interact call for a systematic examination of why tensions arise, and for constructing policy responses that are similarly wide ranging.

Loosening and downplaying of sovereignty

Several case studies show Asian states adopting positions that downplay the importance of sovereignty as an issue in global health, both at the individual state level and at the level of international negotiations. Asian countries such as China and India have willingly engaged with a range of global health institutions when they have been recipients of foreign aid. These global health players and initiatives range from foreign private entities such as the Bill and Melinda Gates Foundation (BMGF) to public–private partnerships like the Global Fund to Fight AIDS, Tuberculosis and Malaria (GFATM). However, these positive engagements are often embedded within a broader strategic context. In his study on the interaction between the BRICS countries (Brazil, Russia, India, China and South Africa) and the international health community on dealing with HIV/AIDS, Gomez (2009) describes a twin dynamic of receptivity and resistance taking place. States such as India and China are more receptive to the international health community when cooperation offers advantages of programme expansion and reputation enhancement, or when there has been a history of collaboration. They have also resisted global health initiatives when there have been clashes with domestic policies, normative structures or pharmaceutical capacity. What these dual practices amount to is a growing strategic approach by these emerging nations. Gomez describes this as a demonstration by these countries that they are capable of dealing with their health issues and as such a stronger exertion of their sovereignty. That said, the definition of sovereignty being asserted here is arguably one that is more flexible (both receptive and resistant depending on circumstances), and which implicitly accepts the legitimacy of engaging with non-state actors and non-traditional initiatives in the global health community.

In global rule-making efforts such as the International Health Regulations (IHR) revision process, various Asian participants raised objections during negotiations on the basis of sovereignty concerns. However, these concerns did not impede the successful revision of the IHR, as described by Kamradt-Scott, Lee and Xu in Chapter 5 of this volume. The IHR (2005) represent a significant revision of outdated rules surrounding the governance of international disease threats. The new regulations expand the scope of diseases covered, strengthen the way in which information on disease events is collected, used and shared, clarify the responsibilities of states in their surveillance and response to potential health threats, and gives added authority to the World Health Organisation (WHO). The WHO can seek verification from state parties on disease events, and state parties are obliged to respond to the requests. Finally, the WHO is also able to share information from non-governmental sources with both state parties and intergovernmental organizations (Fidler and Gostin, 2006).

During negotiations, the Chinese government objected to the IHR text on grounds of sovereignty in two areas: disease surveillance, reporting and investigation mechanisms, and the status and representation of Taiwan. Chapter 5 details the successful revision process of the IHR negotiations despite these concerns, providing evidence of the 'loosening' or reconfiguring of the sovereignty principle vis-à-vis the need to formulate new rules for governing global health.

The Framework Convention on Tobacco Control (FCTC) negotiations also provide hints of how Asian countries can, and have, actively shaped new understandings of how to balance sovereignty and global health needs. As described by Lee and Kao (Chapter 7 this volume), the positions of Asian participants were highly diverse. The Japanese government, which owns half of the manufacturer Japan Tobacco International, for example, argued for national governments to retain control over what forms of regulation were best suited to their respective countries. In contrast, Thailand and India played leading roles in negotiating a framework that moved state parties away from interests defined by territorial boundaries, towards transboundary notions of public health protection. The FCTC therefore represents an interesting case of some Asian states not just acceding to, but actively shaping, new rules of global governance that reflect a more flexible understanding of sovereignty.

Sovereignty as a tool to advance national interests

For the issue areas analysed for this project, there appears to be a preference in Asia for promoting state-centred forms of cooperation. The clearest evidence for this comes from the behaviour of countries such as Japan, China and India as donors in development assistance for health (DAH). Foreign aid is an area where the state has a high degree of control and discretion in setting the rules of engagement. As shown in Chapters 2, 3 and 4, Japan, China and India have all adopted DAH policy rhetoric that reflects sensitivity towards respecting the sovereignty of recipient nations. Moreover, the three countries' management of DAH is strongly driven by their respective foreign ministries, thus highlighting the increasingly close connection between foreign policy and health matters. These agencies, in turn, have formulated policies to advance state sovereignty rather than global health goals. The institutions and mechanisms that the three countries have chosen to channel DAH underscore preferences for state-centred modes of cooperation that further national objectives. What these objectives are, however, varies according to domestic context.

Given the above, the project found the environment for emerging donors to be highly dynamic, with the DAH strategies of the three countries rapidly evolving although in potentially different directions. In Chapter 2 Christine Pilcavage describes how Japan has revised its foreign aid principles, which are today framed under the concept of human security, less by territorial boundaries and more by universal human needs. Japan has also played a leading role in promoting health in different high-level multilateral fora such as the Group of Eight (G8) countries. In contrast, China's White Paper on Foreign Aid, issued in April 2011, staunchly upholds the principles of non-interference and equality (Information Office of the State Council, People's Republic of China, 2011). These developments suggest the non-linear and complex ways in which emerging Asian powers will challenge, influence and be shaped by current development discourses. The future role of China and India, in the context of the emerging economies of the BRICS countries, is also worth observing amid indications of closer coordination in a strategic manner (Global Health Strategies Initiative, 2012; Glennie, 2012).

Sovereignty as a tool to challenge global rules

The sovereignty principle was also found to be employed, in some cases, to challenge global rules perceived to be unfair and detrimental to public health outcomes. For example, the Agreement on Trade-Related Intellectual Property Rights (TRIPS) severely constrained the national policy space for access to medicines for low- and middle-income countries (LMICs) in the 1990s. Moon and Szlezák point out in Chapter 8 that, while the formal TRIPS regime allowed governments flexibilities such as compulsory licensing, in practice the political space for exercising such options was restricted by external pressure and trade interests. They further detail how the actions of governments and civil society groups in Malaysia, Thailand and India championed new rules that challenged TRIPS and reasserted health-centred interests. However, the authors carefully note that it was not simply governments fighting to re-establish national policy space. Instead, efforts were made in collaboration with civil society groups, transboundary coalitions, international organisations and the scientific community to reassert the right of World Trade Organisation (WTO) member states to use flexibilities on the grounds of protecting national public health interests.

In another example, Kamradt-Scott and Yoon discuss in Chapter 6 how Indonesia announced in 2007 that it would withhold H5N1 influenza virus samples from the WHO on the grounds of inequities in rules surrounding access to antiviral drugs and vaccines (*Jakarta Post*, 2007). The government's framing of its protest around the notion of 'viral sovereignty' sparked worldwide controversy, notably for being based on traditional notions of territorial sovereignty that dangerously undermined collective global health security (Holbrooke and Garrett, 2008). However, the country's stance highlighted fundamental inequities in the system of vaccine production and consumption which many LMICs identified with. This challenge to existing virus-sharing norms led to the negotiation of new rules, under the Pandemic Influenza Preparedness Framework (PIPF), regarding virus sharing, intellectual property rights (IPRs), and revised responsibilities for drug manufacturers (Fidler and Gostin, 2011), and in the ongoing movement urging the WHO to start the process of developing a research and development treaty.

Sovereignty as the lowest common denominator

One reason for the strong reliance on state-centred modes of cooperation in Asia appears to be the presence of historically deep political, ethnic, religious and economic divisions within the region that continue to hinder collective action today. The absence of trust, or agreed norms of regional and multilateral cooperation, has hindered the formation of transboundary partnerships and networks. Sovereignty has instead ordered relations between a set of politically, ethnically and geographically diverse grouping of nations. The project considered the governance gaps that have resulted from this state of affairs. For example, pandemic influenza governance has focused on at the border controls, rather than on systemic strengthening of public health systems that transverse territorial boundaries. In addition, the region's deep and historically based adherence to the principle of non-interference in other sovereign states has created a policy environment where transboundary issues of mutual concern are often not discussed.

Understanding sovereignty through multiple lenses

The governance challenges wrought by globalisation bring new tensions to the relevance and application of traditional notions of sovereignty. Indeed, there are plenty of examples of rising Asian countries using sovereignty as a tool to advance their individual national interest – often to the detriment of global governance needs. However, the evidence presented in this book also suggests that a focus only on this clash between sovereignty and globalisation may yield limited insights into how global governance can be strengthened. Indeed, the sovereignty principle can be equally used to address inequities in existing rules and norms, or simply to maintain peace and stability in the absence of deeper institutional arrangements. These difficult tensions point to the need to analyse sovereignty and globalisation through multiple lenses, and to distinguish between different sources of tension.

In cases where global rules and standards are driven by one dominant set of interests, or without participation from critical stakeholders, governance mechanisms can be perceived as illegitimate, inequitable, exclusive and ill-fitted for the world's diversity of socio-economic settings. In such situations, sovereignty remains a useful tool that states can wield to push for a revision of the rules. Moon and Szlezák's chapter shows that, even in such cases as the experience of Thailand, India and Malaysia in influencing new norms for IPRs and access to medicines, assertions of sovereignty under conditions of globalisation are more effective when undertaken with the participation of transboundary networks and non-state actors. In Chapter 6 Kamradt-Scott *et al.* provide evidence that, in other cases, where a lack of trust undermines global governance, the problem lies with an absence of alternative mechanisms that can create incentives for collective action.

As such, recommendations for improving GHG could derive from the motivating factors behind various uses of the sovereignty principle. Rather than acting at odds with each other, sovereignty and globalisation could be understood as 'mutually embedded' (Väyrynen, 2001). A more flexible and multidimensional approach to devising policy responses could be considered. If sovereignty is being used as a tool for advancing individual national interest, an examination of the political economy behind national interest formation could open up avenues to push for a more health-centric and transboundary construction of foreign policy goals. If sovereignty is being used as a tool to challenge existing global rules, an assessment of the process by which these rules are made, and adjustments to include neglected voices and concerns, might be in order. If sovereignty is being used as a last resort principle to order relations in the absence of trust, then confidence-building at the regional level, or greater attention to informal institutions and networks (as we argue in the latter section on regional institutions), might offer progress in improving health outcomes.

Diversity and preferences in institutional design

The above discussion on sovereignty underscores the challenge of designing institutions to effectively take into account the myriad factors, and alignment of interests, involved in governing global health. On the one hand, allowing space for innovation in governance structures allows for experimentation and innovation in collective action to manage transboundary problems. On the other hand, the anarchic policy environment with its multiplicity of interests, norms and actors can lead to incoherence and fragmentation. In this book, we examine how Asian actors are engaging with institutional pluralism from two angles: the composition of state and non-state actors across the governance of various health issues, and connections between global, regional and local institutions. The underlying question is whether health outcomes are enriched or weakened by institutional diversity in the GHG landscape, and the roles played by Asian actors – whether acting as 'governors' influencing the shape of various institutions, or acting as the 'governed' in relation to specific health issues.

Horizontal diversity across issues

The degree of institutional diversity and effectiveness in global governance varies according to the subject of regulation and alignment of interests. This project found varying forms of state engagement in Asia across a range of different institutional designs, from DAH to international arrangements such as the PIPF, IHR and FCTC. In DAH, we find a disconnect between the role of Asian actors as recipients versus donors of aid that mirror their, at times, variable positions on sovereignty. As aid recipients, India and China accept and engage with a diversity of institutions and actors, and have provided fairly open operating space to these actors (e.g. the Global Fund to Fight HIV/AIDS, Tuberculosis and Malaria, and the Ford, Clinton and Gates Foundations). As donors, however, India and China prefer to engage bilaterally rather than multilaterally. They tend to be focused on state-to-state partnerships, with contributions tending to be largely material rather than ideational. This balance of priorities begs the question of what other health problems are being neglected, and what opportunities are lost in terms of tapping into the capacity of non-state actors to play governance functions that governments, acting alone and within their territorial jurisdictions, cannot address.

For governing pandemic influenza under the aforementioned PIPF, and governing disease outbreaks under the IHR (2005), there appears to be a disconnect in Asian countries between a recognition of the potentially transboundary nature of infectious disease outbreaks, and the institutional responses that remain based on state-centric mechanisms. The severe acute respiratory syndrome (SARS) outbreak alerted the world to the need to strengthen global governance around pandemic influenza, giving state agencies a much-needed prompt to revitalise efforts to update the IHR. The surveillance aspect of the IHR has arguably been enhanced through the provision allowing the use of non-state sources of information. However, as Kamradt-Scott *et al.* describe, Asian countries did not play an active role in the revision process, and participation was highly state-centric. Similarly with pandemic preparedness, efforts in Asia have revolved around governments and to a lesser extent international or regional IGOs.

In less traditional institutional arenas, that actively engage non-state actors in new forms of decision making, it is difficult to characterise a common approach by Asian states. One example is tobacco control. The FCTC process represented an innovative approach to drafting international health rules, by incorporating participation by a range of stakeholders, notably NGOs with official relations with the WHO as observers and providers of unofficial briefings during negotiations. While Japan and China played the role of spoilers during the negotiations, the enhanced role given to NGOs was central to raising attention and scrutiny over the pro-tobacco stance of these governments, and eventually in pressuring the two states to adjust their positions somewhat. The governments of India and Thailand, in contrast, played leading roles in the successful negotiation of the FCTC, with Thailand pushing strongly for the participation of NGOs (see Chapter 7).

Domestic foundations to global institutions

Our findings suggest that the degree and nature of Asia's role in influencing global health institutions depend very much on domestic decision-making structures, as demonstrated through the leadership roles played by India and Thailand in shaping the FCTC. As Lee *et al.* (2012) point out, the open participation and engagement of civil society in India and Thailand's domestic health policy process was directly related to these countries' support at the global level for the FCTC to include substantive voice and responsibilities for NGOs. Regarding access to medicines, India and Thailand again were leaders in developing national intellectual property institutions that advanced public health interests.

Moon and Szlezák (Chapter 8) attribute India and Thailand's challenging of existing IPR rules to the close networks between their civil societies and governments regarding the access to medicines issue, as well as the political space afforded to civil society groups seeking to influence IPR rules through legal and administrative systems. China's IPR-related institutions, in contrast, have not taken public health concerns into account so far. The authors argue that China's domestic and external policy environment has much to do with this difference: specifically the heightened trade pressure on China to toughen its IPR protections, the narrower space for civil society groups to operate and the weaker ties between domestic NGOs and global public health networks.

In relation to DAH, domestic health needs and the institutional environments in Japan, India and China similarly shape the countries' approaches in addressing public health needs at regional and global levels. Wang *et al.* (Chapter 3 this volume) and Guntupalli and Nachiappan (Chapter 4 this volume) detail how the bureaucratic fragmentation of agencies dealing with ODA in China and India has created DAH policies that inhibit a focused or coherent approach on health. Japan, in contrast, has a more structured inter-agency process and one implementing agency (the Japan International Cooperation Agency). While Japan frequently engages the participation of non-state actors in the formation of state DAH policies, China and India have not allowed non-state actors to play much of a role. The lack of participation by non-state actors – particularly civil society groups – is mirrored by the state-centric nature of resulting policies. The result is that China and India's domestic DAH policy communities are disconnected from broader discourses on GHG.

Regional institutions

The project found that the political diversity in Asia, and lack of consensus about what role the region should play in managing transboundary health problems and thus which institutions work best, has hindered the building of regional institutions. Asian countries (except for China) were largely disengaged from the IHR negotiations, and regional institutions played no role either in the preparatory stages or actual intergovernmental discussions. As Kamradt-Scott, Lee and Xu describe in Chapter 5, 'Asian governments approached the IHR in an individualistic and state-centric manner, declining to form regional alliances'. While the Association of Southeast Asian Nations (ASEAN) and the Asia-Pacific Economic Cooperation (APEC) forum were active in organising cooperative efforts and discussions on pandemic preparedness, they were also heavily criticised for being inefficient and ineffective. Historical mistrust, and socio-economic and political diversity within the region, was cited as hindering transboundary collaboration. In terms of material contributions to global health, the amount of funding that the Asian Development Bank (ADB) channels to health projects has been minimal (1 per cent in fiscal year 2009). As the number of issues requiring collective action grows, the weaknesses of Asia's regional institutions are expected to come under increasing scrutiny. It is precisely because trust appears so weak in Asia, and countries are at such varied stages of economic development, that the core function of regional IGOs is seen as minimising conflict and maintaining stability, rather than fulfilling broader regional governance needs. This is the corollary to the region's attachment to sovereignty as an organising principle to preserve peace.

However, the chapters also reveal some areas where the actual functions of managing transboundary issues are being built within the region, and where historical differences may be being overcome. Evidence suggests that, in some issue areas, elite-level policy negotiations through informal networks play a stronger role in governance than formal regional organisations. For pandemic preparedness, for example, Kamradt-Scott *et al.* observe that

> Many of the new links are based on informal networks between public health and scientific colleagues who share information on a regular basis via email, telephone, or the Internet. Many of these professional networks have not been documented, and have emerged distinct from more formalized intergovernmental processes.

In addition, in Chapter 7 Lee and Kao describe how the FCTC experience demonstrates the potential of regional institutions to play a part in negotiating the heterogeneous preferences within Asia. Lee and colleagues (2012) detail the role that WHO's Southeast Asia Regional Office (SEARO) and ASEAN both played in balancing the wide-ranging tobacco interests in the region, and in building regional consensus prior to discussions at the global level. This example suggests that the enduring hostilities that divide Asian countries might be overcome to address specific issue areas, in the presence of strong leadership and where domestic constituencies are included in policy processes.

Vertical connections – from local to global

It has been frequently observed that the institutional environment in global health is marked by a progression of fragmentation. Mechanisms are heterogeneous across different issues and predominantly operate in institutionalised silos. Policies and actors, as a result, are disconnected at the local, regional and global levels. Above all, the institutional landscape lacks coherence to address health problems that require transboundary responses. One longer-term implication, suggested by the findings of this project, is that the emerging multipolarity in world order may lead to further fragmentation. These disconnections apply not just to the formulation of rules for global health, but also to their implementation. This point is particularly relevant for Asia because, while some countries in the region are rapidly developing economically, institutional development in the social sectors (including health) may lag behind. The result is a greater globalisation of health needs, but not requisite institutional capacity to respond effectively.

In sum, Asia's engagement with and promotion of different institutional designs varies horizontally across issue areas and vertically through global, regional and local levels. As health aid recipients, Asian states have shown a willingness to engage with a whole range of state and non-state actors, and transboundary public–private partnerships such as GFATM. As health aid donors, however, states such as India and China have chosen to focus on state-centric relationships and projects. On the whole, there appears to be a regional preference for using state-centred mechanisms to manage health problems, although as discussed above, the make-up of local political structures matters. Those countries whose domestic processes included participation from non-state actors correspondingly either promoted or were open to institutional designs that afforded greater diversity of partners at the supranational level. The role of regional organisations such as ASEAN or WHO regional offices appears to be highly varying. ASEAN was found to be highly ineffective in managing issues such as pandemic influenza governance and played no role in fostering discussions in the run-up to IHR negotiations. In the FCTC, however, regional-level discussions were critical in resolving differences and consolidating positions in the WHO negotiations.

Conceptions and contributions from Asia

The third analytical theme is conceptions from Asia on global governance and Asia's role in managing global health problems. There has been no lack of interests, ideas and institutions seeking to shape the governance of global health (Dodgson *et al.*, 2002; Lee, 2009). The now substantial GHG literature captures the proliferation of approaches and perspectives formed over the past two decades (Zacher and Keefe, 2008; Buse *et al.*, 2009; Kay and Williams, 2011; Harman, 2012). These include: (a) market-based approaches to the production and consumption of health goods and services; (b) universalist approaches grounded in the equitable right to health as social justice; (c) security-focused approaches to unmanaged global health risks; and (d) biomedical approaches to the control, treatment and prevention of disease (McInnes and Lee, 2012). What is not well understood is how these approaches play out in different geographical or social contexts. In the context of this book, how is global health defined and perceived in Asia, and what approaches shape Asian perspectives on GHG?

Building an inclusive understanding of global health governance

Rather than one 'Asian' conception of GHG, the chapters reveal incoherence. The region's immense political diversity may explain the absence of common approaches to form to deal with shared health needs. The limited engagement of Asian participants in the IHR revision process suggests that regional actors have not recognised the relevance of such negotiations or have been content with letting others shape the rules on some global health issues. Wang *et al.* (Chapter 4), and Guntupalli and Nachiappan (Chapter 3), underscore that China and India's contributions to global health remain largely material rather than ideational to date, although both note the ambitions of the two countries to become more active donors. Nor have regional organisations played a leadership role in bridging existing normative and political divides. Regarding IPRs and access to medicines, for example, Moon and Szlezák point out that the positions of various Asian states appear to have been defined, not by any shared conception of IPRs, or cultural or historical roots, but by their rate of economic growth and degree of political space available for civil society participation.

This gap, between the growing expectations for an emerging Asia to play a more prominent role in GHG, and the nature of engagement to date described in this book, suggests that the region remains governed by rules and institutional arrangements agreed elsewhere. Many countries in the region remain aid recipients and may simply lack the capacity to be rule-setters via existing global health initiatives. Indeed, existing global health institutions remain perceived in the region as the prodigy of a small number of high-income countries, even though the health needs the institutions seek to address are collective. The picture arrived at suggests clear disconnect between emerging conceptions of GHG as debated and promoted by scholarly and policy communities worldwide, and engagement within the Asian region.

Health as a vanguard for global governance?

Analysis of Asia and global governance, of course, goes well beyond the field of health. As described at the beginning of this introductory chapter, there is relative consensus worldwide on the importance of strengthening collective action on a host of shared concerns in an increasingly globalised world. In understanding Asian engagement with GHG, what can we learn about the region's potential contribution to global governance more generally?

Insofar as we can imagine a future where Asian countries are increasingly willing to challenge the status quo, it is not clear what new rules and norms will be put forth. In Chapter 11 Fidler contends that Asian countries' commitment to the Five Principles of Peaceful Co-Existence will shape the nature of their engagement with global governance. Given that sovereignty and non-interference sit as core tenets in the Five Principles, there could be a potential clash with existing discourses in GHG that advocate more flexible interpretations of sovereignty and the role of non-state actors. Alternatively, Wang *et al.* write that as an aid recipient,

China has demonstrated a willingness to engage non-state actors and innovative global initiatives that do not adhere to classical interpretations of sovereignty. The country's ratification of the FCTC, as described by Lee and Kao, despite the political strength of its domestic tobacco industry, may demonstrate a desire to be seen as a responsible emerging power. Asian countries are also slowly becoming more active participants (although not leaders or rule-setters) in some innovative GHG efforts, such as the GFATM and the Global Alliance for Vaccines and Immunisation (GAVI). There are growing examples of Asian countries taking leadership roles to advance health-centred goals. For example, Japan championed health issues at the 1994 Global Issues Initiative on Population and AIDS, and the G8 meetings of 2000 and 2008 (see Chapter 2), while Thailand and India have effectively altered the status quo on the rules governing access to medicines (see Chapter 8). India and Thailand's leadership in the FCTC process, in particular, demonstrates the potential for Asian countries to proactively shape new rules in global health governance (see Chapter 7). It also shows that, in the presence of effective leadership supported by open and participatory domestic decision-making structures, regional solidarity can be built and historical mistrust overcome.

In the area of DAH, however, where states are able to proactively set the rules, the nature of their health assistance is very much entrenched within a worldview emphasising classical notions of sovereignty, utilising traditional tools, and relying mainly on state-to-state cooperation. Yanzhong Huang (2010) suggests that the disconnect, in the case of China, arises out of a fundamental difference in world view:

> Although China recognizes that solutions to global health problems necessitate neoliberal strategies of cooperation over disease prevention and control, its actions on global health problems are still justified from the lens of classical realism that focuses on power, influence, and security.

Asian efforts to strengthen pandemic preparedness further revealed a clear preference for state-based action to deal with what has been accepted as a transboundary issue. Institutional responses have lagged behind conceptual understandings of the transboundary problem at hand. It is important, however, to reiterate that the roots of the region's commitment to state-based responses and to classical sovereignty are not solely about conceptual disconnects. The lack of trust, and historical and socio-economic diversity, remain fundamental barriers to collective action. The lack of institutional capacity to implement basic response and regulatory functions further impedes the establishment of more innovative transboundary solutions.

Health cooperation versus competition

Emerging multipolarity may intensify normative debates on GHG. Where health objectives are poorly defined or articulated, the potential for other policy goals to outweigh GHG will be greater. For example, DAH policy in China and India are largely shaped by ministries such as foreign affairs and commerce. Huang (2010) articulates the risks of this approach to health clearly:

> China's active engagement in global health is primarily driven by a foreign policy agenda that focuses on expanding international influence while improving international image . . . The danger is that when health is placed in the realm of realpolitik, it runs the risk of being 'dependent on the logic of such politics – which is not based on science and not subject to public deliberation and peer review, but on the Machiavellian instincts of those in power'.

Therefore, as long as global health issues are conceived in these countries as an appendage of foreign policy, there is likely to be competition, rather than collective action, across countries.

As Asia continues to develop economically, global health issues may be subsumed by other policy agendas. The existing governance gaps and policy distortions are well-documented. In terms of health aid, while there are severe capacity constraints in many Asian health systems that hamper implementation of the IHR or strengthening of pandemic preparedness, Asian donors are not channelling resources into these needs. Chapters 2, 3 and 4 suggest that the pursuit of regional and global influence, rather than global health need, appears to be defining aid policy. Indeed, competition extends beyond aid policy. As Moon and Szlezák point out, India and China's capacities in pharmaceutical R&D are expanding with active investment from multinational companies, local firms, academic and government institutions. These countries in time seek to be major exporters, with the logic of market competition taking priority over health needs. Insofar as there tend to be less clear state–corporate divisions in some parts of Asia (e.g. those societies that have developed through state corporatist or market authoritarian models), the economic rise of these countries bring interesting implications for how the rules surrounding global health IP issues will be influenced and reshaped. Fidler warns that not only would such competition worsen an already fragmented GHG landscape, but that resulting policies will increasingly serve narrow state interests rather than collective action. In the absence of agreed objectives, rules and enforcement mechanisms about global health needs, in other words, other strategic interests will maintain a dominant role. The fundamental question arrived at is whether emerging multipolarity will make it easier or harder to build a consensus around the objectives and rules of GHG?

Outline of this book

This book seeks to support the search for more effective GHG, to enable collective action on a broad range of transboundary health challenges, by seeking new understandings of the role of a rising Asia. Part I of this book focuses on China, India and Japan as aid donors to global health efforts. Japan has been Asia's leader in the provision of health development aid for many years, but new players are now becoming more significant. It is shown that donor–recipient relationships are becoming more complicated with the arrival of Asian donor countries, bringing with them different approaches to aid policy. The three chapters in this section document the three country's health aid policies and the implications raised for GHG.

Part II examines Asian contributions to the agreement of GHG mechanisms as foundations for governing collective action in global health. The chapters deal with the revision of the IHR (2005), preparedness measures for pandemic influenza and the FCTC, and show that there has been much variation in the degree of engagement in these respective negotiations and the positions taken by Asian state and non-state actors. This is followed by analysis of the governance of global health research and knowledge products in Part III. These are arguably among the most under-governed and contested areas in health. The chapters examine the roles that Asian actors have played so far in either articulating, challenging or implementing the rules governing global health research and knowledge products, and identify areas of potential experimentation as well as contestation. The book concludes with three chapters reflecting on the project as a whole, in terms of what conclusions can be drawn about Asia's role in governing global health.

Note

1 This chapter is adapted from Tan Y, Lee K, Pang T. (2012) Global health governance and the rise of Asia, *Global Policy*, 3(3).

Part 1

Asian countries as global health donors

2 Japan's overseas development assistance in the health sector and global health governance

Christine Pilcavage

Introduction

After World War II, Japan rapidly transformed itself from an Official Development Assistance (ODA) recipient to a major donor nation. This transition reflected Japan's response to its domestic economy and its evolving national and regional security policies. Scholars such as Calder (1988) and Orr (1990) have noted that *gaiatsu* (foreign pressure) from the US influenced Japan's ODA policies and the amount of aid that Japan was giving.

Japan received 31 World Bank project loans from 1953 to 1966 – for US$863 million – to help rebuild after the devastation of war (World Bank, n.d.). All were for infrastructure projects – transportation, communication, and power – the kind of projects that became characteristic of the loans Japan would provide to developing countries. During its years as an aid recipient, Japan also began providing development assistance. Initially, contributions were intended as war reparations and the promotion of trade; Japan needed to strengthen its economy and rebuild ties with its Asian neighbours.

Japan was one of the leading donors and the only Asian country to join the Development Assistance Group (currently the Development Assistance Committee) when it was created in 1960 (Führer, 1996). In 1964, the International Monetary Fund graduated Japan from an aid recipient to an industrialized country, and Japan began responding more to Development Assistance Committee (DAC) norms by increasing their ODA in hopes of being accepted and respected by Western donor community (Arase, 2005). By 1977, the amount of Japanese aid was comparable to other major DAC members (MOFA, 1988); by 1989, Japan had become the world's premiere donor (Yanagihara and Emig, 1991) and held that position until the beginning of the twenty-first century.

Because the Japanese constitution prohibits the use of military power (and thus military assistance), ODA became an important component of Japan's domestic 'comprehensive security' strategies (Drifte, 1996), which linked development to peace and recognized Japan's reliance on foreign countries to secure natural resources. In 1980, the government of Japan produced an unofficial report, 'Philosophy on Economic Cooperation', describing ODA as a 'cost for contributing to the creation of an international order to ensure Japan's comprehensive national security', and identifying 'humanitarian and moralistic' reasons that Japan should provide aid. Japan also reasoned that its ODA contributions should be in proportion to its economic power.

During the 1980s, Japanese ODA was characterized as the 'recycling' of trade surpluses (Ohno, 2003), but also responding and reacting to the US demand to increase security interests in the region. The adoption of the ODA Charter in 1992 was Japan's first step in framing and documenting its development assistance policy. In addition to the political, economic and military principles, the ODA Charter clearly defined geographic and sectoral priorities, such as basic human needs and infrastructure, and provided a practical approach to aid in response to the criticism that Japanese ODA was intended only to promote trade and commerce. However, the underlying mercantilistic nature of Japanese ODA still persisted (Hook and Zhang, 1998).

After the Cold War, with the emergence of the concept of non-traditional security, Japan gradually incorporated human security into its definition of foreign policy and development assistance. The concept of human security draws on Japan's own history: the preamble to the 1947 Japanese Constitution states, 'We recognize that all peoples of the world have the right to live in peace, free from fear and want' (Hook and McCormack, 2001). This concept was ultimately incorporated into Japan's revised ODA Charter in 2003, which explicitly defined the goals of ODA as 'to contribute to the peace and development of the international community and thereby to help ensure Japan's own security and prosperity' (MOFA, 2003a).

By the end of the 1990s, the downturn in Japan's economy meant that Japan could no longer continue to increase its ODA at the magnitude of the past decade-and-a-half. The Japanese public was increasingly dissatisfied with the country's ODA and showing signs of aid fatigue amidst Japan's continued economic stagnation and budget deficits. The annual foreign affairs public opinion polls from 1993–2004 showed declining public support for ODA, and after 1997 there was a substantial decrease in the overall ODA budget. Public support, however, has slowly increased since 2005. Despite declining ODA, Japan's bilateral assistance in volume has continued to rank as one of the largest among government donors. Japan ranked second after the US from 2001–2006, when it slipped to third in 2006, and fifth in 2007.

Decreased funding was accompanied by a change of policy direction. In 1997, Japan began to focus on quality rather than quantity, emphasizing recipient countries' ownership and being responsive to their cultural and economic situations. This was a response to both *naiatsu* (domestic pressure) and *gaiatsu* to become more accountable, and for ODA projects/schemes to be integrated under a clear medium-term ODA plan. Since the ODA Charter was revised in 2003, country studies/plans and Country Assistance Programmes (CAPs) have been created to guide requests from recipient countries and to increase the efficiency and effectiveness of ODA implementation.

During this time, Japanese ODA became increasingly involved with global health initiatives, generally profiled under the rubric of human security. In 1994, the first five-year Global Issues Initiative (GII) was created, followed by the

Okinawa Infectious Diseases Initiative (2000), and the Health Development Initiative (2005). In 2010, Japan's Global Health Policy 2011–2015 was announced. Japan's involvement in global health heightened when it played host to the 2000 and 2008 G8 Summits. Japan's initial contribution to the health sector was small compared to other donors, but its contributions have grown over time; in 2007 and 2008, Japan ranked fifth among major bilateral donors for health assistance.

The majority of ODA is channelled through the Ministry of Foreign Affairs (MOFA) and the Ministry of Finance (MOF): 62 percent from MOFA in FY2006 and FY2007, and 25.4 percent from the MOF in FY2006 and FY2007 (MOFA, 2008). The budgets for Japan International Cooperation Agency (JICA), grant aid and contributions to multilateral organizations are included in these shares. A small share of ODA is also channelled through the Ministry of Economy, Trade and Industry (METI), and through the other agencies and ministries involved in technical cooperation.

Budget trends and categories of health sector assistance

The total amount of Japan's ODA has been trending downwards since the turn of the millennium because of the country's financial crisis and budget deficits. Its health sector assistance, however, has remained relatively constant. Japan's total health ODA budget for 2008 was US$792.9 million, ranking fifth among the donor nations (Government of Canada, 2010). However, when measuring Japan's total ODA contribution as a product of its gross national income (GNI), it was only 0.17 percent in FY2007, well below the UN ODA target of 0.7 percent of GNI, when Japan's total ODA budget was US$7.68 billion. In the same year, Japan's health assistance was only 0.013 percent of GNI, placing it second to last among the 22 OECD–DAC members (OECD DAC, 2008; IHME, 2009).

Japan's assistance in the health sector can be divided into bilateral assistance to recipient countries through loans, grants and technical cooperation; and multilateral assistance to international organizations. Figure 2.1 shows trends in bilateral and multilateral assistance over 17 years.

Japan provides a small percentage of bilateral assistance in the form of loans for projects, but since assistance in the health sector is considered humanitarian in nature, most bilateral support is given through grants and technical cooperation.

Bilateral assistance

Technical cooperation, also known as technical assistance, is the facilitation of transfer of Japanese health technologies and knowledge through health-focused projects. It includes training of health personnel, placement of short- or long-term policy and health/medical expert advisors, provision of medical and other equipment, health-related development studies and placement of health-related Japan Overseas Cooperation Volunteers (JOCV) and Senior Volunteers to work in health-related activities (MOFA, 2009a).

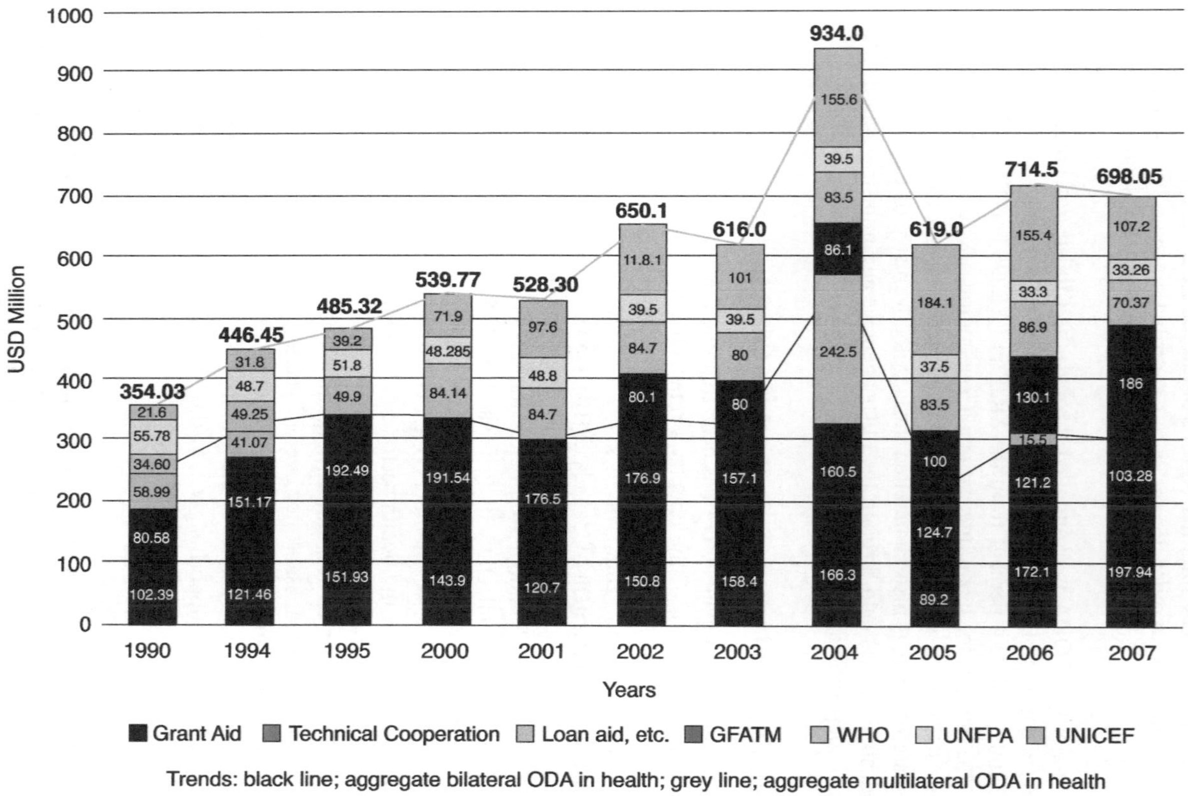

Figure 2.1 Japan's ODA in the health sector (in million US$).
GFATM = The Global Fund for AIDS, Tubereulosis and Malaria
Source: *Japan's ODA White Paper various years: UNICEF annual report 2007*

Table 2.1 Technical Cooperation in the health/medical care sector (number of people; % of shares in respective categories

Fiscal year	*Trainees accepted*		*Experts dispatched (short and long term)*		*Members of study teams dispatched*		*JOCV*		*Other volunteers*	
	N	%	N	%	N	%	N	%	N	%
1986	562	9.4	506	25.6	n/a	n/a	94	11.4	n/a	n/a
1988	646	9.5	429	17.6	n/a	n/a	130	16.5	n/a	n/a
1990	713	9.4	455	18.2	n/a	n/a	83	11.9	n/a	n/a
1992	782	9.4	453	16.6	n/a	n/a	134	14.3	n/a	n/a
1994	971	10.2	510	16.8	n/a	n/a	148	13.1	n/a	n/a
1996	1214	11.1	464	15.4	n/a	n/a	172	14.4	n/a	n/a
1998	2428	12.3	487	14.2	n/a	n/a	185	15.8	n/a	n/a
2000	2184	12.5	558	16.5	n/a	n/a	243	17.7	n/a	n/a
2006	4841	16.0	675	14.9	357	6.2	337	22.0	32	8.1
2007	4605	21.6	757	15.3	398	6.5	316	21.3	28	6.8

Numbers of tech coop persons are new incoming individuals and are not double-counted.

Source: Japan's ODA annual report (1991, 1995, 2001); *JICA annual report* (2008); JICA JOCV data.

As seen in Table 2.1, the allocation of technical cooperation in the field of health has been growing gradually and steadily, signifying Japan's commitment to global health.

Several interviewees from academia, government, NGOs and multilateral communities within Japan indicated that recipient countries often rely on JICA experts or Japanese consultants to assist in proposal development due to *yosei-shugi*, the 'request-based' nature of Japanese assistance. Further, private consulting companies play a large part in technical cooperation: conducting development studies and surveys as well as planning, monitoring and evaluating health-related projects, including health infrastructure (Hyodo and Katsuma, 2008; JICA, 2010). One Japanese politician criticized Japanese 'experts' and JOCV as an expensive way of using ODA and believed that NGOs would be a more cost-effective measure of spending Japanese taxpayer's money. As cited above, Japan has begun to place contingencies on grants and shift away from the traditional 'request basis' approach to aid. MOFA and JICA developed country studies/plans and CAPs in order to prioritize the recipient country's needs; respect its national development strategy; and assure efficient, effective implementation. An interviewee cited this shift as Japan's direct response to domestic politics and public dissatisfaction with the lack of ODA transparency. In addition, the revised ODA Charter of 2003 emphasizes policy dialogue (*seisaku taiwa*) and policy-based lending (*seisaku shien*), which has fostered the more active participation of recipient countries in ODA initiatives.

Grant aid is given to developing countries without obligation to repay. The health sector has different types of grant aid:

- General projects (construction and maintenance of the health infrastructure, provision of medical equipment and supply of vaccines);

- Emergency grant aid (humanitarian relief for natural disasters, conflict areas, refugees and displaced persons);
- Grant assistance for grass roots human security projects (assistance to NGOs, local governments and non-profit organizations, such as hospitals and research institutions).

These grass roots grants are managed through Japanese embassies, and often have health as a priority. Informants have indicated that grass roots grants are more flexible and have a quicker turnaround time from proposal submission to disbursement of funding than other Japanese grant schemes, making this an ideal form of assistance.

Before the mid-1990s, grant aid projects were mainly for physical infrastructure, such as secondary and tertiary hospitals. Japan's ODA budget was increasing from the mid-1980s, and building large-scale health infrastructure was a way to rapidly absorb the funds. By the late 1990s, there was a shift in approved health projects from tertiary to primary health care services, and single large-scale infrastructure projects, like hospitals, were being combined with the 'softer' components of technical cooperation, and included items such as teaching materials and posting of Japanese 'experts'.

Bilateral ODA commitments in health have been officially recorded by the OECD since 1971, when Japan pledged US$3.31 million to health-related assistance. Spending in bilateral health assistance hovered at 2–3 percent of the development budget, but Japan was among the top three sources in health sector programming among bilateral donors from the late 1970s and into the 1980s (Howard, 1989). There was a considerable increase in ODA-provided bilateral health assistance beginning in the mid-1990s. The amount of ODA allocated to bilateral health peaked in 1996 at US$418.02 million, followed by fluctuating decreases in the late 1990s, and reaching another peak in 2004 (US$558.02 million). Since 2004, the bilateral health budget has been fluctuating in the US$200–300 million range.

Should the amount of Japan's ODA continue to decrease, grant assistance to poorer countries, such as those in Africa, will most likely continue to increase while assistance to Asia, where countries are experiencing rapid economic development, will decrease. However, Asia can expect to receive an increase in Japan's ODA in the form of concessional loans.

Multilateral assistance

Japan has been a leading contributor to international organizations since the mid-1980s, when its foreign policy entered a 'spending strategy' (Wan, 1995). Japan views this method of assistance a 'useful form of politically neutral disbursement' (Rix, 1990). The 1990s marked a shift from a bias toward bilateral assistance to a greater emphasis on multilateral assistance (Sasuga, 2007). In 2002, Japan ranked second among DAC members in multilateral contributions (OECD, 2004). During this decade, Japan's subscriptions to multilateral organizations ranged from 24.3 percent of total ODA disbursements in 2001 to 37.7 percent in 2006.

Of the many United Nations (UN) organizations that receive ODA funding in the health sector, three are the largest recipients of Japan's ODA: the United Nations Children's Fund (UNICEF) since 1953; WHO from Regular Budget Funds since 1952, and Extrabudgetary Funds since 1973; and the UN Population Fund (UNFPA) since 1971. In addition, International Planned Parenthood Federation (since 1969) and the GFATM (since 2002) have received a sizable portion of Japan's ODA. The International AIDS Vaccine Initiative has secured a commitment of US$10 million over the next five years from the Japanese government. The money will be channelled through a new trust fund set up in the World Bank.

Multilateral banks are also part of Japan's multilateral strategy. Japan became a member of the World Bank (International Bank for Reconstruction and Development) and IMF during the 1950s. Japan joined World Bank's International Development Association when it was established in 1960, and helped to found the Asian Development Bank (ADB) in 1966. Japan became a member of the Inter-American Development Bank (IDB) in 1976. Japan joined the Africa Development Bank (AfDB) in 1983, having been a signatory member of the Africa Development Fund since its founding in 1973 and one of its top contributors. The World Bank, ADB, AfDB and IDB all have Japan-funded health components in their programs.

Geographic and cultural priorities in health policy

Historically, the concentration of Japanese bilateral ODA has been in Asia. Asia was the focus of Japan's war reparation, and its development assistance emerged as Japan built its relationships and trade partners in the region. In 1970, the Asian region received 98.2 percent of Japanese ODA. Over a quarter of a century later, in 1996, the amount of ODA to the Asian region dropped by nearly one half to 49.6 percent. By the mid-1990s, Africa, Latin America and the Middle East received a larger proportion of Japan's ODA, although certain Asian countries like Indonesia, China and the Philippines still remain the top recipients of Japanese bilateral aid (see Table 2.2).

These trends are mirrored in the health sector. Asia received the largest share of medical and health general grant aid until FY1990, when Africa slowly began to receive a larger share, as seen in Table 2.3. In technical cooperation, Asia has seen a gradual decline since 2004.

According to interviews, these trends were due to several factors:

- Economic growth in Asia decreased need in that region, while pressures from the international donor community, including celebrity attention, increased interest in 'helping' the poorest countries in Africa;
- International security concerns made Africa a focus during the Cold War;
- Japan's interest in a permanent seat on the UN Security Council and the potential for support from the African Union bloc;
- Increased assistance to Afghanistan and Iraq to support its ally, the US, in stabilizing the region.

Table 2.2 Major recipients of Japan's bilateral ODA (total in US$ million)*

	1970		*1980*		*1990*		*2005*	
Rank	*Country*	*Amount*	*Country*	*Amount*	*Country*	*Amount*	*Country*	*Amount*
1	Indonesia	125.84	Indonesia	350.30	Indonesia	867.78	**Iraq**	3502.85
2	Korea	86.76	Bangladesh	215.14	China	723.02	Indonesia	1223.13
3	Pakistan	39.55	Thailand	189.55	Philippines	647.45	China	1064.27
4	India	32.73	Burma†	152.46	Thailand	418.57	Viet Nam	602.66
5	Philippines	19.23	**Egypt**	122.97	Bangladesh	373.57	**DR Congo**	376.26
6	Thailand	16.91	Pakistan	112.42	Malaysia	372.62	Sri Lanka	312.91
7	**Iran**	11.96	Philippines	94.40	**Turkey**	324.21	Philippines	276.43
8	Burma†	11.94	Korea	76.30	Pakistan	193.55	**Zambia**	131.94
9	China	9.53	Malaysia	65.63	Sri Lanka	176.07	**Serbia and Montenegro**	121.58
10	Singapore	5.75	Sri Lanka	44.78	**Poland**	149.85	**Honduras**	103.47
Total amount of net disbursement for 10 countries		**360.2**		**1423.95**		**4246.69**		**7715.50**
Total bilateral ODA						**6939.56**		**10484.61**

* Amount of total ODA includes debt relief.

† Burma officially became Myanmar in 1989; Myanmar became a member of ASEAN in 1997.

Non-Asian countries are in **bold**; Asian countries are in regular font.

Source: Ministry of Foreign Affairs, *Japan's ODA*, 1988, 1991,2006; Ministry of Foreign Affairs, Wagakuni no Sifu Kaihatsu Enjo 1989, vol.1 (in Japanese).

Table 2.3 Geographical distribution of Grant Assistance (GA) and Technical Cooperation (TC) in the health sector (as % of total health sector GA and TC)

Fiscal year	*Asia*		*Africa*		*Oceania*		*Middle East*		*Latin America*		*Europe*	
	GA	*TC*	*GA*	*TC*	*GA*	*TC*	*GA*	*TC*	*GA*	*TC*	*GA*	*TC*
1990	55.7		13.7		19.9		1.0		7.7		–	
1992*	38.1		25.0		16.8		2.7		17.3		–	
1998	49.2		17.1		2.9		5.7		20.0		11.4	
1999		41.7		8.3		–		0.0		50.0		0.0
2000	48.8	50.0	24.4	12.5	0.0	–	4.9	12.5	12.2	25.0	9.8	0.0
2001		50.9		21.1		0.0		10.5		17.5		0.0
2002		52.8		20.8		0.0		7.5		18.9		0.0
2003		51.0		20.4		0.0		6.1		22.4		0.0
2004		46.2		20.0		1.5		7.7		23.1		1.5
2005	39.1	36.8	30.4	30.5	4.3	2.1	4.3	9.5	17.4	20.0	4.3	1.1
2006	29.4	35.7	47.1	27.0	0	3.5	0	13.9	17.6	20.0	5.9	0.0

* Does not add up to 100 percent due to rounding up.

Source: Japan's ODA (1991, 1993); *JICA's Annual Report* (2000–2007).

Japan has been engaged in regional economic cooperation and trade since it began providing ODA, but more recently has been exerting itself to establish regional health initiatives and funds, such as the Japan–ASEAN Integration Fund. The Fund's Plan of Action addresses global issues such as combating infectious diseases and promoting human security.

Japan has been actively engaged with Asia-Pacific Economic Cooperation (APEC), whose regional forums have recently added health as a priority issue in addition to trade and investment. Japan hosted the APEC meeting in September 2010, and has included health as a priority topic under human security. Japan will also chair APEC's Health Working Group and promote its efforts in global health, especially health-systems strengthening for the region. Increasingly, the government of Japan has used its position as chair at influential platforms such as the G8 and APEC to identify itself as a global health leader and advocate for global health governance.

Other elements of Japan's health policy have been influenced by respect for the recipient country's own needs and sovereignty. For example, one of the unique characteristics of Japanese assistance has been the 'request basis' or *yosei shugi*, where the developing country would request the type of aid they wanted to receive. Kohama (1995) noted that this principle enabled Japan to be passive in development assistance and place the initiative on the recipient side. The development community has criticized the principle for being unclear and 'too broad', but the underlying purpose was to ensure the long-term development of recipient countries' economies, promoting the ODA policy of self-help and thus ensuring Japan's trade partners and its own economic growth.

Another example is Japan's focus on human security as a main feature of its foreign policy and diplomacy. In 1998, then Foreign Minister Keizo Obuchi, who became prime minister later that year, first described human security as part of Japan's foreign policy in his speech, 'Japan and East Asia: outlook for a new millennium', in Singapore. He stated that Japan's ODA should be used in the context of 'health and employment' and that Japan 'must seek new strategies for economic development that attach importance to human security, with a view to enhancing the long-term development of this region'. To support this, Prime Minister Obuchi created the UN Trust Fund for Human Security, and Japan included human security as part of its ODA policy in 2003. By the end of 2008, a cumulative total of 191 UN Trust Fund human security projects with a budget of US$303 million had been approved, of which 25 percent were health projects (MOFA, 2009b). Further, 'human security' language can be found in most Japanese foreign policy documents.

The Japanese approach to development assistance focuses on the grass roots level. Japanese experts use a bottom-up approach to empower and protect the communities they work with, and to foster sustainability. Field-based 'learning-by-doing' guides Japan's technical transfer, and is consistent with the human security approach to health. One high-level Japanese official noted, 'JICA experts don't have a paternalistic attitude; they work on equal footing with their counterparts.' Another interviewee from the NGO sector offered a cogent summary of the approach:

> Japan's strength in development assistance is with projects – in implementing – and not at the policy level. Japan is not necessarily good at developing large policy or strategy with short-term and mid-term goals, like the US and UK. However, Japan is better at mid-term/long-term goals like human resource development and working within the framework of human security. Japan is good at working at the grassroots level – face to face with local people and on sustainability. It's part of Japan's personality.

This is one of the great strengths of Japanese ODA.

Japan's institutional mechanisms for global health policy

Government and quasi-governmental agencies

Japan's ODA is administered among the Cabinet Office and 12 ministries and agencies, which provides a fragmented relationship due to the large numbers of ministries and agencies involved. As stated earlier, the governmental ministries most directly involved with Japan's ODA in the health sector are MOFA and the MOF, with substantial involvement of the Ministry of Health, Labour and Welfare (MHLW). Currently, there is no independent international development agency that manages all of Japan's ODA.

MOFA plays the major coordinating role and oversees the policy aspects of Japan's ODA. The MOF deals with international financial institutions. MOFA, MOF and the Ministry of Economy, Trade and Industry, along with the Cabinet

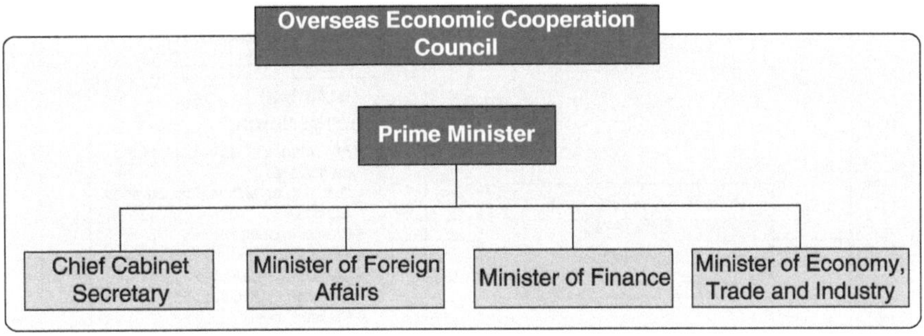

Figure 2.2 Strategic planning of Japan's ODA.

Office, which make up the Overseas Economic Cooperation Council that is chaired by the Prime Minister, oversee strategic planning of Japan's ODA. The MHLW is involved with health-related technical cooperation and not directly involved with the ODA decision-making process.

Within MOFA, the Global Issues Cooperation Division (which is under the International Cooperation Bureau) deals with health-related projects and the policy planning functions of bilateral assistance. Health is a weak area for MOFA due to the limited number of people with an advanced degree in health or development working in the area. As a positive step for strengthening strategies and decisions in global health, after the 2000 G8 Okinawa Summit, MOFA created a fixed-term position and hired a person with an advanced health degree to provide technical assistance and guidance on global health issues.

Several governmental-related organizations are also principal players in ODA in the health sector. The most important is JICA, which serves as the main implementing agency for Japan's ODA. JICA became an independent administrative institution in 2003, and the government appointed Sadako Ogata as president, who was not from the traditional Japanese bureaucracy. She was a leader with many years of experience at the UN, including ten years as UN High Commissioner for Refugees. To more effectively implement JICA's new country-specific approach, JICA's budget and departments, which were previously scheme-based, were reorganized around regions and issues (see Figure 2.3). In 2008, the Overseas Economic Cooperation Operations, the part of the Japan Bank for International Cooperation (JBIC) that provides ODA loans, merged with JICA, making JICA the largest bilateral development organization in the world.

The number of development professionals working at JICA has increased over the years, more than doubling from 1977 to 1997, and the allocation of field staff increased nearly five times during that period. Madame Ogata has made a concerted effort to dispatch more JICA staff to field missions and placed fewer at JICA headquarters in Tokyo. In April 2008 JICA had 55 overseas offices, 6 regional support offices and 17 domestic offices. These figures do not tell the complete story: the number of non-bureaucrat/non-JICA staff (short- and long-term experts) has increased: from 2,946 experts in 2003 to 4,597 experts in 2008. Although these

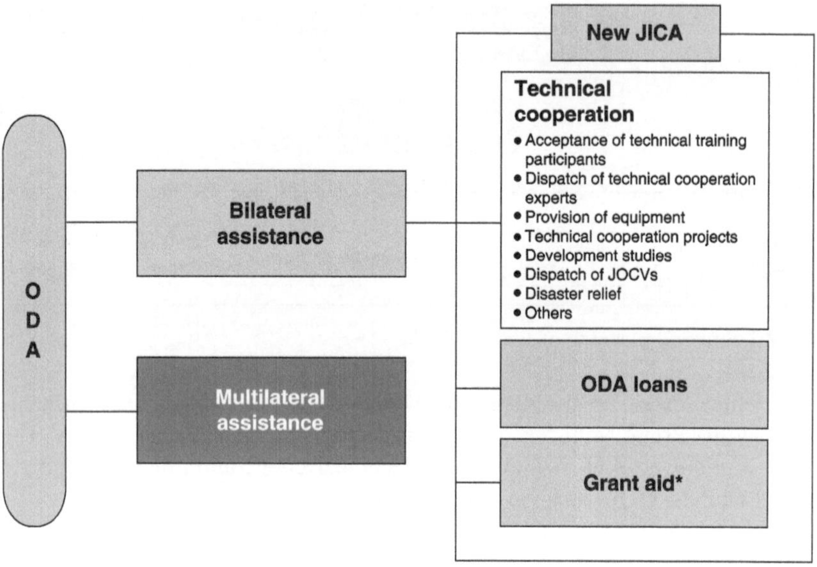

Figure 2.3 JICA's new role in Japan's ODA.

* Does not include the portion of grant aid administered by MOFA for diplomatic reasons.
Source: Adapted from *JICA annual report* (2008) and JICA's webpage.

people are JICA-employed, they are not counted as part of JICA staff and thus not included in Table 2.4.

Several other organisations play a role in Japan's health-sector ODA. The Japan International Cooperation Center (JICE), a non-profit foundation that was formerly the International Cooperation Service Center, was created in 1977 to assist JICA in the implementation of Japanese technical cooperation projects. The Japan International Cooperation System was created by MOFA in 1989, when Japan's ODA budget was growing, to be a procurement agency for grant aid and technical cooperation. Under MHLW, the Bureau of International Cooperation of the International Medical Center of Japan (IMCJ) has been providing technical cooperation and sending 'experts' to developing countries since 1986. IMCJ also

Table 2.4 Number of JICA Staff

	1977	*1982*	*1987*	*1992*	*1997*	*1998*	*2003*	*2009**
JICA Total staff	579	741	867	1023	1173	1180	1213	1664
Posted at overseas offices	57 (9.8%)	111 (15%)	156 (18%)	254 (24.8%)	324 (27.6%)	329 (27.9%)	369 (30%)	413 (24.8%)

* In 2008 a part of Japan Bank for International Cooperation dealing with Overseas Economic Cooperation Operations (concessional loans) merged with JICA, and 214 JBIC employees were added to JICA.

Source: MOFA, JICA and OECD (2004).

provides health-related training courses and conducts surveys and research. In April 2010 IMCJ became an independent agency, and changed its name to the National Center for Global Health and Medicine. The MHLW established the Japan International Corporation of Welfare Services in 1983, to provide health-related technical cooperation similar to that of IMCJ.

Professional staff

The number of global health professionals in Japanese governmental organizations is small compared to comparable institutions in the US and Europe. In 2009, JICA had an estimated 29 staff with health-related advanced degrees. The number of Japanese personnel at international organizations is equally slim.[1] For example, only 0.8 percent of WHO professional and general employees in 2007 are Japanese, a dire under-representation given that Japan was the second-largest contributor to the WHO and provided nearly 20 percent of the total contribution (WHO, 2009b, 2010e). Many of those interviewed from universities, multilateral organizations and the Japanese parliament also noted the dearth of Japanese in senior/leadership positions at international organizations. There is currently only one Japanese senior management-level staff member at the WHO, a few at UNDP, and none at the Global Fund. One interview suggested that without high-level leadership participation, there is no advocate to articulate and rationalize the benefits of Japan's continued significant financial contributions to these organizations to Japanese citizens and its government.

One reason for this lack of health and development professionals is the *ido* (transfer) system, under which Japanese bureaucracies rotate employees among divisions in order to give them an understanding of how the overall system works (Rix, 1980). As a result, the Japanese bureaucracy cultivates generalists, not specialists. This poses a challenge for people working in global health and officials seconded to multilateral or international organizations. It takes time to understand the local situation and to develop contacts and nurture relationships, and short assignments do not allow staff to fully understand technical issues. One interviewee in a senior position at a multilateral organization said the *ido* system produced 'lots of waste and was not an efficient way of using human resources . . . and placed Japan at a disadvantage'.

Another challenge is the rigid Japanese traditional lifetime employment and single-track seniority system, which discourages Japanese government officials from training via placement at international organizations on a health project in a developing country. An extended leave of absence (more than two or three years) to work on a development project or at an international organization, such as the WHO, is often difficult and harms career advancement and job security. Furthermore, the current bureaucratic structure favors individuals directly from college, especially from top universities. College graduates who opt to spend time overseas on a development project may find that their experience does not add value to their résumé or translate into a job in Japan.

Finally, some interviewees mentioned the lack of proficiency in languages other than Japanese – especially English – as an obstacle attracting Japanese professionals to global health as a profession. The Japanese language can be both subtle and vague, and native Japanese speakers talking in their second or third language can create ambiguity or misunderstanding of Japan's policies and goals. However, this is changing as younger individuals who have had opportunities to study abroad and are more fluent in English join the ranks of ODA professionals.

These risks help explain the limited number of Japanese in leadership positions at health-related international organizations and projects (Wagatsuma, 1989; Kasai and Lee, 1997). Although there are a limited number of Japanese global health professionals, there is a large pool of talented Japanese working on domestic health topics, such as maternal and child health. One interviewee in Japanese academia pointed out this serious disconnect between Japan's domestic public health experts and global health experts, despite the critical relationship between these policy areas. He mentioned that it was his personal mission to promote/nurture young talent in Japan and expose domestic experts to global health, because ultimately global health is part of Japan. He believed this was his role in global health governance.

Non-governmental organizations

The role of Japan's civil society in global health policy is expanding. Japanese non-profit organizations started work in international development and health about the same time as the government began providing ODA. The Japan Overseas Christian Medical Cooperative Services (JOCS), the oldest international NGO registered in Japan, was created in 1960 by Japanese Christian physicians to care for the victims of the Sino-Japanese War. The Japanese Organization for International Cooperation in Family Planning (JOICFP) was established in 1968. At first, new NGOs in Japan were devoted to domestic issues, but by the 1970s NGOs such as the Japan International Volunteer Center (JVC) began to form with specific causes 'in response to the needs of the developing world' (Kuroda, 2003). By the 1980s, international NGOs such as World Vision, Plan International and CARE began to create partner organizations in Japan (Itô, 1998; Kuroda, 2003). Currently, there are about 30 Japanese NGOs working in the field of global health.

Unlike the US and Europe, the Japanese government did not call on NGOs to implement international health aid until the 1990s. According to some NGOs and Japanese politicians, MOFA underestimated NGOs' professional capabilities and did not see them as real partners. In 1994, MOFA began to incorporate NGOs more actively in their ODA discussions through the 'Dialogue between MOFA/NGO on GII/IDI', a forum which continues today.

The proportion of health-sector ODA implemented by NGOs and civil society organizations (CSOs) is much less for Japan than for other major donors. For example, in 2008, only 0.86 percent of Japanese ODA dispersed in the health sector was carried out by NGOs, compared to 11.83 percent in Australia, 16.95 percent in the US and 27.84 in Norway.[2] The leading donors for Japanese NGOs working in global health are MOFA and JICA. Public funding, however, remains biased towards larger, more familiar organizations, like UNICEF.

Japanese NGOs are growing and establishing a stronger presence in global health, but they are not comparable in number or scale to their counterparts in the US or Europe. One of the main constraints of Japanese NGOs is their financial status. Japan has few religious charitable organizations. The Japanese public is not accustomed to donating funds to NGOs; nor is the Japanese business sector accustomed to philanthropy, especially in the global health field. Public awareness of Japanese NGOs as professional organizations is still very low and many Japanese characterize NGOs as volunteer organizations. However, acceptance of non-profit organizations as professional organizations has risen considerably since the 1995 Kobe earthquake. The Law to Promote Specified Non-profit Organization Activities, adopted in March 1998, established a legal framework for Japanese NGOs. It also helped improve public awareness and increase the credibility and tax status of NGOs.

Other influential non-governmental groups have connections to academia. The best-known example is the Working Group on Challenges in Global Health and Japan's Contributions, informally known as the 'Takemi Working Group' (TWG). The 2008 G8 Summit in Japan it brought together Japanese experts in academia, civil society and the private sector to discuss Japan's role in and contributions to global health, along with government officials under the leadership of two important individuals: Keizo Takemi, an academician and politician who served as State Secretary for Foreign Affairs and Senior Vice Minister of Health, Labour and Welfare, and Tadashi Yamamoto, President of the Japan Center for International Exchange (JCIE). The TWG also tapped into the resources of Harvard School of Public Health, where Takemi was a research fellow. Independent Japanese think tanks, such as the Health Policy Institute, Japan and JCIE, are also actively involved in Japan's health policy.

Japan's expanding profile in health assistance

In the 1990s, Japan's profile in health assistance began to grow. In 1994, Japan announced the Global Issues Initiative on Population and AIDS, the first of Japan's five-year health initiatives, and allocated US$3 billion to it over the next five years. This initiative also stressed a collaboration with the US in tackling global health challenges, building on the strengths of both countries, and making it a trilateral cooperation with the developing country.[3] In the same year, Japan hosted the Tenth International Conference on AIDS in Yokohama. These two events were a turning point for Japan that has become more pronounced since the new millennium with events surrounding the G8 Summits, other major conferences, the USAID–JAPAN Partnership for Global Health, and the incorporation of human security in the revised ODA Charter.

2000 G8 Summit in Okinawa

Under the Japanese leadership, the 2000 Kyushu-Okinawa G8 Summit established global health as an important agenda (Kirton and Mannell, 2007; Kurokawa,

2009). Japan also allowed the voices of other Asian countries, such as China, India, Indonesia and South Korea, to be heard (Dobson, 2005). The government of Japan strongly supported initiatives to combat parasitic and infectious diseases, with an emphasis on HIV/AIDS, malaria and tuberculosis, and also announced its own Infectious Diseases Initiative (IDI), which pledged US$3 billion for infectious and parasitic diseases over five years, and actually spent more than US$4 billion over the first four years (Kunii, 2007).

The Summit produced a firm commitment for global health from the G8 leaders. It was a venue where Japan exhibited leadership, cementing its role of global health governance, galvanizing new resources for global health, and encouraging the creation of the Global Fund to Fight AIDS, Tuberculosis and Malaria two years later – a contribution that is not widely known. This is largely because of Japan's resistance to publicity and its preference for low-profile leadership and consensus-building behind the scenes (Rix, 1993, Drifte, 1996). This subtle style of leadership is rooted in Japan's history as an aggressive nation and the uneasiness felt by its East Asian neighbors (Dent 2008).

A new type of global health diplomacy developed in Japan as a result of Japan hosting two major international events: the 2008 G8 Summit in Toyako and The Tokyo International Conference on African Development IV.

The 2008 G8 Summit in Toyako

In 2008, Japan hosted the G8 Summit again in Toyako as the world was facing financial crises, disastrous food shortages and climate change. Global health was at risk of being dropped from the priority list, given the various competing crises. However, as host nation, Japan created the agenda and topics for the meeting and placed global health – specifically health-system strengthening and continued support for Millennium Development Goals (MDGs) 4, 5 and 6 – on the priority list. These topics were featured in the Summit Leaders Declaration and the Toyako Framework for Action. Although some critics were pessimistic about the lack of financial pledges for health, the Summit did produce some notable achievements. First, the Government of Japan arranged the first separate Health Experts Group before the Summit. Another achievement was the approval of a mechanism to track and evaluate the extent to which the G8 countries met the commitments in their health pledges (McCurry, 2008). The G8 2010 Muskoka Accountability Report's executive summary outlined three intentions of the report:

- A performance report of G8's commitments related to development assistance
- An assessment of the results of G8's actions
- A venue to create lessons learned for future opportunities.

In this context, the report fostered transparency in identifying the achievements and failures of the countries to meet their commitments.

The Tokyo International Conference on African Development IV (TICAD)

TICAD is a conference for the promotion of African development that was first held in 1983 co-hosted by the Japanese Government, the UN and the World Bank, and that has been held every five years since. TICAD aimed to help reduce poverty in Africa through economic development, promote trade and investment between Africa and Asia and, more recently, help achieve the MDGs within the framework of human security (TICAD/UNDP Africa Bureau, 2012).

Hosting TICAD IV and the G8 Summit presented Japan with unique opportunities to contribute to global health policy making. The Summit was the first time that Japan used a participatory planning process, creating a multi-stakeholder group to set the agenda for the meeting. The decision-making process involved public–private and intergovernmental partnerships, drawing on the global health expertise of participants from academic, private sector, public, and non-governmental organizations. This was the first time that the Japanese bureaucracy joined beyond purely sectional interests on behalf of a broad health agenda. MOFA, MOF and MHLW came together to discuss health matters that extended beyond domestic borders and position, and to prepare Japan to take its place at the international health policy dialog table. The inclusion of civil society and other actors beyond the traditional ministries in decision making was made possible by aligning the right people at the right time. The strong leadership of Keizo Takemi, who headed the TWG, with Tadashi Yamamoto of JCIE, played a crucial role in this carefully prepared process. In effect, the TWG worked outside formal governmental channels and functioned as Track II diplomacy, enabling multi-stakeholder participation in global health governance, fostering the free exchange of ideas amongst members of the bureaucracy and civil society, and creating a new way of developing policy in Japan.

The future of Japan's engagement in global health and global health governance

The new global health agendas that are emerging are population aging, non-communicable diseases, policy cooperation to middle-income countries, and universal health coverage. Japan's wealth of knowledge and experience in these areas will inevitably place the country in a leadership position in setting the global health agenda in the near future. When interviewees were asked to define Japan's comparative advantage in global health, the most common response was its postwar experience in improving health, including health system management. From a policy point of view, considering Japan's financial limitations and its relationship with East Asia, Japan can best share its experience in the area of health systems. Japan's health care system evolved from the pre-war period and was implemented when it was a middle-income country in the 1960s. Japan has fine-tuned its own system, and the health insurance scheme that is a crucial aspect of it, learning what works and what to avoid – knowledge that can be shared with today's middle-income countries. Given geographic proximity and historic relationships, Japan can provide both funds and policy leadership to middle-income Asian countries in the next five to ten years.

Japan's population has the highest life expectancy in the world and is the fastest-aging society. These demographics have inevitably increased the prevalence of chronic diseases: primarily cancer, cardiovascular disease, chronic respiratory disease and diabetes. In response, Japan has instituted several policy measures. The Health Promotion Law that passed in 2002 established an annual check-up (waist measurement, blood pressure and cholesterol level) for the entire population. A scheme for long-term nursing care insurance has been added to national health insurance. Japan may not be a leader in tackling HIV/AIDS or malaria, but looking ahead 20–40 years, it can make a meaningful contribution to addressing the non-communicable diseases that may be the biggest problem in global health.

However, the extent of Japan's role will depend on the domestic political situation and the leadership taken in ODA policy. In August 2009, the Democratic Party of Japan (DPJ) won in a landslide victory over the ruling Liberal Democratic Party (LDP). The DPJ's campaign platform focused on domestic issues, such as subsidies for child rearing and education allowances, with very little attention to ODA, except for the slogan of *nyua nyuou* ('enter Asia, enter the West'), implying closer ties with both the US and the Asian countries (Funabashi, 2009). Aside from that statement, the DPJ has not engaged in major discussions on global health or how to align ODA with national or regional interests. More positively, the party has recognized ODA as an important tool of foreign policy. Further, they have stated that they will engage civil society more and provide more support for non-profit organizations by reforming the tax law to allow deductions for donations. Some NGOs working in global health have noted an increase in the pool of resources available to them since 2010, and more participation of senior bureaucrats at meeting with NGOs.

An important priority for the DPJ is the elimination of 'inefficiency and unfairness'. JICA has been one of the government agencies charged with eliminating waste and its budget has decreased along with the decreasing ODA budget. Some NGOs see this cost-cutting as forecasting an even bleaker outlook for their funding opportunities. Further, the 2010 election did not produce the support the DPJ was anticipating, despite *jigyo shiwake* (waste-cutting measures) as a political strategy. Although the DPJ has broadly mentioned ODA in their focus area, the ODA budget could be jeopardized in favor of funding domestic priorities and increasing public support. In addition, the frequently changing prime ministers – five in the past three years – makes developing consistent policies from the cabinet office difficult.

The Japanese development community has been experiencing 'aid fatigue' and there has been mounting pressure from citizens to decrease ODA. At the same time, there are demands for increased accountability and transparency in the foreign aid bureaucracies. Past public criticism of lack of ODA transparency (including a bribery scandal using ODA funds in Vietnam and the public outcry against the *amakudari* system, where Japanese senior government officials retire into distinguished, high-paying public or private sector positions) have been major sources of institutional reform.

Japan is experiencing an extended recession. In July 2009, unemployment reached an all-time high of 5.7 percent. As a result, the country is becoming inward-looking, and prejudice against ODA is increasing. For the first time in years, the trend of high school students wanting to go abroad has reversed. Further, youths felt 'dark' about the future. Unemployed or irregular workers are questioning why the government is giving large sums of money to developing countries when there are needs within the country.

However, opinion polls have found that support for overall ODA has been slowly increasing since reaching a nadir of 19 percent in 2004 to 29 percent in 2009, with the public especially favoring the health sector for development cooperation. Health (73 percent), followed by water/sanitation (68 percent) and education (55 percent) were the areas the public approved in this June 2010 public opinion poll (www8.cao.go.jp/survey/tokubetu/tindex-h22.html).

There is a huge gap between public opinion and the discussions that take place at international forums like the G8. Greater public awareness of global health and global health governance may help to generate further support for ODA. Japanese media regularly cover health-related topics, such as tuberculosis and malaria, but rarely global health.[4] Thus the public may be confused about what global health is and why it is important for Japan to continue to play a leading role. Until the general public understands and appreciates these issues, it will be a struggle to encourage the government to make ODA a priority.

Many of the Japanese interviewed for this chapter questioned its government's interest in establishing itself as a leader in global health. With the exception of hosting the G8 Summits in 2000 and 2008, they noted Japan's otherwise passive participation at international conferences and limited involvement in setting global health trends. Nonetheless, they are hopeful that Japan can reverse this trend and become a more active partner by applying its postwar experiences in improving health to place the country in a leadership position in global health.

Conclusion

When Japan began providing ODA, health was not a priority area, but it has evolved into an important sector of Japan's ODA and foreign policy under human security. Japan's profile in health assistance began to grow with the formulation of health initiatives in the 1990s. In the past decade, Japan took a global health leadership position by introducing infectious diseases and health for developing countries at the 2000 G8 Summit in Okinawa. And eight years later, at TICAD IV and the G8 Summit in Toyako, Japan was a leader in making health system strengthening; MDGs 4, 5 and 6; and other health issues a priority.

Traditionally, the central government – mainly bureaucrats – dominated global health policy making, but civil society is increasingly playing a role in global health. Further, Japan is engaging in new global health diplomacy through a public–private collaboration that has incorporated the suggestions of many stakeholders into global health policy making. However, prolonged economic stagnation, budget deficits and debt, the insecurities of lifetime employment and rising unemployment and poverty are putting pressure on the Japanese government to cut its budget. Other competing priorities, such as the Afghanistan/Pakistan assistance package and climate change, have entered Japan's foreign policy.

Japan now ranks as the third-largest economy in the world, down from second place. The era of Japan as the 'number-one' donor ended with the new millennium, and ODA continues to decrease. Although the ODA budget is small compared to other areas of spending within the national budget, foreign assistance is an easy target for budget cutting. There are no champions of global health within the Japanese parliament and no strong domestic constituents advocating for global health funding. However, recent polls revealed the Japanese public's continued support of health aid within the shrinking ODA budget.

The Takemi Working Group is a strong advocate for global health, but it lacks sufficient visibility and media coverage. Japan's leadership in global health and global health governance is growing, but the current administration's strategy on global health is uncertain given the instability and confusion of the current political scene, and the absence of consistent political leadership. In addition, Madame Ogata's leadership at JICA will eventually come to a transition, given that she has already held her position for over seven years and turned 83 this year. Further, with the decreasing ODA budget, Japan will need to turn to other areas – mainly the wealth of knowledge from its postwar experience in improving health to place the country in a leadership position in global health. As one government official noted, 'Japan slowly follows the trend, but is eventually leading and resetting the agenda. Japan has its own pace and the pace is not as quick as the American or European donors.'

The Japanese way of doing politics is 'leadership from behind' – being a facilitator without encouraging a huge reaction from the rest of the world. Leadership is not a traditional national character of Japan, but Japanese leadership is developing, just as Japan's future role in global health and global health governance are emerging.

Notes

1 As per an email from a staff at JICA on 8/24/2009 indicated a rough estimate of 29 JICA staff with advanced health degrees: nursing (6), medicine (2), demographics (2), public health (15) and veterinary medicine (4).

2 Percentage was computed using OECE.StatExtracts (http://stats.oecd.org/index.aspx) for total "Health" and "Population and Reproductive Health" ODA channeled to NGOs and civil society for 2008. DAC member average was 17.86%.

3 This trilateral collaboration was known as the US-Japan Common Agenda, which began in July 1993. After a review in 2001, the collaboration was transformed to USAID-Japan Partnership for Global Health.

4 A search in Japanese using Nihon Keizai Shimbun's (Japan Economic Times Company) Nikkei Telcom on major national Japanese newspapers was conducted on 4/25/2009. Search using key work "global health" for the past year produced no results.

3 Global health governance in China

The case of China's health aid to foreign countries

Jenny Qu Wang, Minquan Liu, Aming Liu, Tao Wei and Hang Li

Introduction

Despite being a developing country itself, China has provided considerable aid to other developing countries over the past half-century. As the world now becomes more globalized and China's role in this world expands, its aid to foreign countries has gained a unique significance in the ongoing discourse of global governance.

There is a growing body of Chinese and English literature that studies China's general aid to foreign countries. However, as an important part of China's foreign aid, its health aid to other developing countries has been less actively and systematically studied due to the limited amount of publicly released data and information. Existing research on China's health aid to foreign countries (CHAFC) has focused on one particular form – the deployment of Chinese Medical Teams (CMTs). Obviously this research cannot indicate the scope, extent, and target of China's overall engagement in this field, nor does it link China's activities in this area to its role in improving global health governance. There is a clear need, therefore, to better understand the overall picture of CHAFC and its potential in shaping China's emerging role in global health governance.

By 'global health governance', this paper adopts the definition as given in the paper by Koenig-Archibugi in this volume, that is, global health governance may consist of a web of relationships that

> can have one, two or all three of the following dimensions: regulative relationships, through which rules are developed, agreed and enforced; discursive relationships, through which ideas are generated and diffused; and allocative relationships, through which material resources are extracted, transferred and distributed.

While global governance thus defined covers a wide range of aspects, in this chapter we shall only focus on health aid as a vehicle of global health governance-building, more specifically, China's role in it.

The paper begins by outlining the political and institutional context of CHAFC, emphasizing its strong link to the country's overall foreign policy stance in general, and foreign *aid* policy stance in particular, and its dependence on multisectoral cooperation within China (in the second section). Specific forms which this aid has taken and the likely magnitudes of the flows involved are reviewed in the third section, while the fourth provides discussions of the principal characteristics of CHAFC, based on the information provided, and the role it has played and it is likely to continue to play in the coming decades in shaping global health governance. A final section provides broad conclusions of this report.

At the outset it is important to state that while there is some information on the forms of CHAFC, little is actually available on the financial flows involved, and the impact of these flows on health development of recipient countries. In spite of this, strenuous effort was made to piece together whatever information could be found from diverse sources. The quality of such information may be open to question. However, in the absence of anything better, this is what we shall present and what we shall base our discussions on.

This research makes a systematic attempt to study the existing work available on China's foreign aid and CHAFC through literature review, historical records analysis and analysis of focused interviews. In particular we systematically searched the database CNKI, one of the largest Chinese language databases in China, and PubMed, as well as through Google Scholars and Baidu, the largest Chinese language search engine. The information collected has served as the basis for piecing together a record of China's engagement in health aid to foreign countries.

Three important sources are especially targeted in our search. One is the information released by the Office of the Preparatory Work for the 30-year History Exhibition on China's Opening Up, an exhibition organized by the Ministry of Commerce (MOC), International Communication Office of the Communist Party of China (ICOCPC), Party Literature Research Center of the CPC (PLRC), and the Xinhua News Agency (XHNA). Many line ministries, including the Ministry of Foreign Affairs (MOFA) and Ministry of Finance (MOF), were co-organizers. Most importantly, the exhibition provides a detailed 30-year history of the bilateral economic and trade cooperation between China and 171 countries, prepared directly by the Economic and Commercial Counselor's Offices of the Embassies in various recipient countries. In the materials gathered for that exhibition, activities of health aid were well represented.

A second important source is a solid piece of research on CMT, published as recently as the end of 2009. This study provides rich details on the history of CMT, including information on the year and responsible province of, and major changes subsequently made to, each health aid project. It has helped to shed much light on the scope and range of CHAFC, and the diverse participants involved, from its very beginning.

A third source is the websites of major international organizations, especially those of the UN system related to health. Principally, five organizations were covered, including WHO, UNICEF, UNFPA, Joint United Nations Programme on HIV/AIDS (UNAIDS) and International Committee of the Red Cross (ICRC). Additionally, the Global Fund to Fight AIDS, Tuberculosis and Malaria was also targeted.

In order to explain the likely factors responsible for the forms and trends of CHAFC that we have identified, as well as the likely contributions they have made to engaging China in global health governance, this research also conducted focused interviews. Two groups of experts were interviewed: experts in the field of health and experts in international relations. Participants included policy makers, social practitioners and academic scholars. In total, nine interviews were conducted. The information collected through these interviews has been systematically analyzed and integrated into this report (see Appendix 6 for a list of the interviewees).

Political and institutional context of China's health aid

A country's aid policy is naturally closely related to its foreign policy, and CHAFC has never been independent of general foreign policy since its inception in the 1960s. This dependence is amply illustrated in three main respects. First, all strategies and actions of CHAFC have been conditioned by the general principles governing the country's foreign policy, collectively known as the 'Independent Foreign Policy of Peace'. In other words, CHAFC has always adhered to these general principles of foreign policy as pursued by China, and that, to a large degree, has given it its reputation as 'health diplomacy'. Secondly, policies on health aid have been subject to China's general policy on foreign aid, and hence strategies that have underpinned CHAFC have closely conformed to those of foreign aid generally. Thirdly, the internal processes of CHAFC decision making and operation have been closely based on a model of multisectoral cooperation.

Health aid policy as part of foreign policy

According to the principles of the Independent Foreign Policy of Peace, the fundamental goals of foreign policy for China are: to preserve its independence, sovereignty and territorial integrity; to create a favorable international environment for its reform, opening up and modernization; to maintain world peace; and to promote common development. The fundamental basis for this foreign policy is the 'Five Principles of Peaceful Coexistence', which were first proposed by Premier Zhou in 1953 when he met with a visiting Indian delegation, and which have since gained widespread acceptance internationally as the key criteria for bilateral cooperation with China. These five principles are:

1 mutual respect for sovereignty and territorial integrity,
2 mutual non-aggression,
3 mutual non-interference in each other's internal affairs,
4 equality and mutual benefit, and
5 peaceful co-existence (China Ministry of Foreign Affairs, 2000).

Within this framework of foreign policy and as a developing country, China has held a positive stance on South–South cooperation. It has pursued the development of extensive and in-depth cooperation with other developing countries in economic, scientific and technological, educational and cultural fields on the basis of the principle of equality and mutual benefit, with an emphasis on results, diversity of forms, and common development (Lv, 2003). In accordance with this stand, China has continued to offer assistance within its capacity to other developing countries in the past half a century with no conditions attached.

As an embodiment and extension of foreign policy, and in accordance with the Five Principles of Peaceful Coexistence, CHAFC has been an important part of China's engagement in South–South cooperation. This has implied that the conduct of CHAFC has had to respect other countries' sovereignty and steadfastly follow the principle of non-interference in the recipient countries' internal affairs, with no conditions attached to the provision of health aid. This 'no-strings-attached' aid was distinctly different from the Western style of foreign aid that has openly sought to exert influence over the internal affairs of recipient countries through aid (Thompson, 2005). It may well be true that these principles have not been fully adhered to by China in every case. Nevertheless, they have served as a crucial point of departure from similar Western aid, paving the way for China to gain trust and confidence from various recipient countries, according to Chinese publications (e.g. Li, 2009; MOH, 2009). In so doing, China has become an attractive partner for recipient countries in many parts of the world, in particular Africa.

Health aid policy as part of foreign aid policy

Health aid policy as part of general foreign aid policy means that strategies of health aid must follow both the principles of general foreign aid and general foreign policy, and that the conduct of health aid be part of the general foreign aid strategies and plans.

Before the opening up,[1] health aid policy adhered to the so-called 'Eight Principles of China's Economic and Technical Aid to Foreign Countries', which was originally drawn up by Premier Zhou Enlai in 1964 when he visited 14 Asian and African countries. These principles included: equality; mutual benefit and non-interference in the recipient countries' internal affairs; improvement in the ability of self-reliance of recipient countries; ensuring real benefit for the recipient countries; minimizing the burden on recipient countries; and strictly complying with obligations. This may be seen as a manifestation of the basic foreign policy principles in the work of foreign aid. As a result, China's aid to foreign countries has had a strong political priority, and this has also been fully reflected in the work of CHAFC (Huang, 2007).

The connection between foreign policy and foreign assistance raised suspicions among some aid recipients, notably certain South East Asian countries.[2] Historically, it is not possible to know the motivations behind Chinese foreign aid, however the principle of mutual benefit seems to imply that China's foreign assistance was not entirely altruistic. Indeed, an important function of China's foreign aid was to help the new government develop as large a net of potential international support as possible. This might explain why in the first 30 years of the People's Republic of China (PRC) CHAFC predominantly targeted newly independent and socialist countries, which were then regarded by the Chinese government as potential allies.[3] This same motivation undoubtedly explains why China had a disproportionally high ratio of foreign aid to state financial expenditure, despite its own low level of economic development.[4]

In the late 1970s concurrent with the China's new policy of opening up, the fundamental principles of foreign aid became more pragmatic. New policy guidelines called for, among others, equality and mutual benefit, real results, diversity of forms and common development. Subsequently, in 1996, China announced five principles of cooperation with African countries, which included friendship so as to become 'all-weather friends'; equality; mutual respect for sovereignty and non-interference in each other's internal affairs; mutual benefit to achieve common development; strengthened consultation and closer cooperation in international affairs; and a vision of the future (Huang, 2007). These new working guidelines for foreign aid naturally applied to CHAFC, too.

These changes in the fundamental principles of foreign aid were reflected in significant extensions of CHAFC, from the deployment of traditional CMTs to new forms of assistance such as personnel training, humanitarian aid, governmental free aid, interest-free loans and discounted interest loans. These new pragmatic forms helped to better cater to the interests of Chinese domestic parties, such as enterprises, research institutes and overseas companies, in the cause of health aid. At the same time, the immediate aim of CHAFC also underwent a significant change. While CHAFC was and still is looked at as an important tool serving certain specific national interests, enhancing China's international reputation as a responsible big power has become a major consideration conditioning the conduct of CHAFC.[5]

While CHAFC has exhibited different features in different periods, the principles of equality, mutual benefit, common development, and no strings attached have always been among its key guidelines. From 1997 onwards, China began to expand its CHAFC, both in terms of its flow and in terms of the number of recipient countries. At present, China provides foreign aid to more than 160 countries, reflecting its rising status as a responsible power in international affairs. Of this, CHAFC has been an important part.[6]

Structure and implementation of Chinese foreign aid

As part of China's general foreign aid policy, CHAFC has been under the centralized management of the MOC. The direct unit responsible for health aid within MOC is the Department of Aid to Foreign Countries (DAFC). DAFC is responsible for formulating and implementing foreign aid policy, drafting the related laws and regulations, promoting reform of the foreign aid sector, making foreign aid plans, developing country-specific aid programs, making decisions for and implementing aid projects and so on. A second department within MOC, the Department of International Trade and Economic Affairs (DITEA), takes charge of foreign aid donated to international organizations within a multilateral framework.[7]

In addition to MOC, another 22 relevant ministries and commissions under the State Council also take part in relevant foreign aid programs according to its specialization. Among the 22 ministries, MOFA and MOF are the two bodies generally involved in foreign aid. The MOFA plays an important role in aligning the practice of foreign aid with the general political and diplomatic considerations of the country and, through its Economic Counselor's Office (ECO) in various countries, it is also involved in the actual operations of processing and managing aid in recipient countries.

The MOF is, on the other hand, directly in charge of the budgeting and allocation of the overall foreign aid funds to each ministry and program. These two ministries, together with the MOC and a specially appointed technical team, provide the inspection of foreign aid programs and projects. Other ministries may be engaged in specific aid programs or projects falling within their specialization. Thus the Ministry of Health (MOH) is entrusted with the responsibility of CMT deployment. Within the MOH, the unit directly in charge of the deployment of CMTs is the Department of International Cooperation (DIC). More specifically, it is the Division of Asian and African Affairs and the Division of Medical Aid to Developing Countries of DIC that execute the responsibility. Likewise, the Ministry of Agriculture (MOA) takes charge of the execution of various agricultural foreign aid programs and projects; the Ministry of Science and Technology (MOST) does the same for science and technology ones; the Ministry of Education (MOE) and China Women's Federation (CWF) play a similar role for those belonging to their line of specialization; the People's Bank of China (PBC) takes charge of the relations with various multilateral development banks, and the Export–Import Bank of China (EIBC) of projects involving preferential loans.

The general system of Chinese foreign aid is multi-sectoral in nature (see Figure 3.1). Since many aid projects and programs are comprehensive packages involving economic development, health, agriculture, education, etc., their operation inevitably require joint actions of all the related ministries (Huang and Hu, 2009).

Chinese foreign aid also has key players from local levels. Generally, local foreign aid affairs are conducted under the centralized management of the Department of Commerce at the level of province, municipality and autonomous region. At the same time, specific line departments at this level would be put in charge of the operation of particular foreign aid programs or projects belonging to their line of responsibility. Thus the Department of Health in each province is directly responsible for organizing provincial CMTs to be dispatched to various recipient countries. Our discussions in the third section of this chapter will provide further details on this.

For health aid, as is outlined in Zhou (2008) and Davies *et al.* (2008), the process normally begins with a request for specific health aid from a recipient government to the Chinese diplomatic mission in its country.[8] Through the ECO, the embassy screens these requests, and then passes them onto the MOFA and MOC in Beijing. The MOC (and MOH) then appoints a technical team to carry out an evaluation of the proposal and to arrive at a preliminary budget. With these detailed reports from the technical team, the MOC then consults various parties concerned, including the MOH and MOF, the various line ministries of relevant specialization, and the embassy in the recipient country. If the project is deemed viable, the MOC then submits the proposal and its recommendation to the State Council for a final decision. If the project is approved for implementation, the MOF then releases the budgeted funds to the MOC or MOH, or both, depending on the case, under the instruction of the State Council. For the deployment of CMTs, the MOH will be responsible for selecting the necessary CMT members and teams from the provinces that it chooses, and will carry out necessary trainings before deployment. For other health projects, such as hospital construction, a tendering process will be initiated by the MOC first, and the companies that win the contracts will then be entrusted with project implementation, under agreement with the MOC. Once work in a recipient country starts, the Chinese Embassy in that country is then put in charge of managing the work, while another body, the Executive Bureau of International Economic Cooperation (BIEC) under the MOC, would execute the work at the project level. The BIEC, DAFC and MOH usually jointly undertake on the spot visits to carry out monitoring.

Although the process of foreign aid (and health aid) approval and execution has been studied by Chinese and Western scholars, little has in fact been uncovered about the magnitude of the health aid undertaken in the past 50 years, especially in regard to its country distribution, time trends, and its contribution to global health governance. Below, we present the limited data that we were able to uncover in the process of writing up this report, which we hope will contribute to a better understanding of China's record and profile of health aid in the past half-century, and its contribution to global health governance.

Forms and flows of China's health aid

Bilateral aid as strategy of CHAFC

Deployment of Chinese medical teams

The deployment of Chinese medical teams (CMTs) to developing countries has been one of the main characteristics of CHAFC, and is a feature that distinguishes Chinese health aid from assistance provided by other countries.[9] China dispatched its first medical team in 1963, at the invitation of the then Algerian government, and has continued to do so for 50 years. A recent study estimates that between the years 1963 and 2008, China had cumulatively dispatched over 20,000 medical workers to 71 countries (Li, 2009). In total, 26 Chinese provinces, autonomous regions and municipalities participated,[10] including several of the least-developed Chinese provinces, such as Shanxi, Shaanxi, Gansu, Qinghai and Guizhou. Of the 71 recipient countries, deployment of medical teams in 68 countries constituted long-term aid, while the three others were short-term aid (such as tsunami aid). Deployment in 44 out of 68 countries continued without a break from 1963 to 2008, while in 24 remaining countries it was interrupted for various reasons, including the

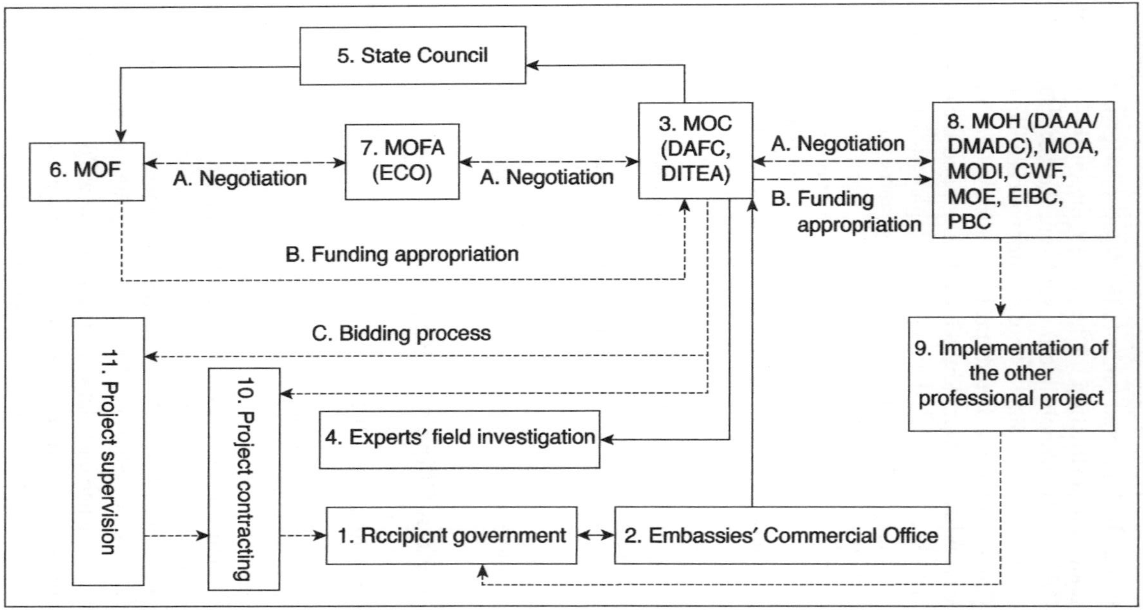

Figure 3.1 Decision making and implementation processes of CHAFC.

Source: Modified according to Zhou (2008: 41).

breakdown of diplomatic relationships. However, in 13 of these 24 countries, deployment has already been resumed. In 2008, there were 47 CMTs working at 122 sites in various recipient countries (Li, 2009: 30–32). The table in Appendix 1 lists all the CMTs deployed by responsible province, recipient country and year.

Of five major geographical regions (Africa, Asia, Oceania, South America and Europe), Africa accounts for the highest share of countries that either have accepted or are accepting CMTs. In total, 47 African countries have received or are receiving CMTs, representing 66.20 per cent of all recipient countries. The second highest share, or 25.35 per cent, are sent to 18 Asian countries. Oceania, Europe and South America account for a comparatively very low 4.23 per cent, 2.82 per cent and 1.41 per cent, respectively. Table 3.1 summarizes this breakdown.

The time profile of CMTs is also of interest. Table 3.2 provides a decadal comparison of CMT deployment. As we can see, after its start in the 1960s, the 1970s heralded the peak of deployment. In total, China deployed CMTs to 28 countries in the 1970s, amounting to 40 per cent of the total number of countries that received CMTs between 1963 and 2008. Most of these deployments continued to the 1990s and 2000s. However, the 1980s and especially the 1990s saw a sharp decline in the number of new deployments. Only fourteen and six new teams were dispatched in these two decades, respectively. This indicates that China had really been most active in pursuing its CMT-type health aid only in the first two decades of its health aid history.

The 1960s–1990s witnessed the withdrawal of 14 CMTs, of which 7 were then re-dispatched to the countries concerned. Among the reasons for these withdrawals, two factors were most important. First, serious civil war broke out in

Table 3.1 Deployment of CMTs by region (1963–2008)

Region	*Number of countries*	*Share (%)*
Africa	47	66.20
Asia	18	25.35
Oceania	3	4.23
South America	1	1.41
Europe	2	2.82

Source: Calculated according to Li (2009: 30–32).

Table 3.2 Cross-time comparison of the number of CMTs deployed (1963–2008)

Time	*New CMTs deployed*	*CMTs withdrawn from recipient countries*
1960s	11	–
1970s	28	7
1980s	14	2
1990s	6	12
2000s	12	1

Source: Calculated according to Li (2009: 30–32).

several African recipient countries in the 1990s. As a result, CMT deployment in these countries was halted. Between 1991 and 1997, China withdrew CMT deployment from five African countries – Algeria, Somalia, Congo (Brazzaville), Congo (DRC) and Sierra Leone. Typically, however, such halts did not last long, with CMT deployment resuming when the civil war ended.[11]

A second reason for the discontinuation of CMT deployment is a break in diplomatic relations between China and a recipient country. From the late 1980s to the late 1990s, diplomatic relations between China and eight African countries that had received CMTs since the 1970s – Burkina Faso, Guinea-Bissau, São Tomé, Niger, Gambia, Central Africa, Chad and Liberia – were severed, leading to a discontinuation of CMT deployment in those countries. However, with the exception of Burkina Faso, São Tomé and Gambia, after a few years CMT deployment resumed with the normalization of diplomatic relations.

The 2000s saw another upsurge in CMT deployment, after a long period of decline in the 1980s and 1990s. Twelve new CMTs were deployed, one was suspended for housing reasons, and six CMTs returned to their former recipient countries.

Construction of health facilities

Aid in the form of the construction of health facilities, such as hospitals, dates to the late 1960s. In 1967, at the request of the Tanzanian government, China donated 0.8 million RMB for the construction of the Abdallah Mzee Hospital in Zanzibar. Shanghai municipality was responsible for the construction, while Jiangsu Province contributed health equipment. On completion of the construction in 1970, this was the second-largest hospital in Zanzibar (Wang, 2009: 20).

In the three decades that followed the opening up policy in China (1978–2008), health aid through construction of hospitals and other health facilities continued, especially in African countries. In all, among the 171 countries that have had economic and commercial relations with China, 26 of them hosted 36 projects of health facility construction, including five centers for malaria prevention. Appendix 2 provides further details of this form of health aid.

While the first ten years immediately following the opening up witnessed a sharp decline in the number of hospitals and other health facilities built – during the 1980s, only one project was undertaken and completed, the Health School of Kibungo in Rwanda in 1989 – by contrast, in the 1990s, eight projects of health facility construction were undertaken in seven countries: Rwanda, Togo, Malta, Mauritania, Benin, Angola and Botswana. The 2000s saw another upsurge in health aid through facility construction. There was at least one such construction project signed or completed in each year of the decade. Altogether 24 hospitals were built or under construction in that period, of which 13 were signed or completed between 2007 and 2008, accounting for over 50 per cent of the total number of projects completed or undertaken in the decade by 2008. Figures 3.2 and 3.3 provide a summary of the time profile of health facilities completed and/or undertaken by China since its opening-up policy.

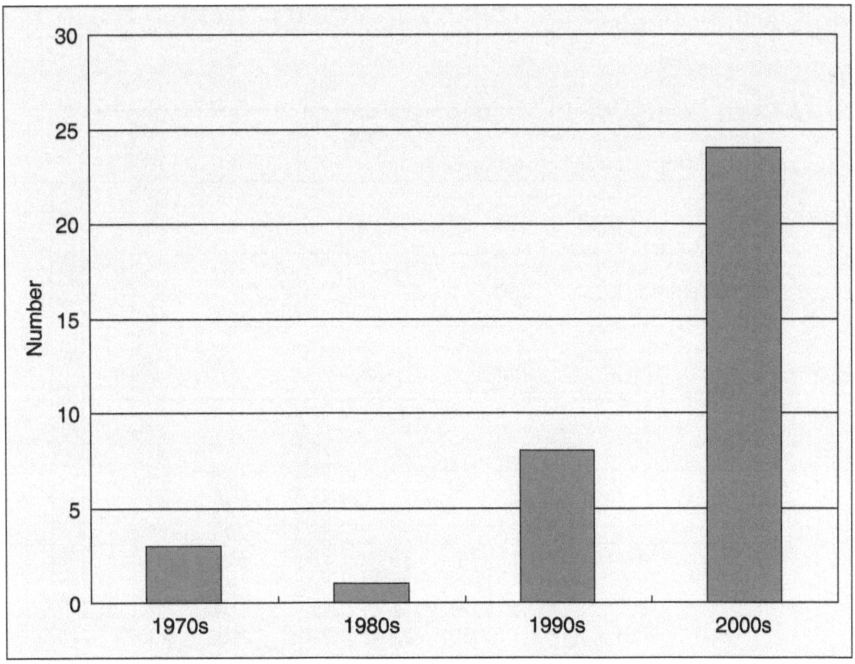

Figure 3.2 Number of facilities built with CHAFC (1978–2008).

Source: Calculated on the basis of Appendix 2.

An analysis of the geographical spread of the health facilities built by China in foreign countries in 1978–2008 indicates that African countries account for the majority (29 of 36). Four were in Asian countries – Afghanistan, Indonesia, and Laos. One was in Europe – the Chinese Medicine Center in Malta. One (including the construction of two health-care centers and one hospital) was in an Oceanic country, Tonga, while one was built in South America, Peru. Figure 3.4 summarizes the data.

Health equipment and medicine

In the past three decades, China provided health aid to 24 countries in the form of health equipment and medicine. Of the 38 projects, 33 were undertaken in the 2000s (89 per cent), 2 in the 1980s, and 3 in the 1990s. Among these, 19 concerned malaria prevention. Appendix 3 provides details of these projects by year of donation and recipient country.

Four countries topped the list for this type of aid: Burundi, Niger, Papua New Guinea and Togo. Burundi and Niger received five rounds, Togo and Papua New Guinea three rounds of this form of aid. Two other countries, Peru and Seychelles, each received this aid twice. The remaining 18 countries each received this form of aid once in the past 30 years.

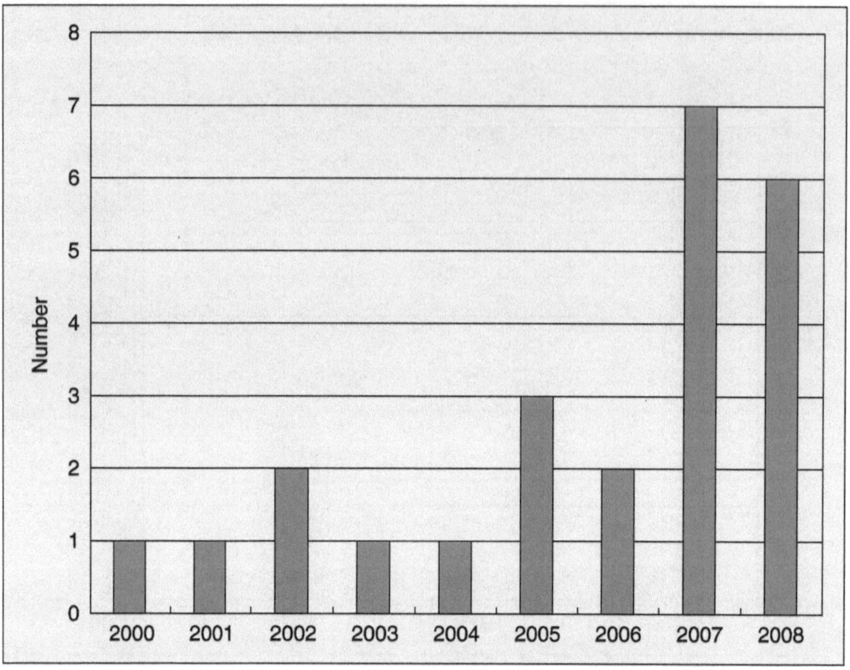

Figure 3.3 Number of facilities built with CHAFC (2000–2008).

Source: Calculated on the basis of Appendix 2.

The 38 projects fall into 6 general categories: malaria prevention, SARS prevention, measles vaccinations, venereal disease and HIV/AIDS, non-categorized medicine and general health instruments and equipment. Among these six categories, malaria prevention ranks first with 19 projects, exactly half of the total. Other projects targeting specific diseases (prevention or otherwise) include: one project for SARS prevention in Seychelles in 2003; two projects for venereal disease and AIDS prevention respectively in Botswana in 2000 and Papua New Guinea in 2005; and one project that provided measles vaccinations in Niger. General health instruments and facilities accounted for 12 more projects, and non-categorized medicine accounted for 7.[12] Table 3.3 further provides information on the number of recipient countries accounted for by each category.

The Chinese aid in health equipment and medicine also betrays heavy regional concentration, with Africa attracting most of the aid: of 38 projects, 29 went to 18 African countries, accounting for 76 per cent of the total number. Of the remaining nine projects, only one was for an Asian country (East Timor), two for a South American country (Peru), another two for two European countries (Belarus and Malta), and the last four went to two Oceania countries (Papua New Guinea and Tonga). Table 3.4 summarizes the information.

Table 3.3 Categories of Chinese assistance in the form of equipment and medicine (1978–2000)

Targets	*Number of projects*	*Number of recipient countries*
SARS prevention	1	1
Measles vaccine	1	1
Venereal disease and AIDS	2	2
Malaria prevention	19	17
Non-categorized medicine	7	6

Source: Calculated on the basis of Appendix 3.

Table 3.4 Chinese aid of equipment and medicine to foreign countries by region (1978–2000)

Regions	*Number of projects*	*Number of recipient countries*
Asia	1	1
Africa	29	18
South America	2	1
Europe	2	2
Oceania	4	2

Source: Calculated on the basis of Appendix 3.

Health human resources training

Providing training for health workers and officials from developing countries has been yet another common form of CHAFC, often undertaken at various local sites in the recipient countries through the work of CMTs.[13] Indeed, this type of 'learning by doing' was widely practiced in recipient countries where CMTs are stationed. China supports sustainable development of local health care systems through various programs of health human resources training, most often in African countries.

In the past, course training was largely centered on traditional Chinese medicine.[14] However, Chinese health aid to African countries has undergone a substantial expansion in the area of human resources training since 2005, especially in respect of the training of health officials at a higher level. This training covered many fields such as poverty alleviation, education, health, economic reform and public administration (Li and Wu, 2009: 51). This reflects a major shift in thinking, with the Chinese government regarding the broad determinants of health, beyond the role of medical care and medical infrastructure.

As a major mechanism of promoting comprehensive cooperation between China and African countries, the Forum of China and Africa Cooperation (FOCAC) has played a key role in promoting health training projects. At the third Summit of FOCAC in 2006 (Ministerial Conference), China launched the plan to provide 62 rounds of training courses to 1600 health personnel in African countries, covering the subjects of Chinese acupuncture, health care technology, nursing skills, HIV/AIDS prevention, malaria prevention and control, and rural health care (Chen, 2008). At the fourth Summit of FOCAC in 2009, China announced a new plan to train African doctors, nurses and managers with the goal of training 3000 health personnel between 2010–2012.

Through the framework of FOCAC, a series of training courses has already taken place. In 2002, 2006 and 2007, at least five major training courses were held in Shanghai, including the FOCAC International Workshop on Malaria Prevention and Treatment, the Workshop on Infectious Diseases for African Countries, the Seminar on Control and Prevention of Parasitic Diseases in Developing Countries, and the Seminar on Evaluation of the Burden of Parasitic Disease. These seminars and workshops have served to provide important in-depth training to health officials and workers from African countries in the field of malaria prevention in particular and disease control in general (MOH, 2009).

Besides Africa, training courses were also held for health workers and officials from ASEAN countries. For example, in October–November of 2007, specific training on the Diagnosis Technology of Avian Influenza Gene was held by China for ASEAN countries. Various seminars in related fields were also held with a view to promoting cooperation between China and ASEAN countries in the field of public health (MOH, 2009).

Bilateral agreements on health cooperation

A fifth form of CHAFC is bilateral health cooperation agreements between China and recipient countries. These agreements cover a wide range of areas of health cooperation including: medicine and medical research; health services; drug abuse prevention; animal and plant health inspection service (APHIS); public health; and veterinary inspection and quarantine. In the last 30 years since the opening, China signed 16 health cooperation agreements with 12 developing countries. All these agreements were signed between 1992 and 2007, of which nine were signed in the 1990s, and the remaining six in the 2000s (see Appendix 4 for details).

Compared with other forms of CHAFC, a distinctive feature of this type of health cooperation has been that agreements are predominantly between China and Asian countries, with a few signed with non-Asian countries, but none between China and African countries.[15] These cooperation agreements helped expand China's health assistance beyond African countries, and allowed it to gain additional influence in other parts of the world. Table 3.5 summarizes the information.

Financing flows in bilateral aid

Since China has not yet publicly released statistics on CHAFC financing flows, it is not possible to estimate the total flow or create a detailed breakdown.[16] The most that can be done is to use whatever available data can be gathered to broadly indicate the likely magnitudes. This is what we attempt to do in this subsection.

Table 3.5 Number of Bilateral Health Cooperation Agreements signed by region (1992–2007)

Regions	*Number of agreements*	*Number of countries*
Central/South America	2	2
Asia	9	6
Europe	5	4
Total	16	12

Source: Calculated on the basis of Appendix 4.

Against the general paucity of data, some information is available to indicate the magnitudes involved in the case of CMTs. According to one source (MOH, 2003), an annual fiscal budget of 100 million RMB (US$14.7 million)[17] was allocated in the 1990s for CMT deployment. This amount gradually increased to an annual budget of 200 million RMB (US$29.4 million) by 2003. This budget mainly covered subsidies to CMT workers during their time abroad, training for these workers prior to their departure and the cost of improving their working and living environments aboard. At the same time, the government also requested the work units that employed the seconded CMT workers to continue to pay their salary at home, and to provide various welfare benefits that they had originally enjoyed. Additionally, an annual budget of 0.3 million RMB (US$44,052) was provided for each CMT, mainly for use of purchasing medicine and other basic consumables, which are given to local patients free of charge.[18]

According to Xinhua Net, by 1998 about 2 billion RMB (US$294 million) had been spent for CMT deployment, involving 16,000 health workers dispatched to over 60 countries in Asia, Africa, Latin-America, South Pacific and Mediterranean regions (Xinhua Net, 2009). However, it is not clear how this total is calculated, and how it breaks down into constituent sub-flows. Nor has there been publicly released information to indicate the total flows since then.

It is not clear whether the total amount reported by the Xinhua Net includes the financial contributions made by participating local governments. Typically, the contribution of a province (municipality, autonomous region) is channeled to improving the working and living environments of the CMTs directly dispatched by that province. Some provinces also provide money for purchasing medicine and equipment. Generally, the amount met by local budgets has varied according to the level of public resources available in the provinces concerned.

Just as there is little information on national magnitudes, there is little information on how much each province may have contributed to CHAFC. Here we present the case of Zhejing Province, one of the richest provinces from coastal China, to indicate the possible magnitudes of local contributions involved. According to Yang (2009), in 2008, the Zhejiang Provincial government set aside an annual budget of 3 million RMB (US$0.44 million) for improving the working and living environments of its CMTs. Additionally, it gave various donations to recipient countries, for example, in 2008, health equipment worth 2 million RMB

(US$0.29 million) was donated to Mali when the provincial delegation visited there. Previously, in 2007, the Zhejiang Provincial government had donated three ambulances to Namibia, at a total cost of 1 million RMB (US$0.15 million).[19]

Still less information is available on the financial flows for other forms of health aid. Information for projects since the turn of this century that the authors were able to collect is presented in Table 3.6. On the basis of this limited information, it appears that a typical donation of medical equipment and medicine amounts to a relatively modest sum, 0.20–5 million dollars each, while the construction of a health facility (hospitals, various health centers, etc.) typically costs more. It appears that much more has been given out in that form.

Table 3.6 also indicates the role FOCAC has played in contributing to a substantial expansion of the scope and level of China's health aid to African countries in more recent years. In keeping with the action plans of the four FOCAC Summits, China stepped up its aid to African countries in health. For example, in the Beijing Action Plan (2007–2009) reached at the third FOCAC Summit in 2006, China announced its 'eight policy measures' to expand its cooperation with Africa, according to which health aid worth 300 million RMB (US$43 million) would be provided to African countries. Specifically, it would assist the African countries with anti-malaria drugs and help them to build 30 demonstration centers for the prevention and treatment of malaria. With this money, a number of anti-malaria centers have already been established in some African countries, as shown in Appendix 2 (FOCAC, 2006).

Following the Beijing Action Plan, the fourth FOCAC Summit in 2009 pushed China's health aid program to Africa even further forward. The Sharm el-Sheikh Action Plan announced that China would provide medical equipment, and malaria-fighting drugs and equipment to 30 hospitals and 30 malaria prevention and treatment centers to be built by China for Africa in the year 2010–2012. The total amount of this aid will reach 500 million RMB (about US$73 million) (FOCAC, 2009).

Growing multilateral aid

Although China's health aid to foreign countries has mainly followed the strategy of bilateral aid, this does not mean that China has not made any contribution to multilateral aid. China has been donating to a number of organizations within the UN system since the 1980s. For instance, China made, on average, an annual contribution of US$0.31 million to UNICEF and US$0.32 million to UNFPA in the first part of the 1980s. In total terms, its contributions to UNICEF in the 1981–1985 period amounted to 1.53 million US$, and those to UNFPA in 1980–1985 totaled US$1.93 million (OECD, 1987: 14). The 1990s saw a gradual increase in its donations. Thus in 1999, its contributions to UNICEF and UNFPA rose to US$6.89 million and US$0.82 million respectively (see Table 3.7).

From the year 2003, China began to make an annual donation of around US$2 million to the Global Fund to Fight AIDS, Tuberculosis and Malaria, making a total contribution of US$14 million in the years 2003–2009. In the 2000s, China

Table 3.6 Monetary amounts of CHAFC given to selected countries (2002–2010)

Country	*Year*	*Amount (US$)*	*Target*
1. Nigeria	From 2002	6–10 million annually	Medicine for malaria prevention, medicine for avian flu, mosquito net, and well-sinking in poor areas
2. Tanzania	Recent years	0.43 million (3 million RMB) annually	Medicine for malaria prevention
	2006	0.25 million	Malaria treatment
3. Ghana	2006	66 million	Expansion and upgrading telecommunications network; construction of a primary school and a malaria prevention centre
4. Zambia	2006	0.2 million	Anti malaria medicine
	2007	60–70 million (estimated)	Aid agreements – construction of a sports stadium in the city of Ndola, and agricultural technical demonstration centre, 2 rural schools, 1 hospital, and an anti-malaria centre
5. Ethiopia	2007	0.25 million	Donation to assist people affected by HIV/AIDS
	2008	0.43 million (300 million RMB)	Anti malaria medicines
6. Uganda	2008–2011	0.43 million (300 million RMB) (estimated)	Establish an anti-malaria center (medicine, training, technical support)
	2009	0.3 million	Medical facilities for reproductive health
7. Six countries: Uganda, Mali, Nigeria, Zimbabwe, Kenya, Bangladesh	2007–2010	3 million	Capacity building for regional reproductive health service center (facilities, training, technical support)
8. African countries	2007–2009	43 million (300 million RMB)	Grant for providing anti-malaria medicine and building 30 demonstration centers for malaria prevention and treatment
9. Africa countries	2010–2012	73 million (500 million RMB)	Providing medical equipment and malaria-fighting materials to 30 hospitals and 30 malaria prevention and treatment centers built by China for Africa

Source: 1, 2: Li and Wu (2009: 49, 50); 3, 4, 5: Davies et al. (2008: 44, 50, 36); 6, 7: Datong Party (2008); NPFPC (2009); 8, 9: FCAC Beijing Action Plan (2007–2009) and FCAC Beijing Action Plan (2010–2012).

has been contributing annually to most of the major international organizations in the UN system that are related to health, including WHO, UNICEF, UNFPA, UNAIDS and ICRC. In the year 2007, the total amount China donated to these five UN organizations and the Global Fund was more than US$24 million, indicating that its contribution to multilateral health aid has substantially risen in recent years compared with the former levels (see Table 3.7).

Nevertheless, China's contributions to multilateral aid have been much less than those from many other countries, especially the OECD countries. A comparison between China and Japan shows this point well (see Table 3.8). Thus Japan's contribution to the WHO in 2006–2007 was about 10 times that of China. Generally, China's contributions to UNICEF, UNFPA, ICRC and the Global Fund have fallen far short of those from Japan.

However, such a comparison may be inappropriate because China is still very much a developing country, despite its 30 years of rapid economic development. A better comparison to make may be between China and India. Table 3.8 presents

Table 3.7 China's annual contribution to Health-Related International Organizations (1996–2009, in USD)

Year	*WHO*	*UNICEF*	*UNFPA*	*UNAIDS*	*ICRC*	*Global Fund*
1996				99,985		
1997			400,000	99,985		
1998			820,000	99,979		
1999		6,889,345	820,000	99,985		
2000		6,853,176	820,000	100,000		
2001		7,103,116	820,000	99,980		
2002		8,358,878	820,000	100,000		
2003		8,515,393	820,000	100,000		2,000,000
2004	15,282,580	8,672,126	900,000	100,000	653,962	2,000,000
2005		37,443,680	900,000	100,000	2,363,520	2,000,000
2006	18,335,660	13,115,082	937,547	99,980	638,828	2,000,000
2007		15,586,004	900,000	100,000	666,121	2,000,000
2008		36,548,820	900,000	100,000	715,858	2,000,000
2009		17,705,405		100,000	732,664	2,000,000

Contributions to WHO, UNFPA, ICRC and the Global Fund are all government contributions. Contributions to UNICEF include both government contributions and private donations; contributions to ICRC include both those from the government and those from national societies.

Contributions to ICRC are quoted in Swiss Franc (CHF), here converted to US$ at the rate 1 CHF = 0.978 US$ that was prevailing at the time.

The contribution to WHO is assessed contribution.

UNICEF lists the contribution of China and Hong Kong separately. The data in this table adds up the contribution from China and Hong Kong. Same is for ICRC, 2004.

Source: The websites of each international organization, including:
www.who.int/about/resources_planning/en/index.html;
www.unicef.org/publications/index_pubs_ac.html;
www.unfpa.org/public/publications/annual_reports;
http://data.unaids.org/Governance/PCB01/Core_1995-2005_en.pdf?preview=true;
www.unaids.org/en/KnowledgeCentre/Resources/Publications/default.asp;
www.icrc.org/web/eng/siteeng0.nsf/htmlall/section_annual_report?OpenDocument;
www.theglobalfund.org/documents/pledges_contributions.xls

Table 3.8 Annual contributions to Health-Related International Organizations by China, Japan and India (2006–2007, in USD)

Organization	*Country*	*2006*	*2007*
WHO	China	18,335,660	
	Japan	173,874,020	
	India	3,760,020	
UNICEF	China	13,115,082	15,586,004
	Japan	289,339,175	231,450,165
	India	3,501,512	5,293,225
UNFPA	China	937,547	900,000
	Japan	33,257,124	33,257,124
	India	199,159	222,222
ICRC	China	638,828	666,121
	Japan	25,906,074	13,604,020
	India	–	–
Global Fund	China	2,000,000	2,000,000
	Japan	130,148,228	186,006,798

Source: The websites of each international organization (see the sources listed for Table 3.7).

data on the financial contributions made by China, Japan and India to these same international organizations. As can be seen, the total donations to these five international organizations made by China in the years 2006–2007 amounted to US$54.18 million, while those from India totaled US$16.98 million, a much smaller amount. So while China compares rather unfavorably with Japan in its total contributions to health-related international organizations, it compares rather favorably with the more comparable country, India.

The significant financial contributions China has made to various multilateral international health organizations are certainly an important measure of its commitment to international cooperation in health and in global health governance building. At the same time, it needs to be pointed out that China's involvement in these organizations does not simply stop at making financial contributions. Indeed, it has also been home to 60 WHO collaborating centers (Appendix 5). Located in 13 cities in China, these centers have played a very important role in supporting various WHO programs. China also hosted the first ever official WHO meeting on traditional medicine in 2008.

Discussion

The information presented above provides a multi-faceted profile of CHAFC. Despite being a developing country itself, China has consistently engaged in providing health aid to many developing countries, especially African countries, in the past half-century. Numerous CMTs dispatched, hospitals and health centers built and personnel trained have undoubtedly brought immense benefits to the populations of the recipient countries, but they have also substantially increased China's 'soft power' in the regions where this aid occurred. Below, we explore issues that have surrounded this aid: the altruistic vis-à-vis self-interested nature of such aid, the controversy over sovereignty, relative roles of bilateral and multilateral aid, the regional perspective and regional cooperation and system- and capacity-building for CHAFC.

Altruism and self-interest

While one would expect CHAFC to have brought benefits to the recipient countries, the act of providing such aid need not be entirely altruistic. Indeed, the principles that have governed CHAFC have themselves stressed mutual benefit. So, clearly, when it decided to provide a particular type of aid, be it dispatching a CMT to or building a hospital in a recipient country, China must have viewed it to be ultimately in its interest as well. Recognition of this should not make such aid morally unattractive. If one accepts the grand objective in everything we do to be enhancing some 'global good', then a win–win situation surely is better than one where interests clash, unless one thinks entirely in zero-sum confrontational terms. Indeed, self-interested motives in the act of giving are not only true of China, but are generally true of all countries in the world when they provide foreign aid.

The most conspicuous benefit for China through providing health and other aid has been the enhancement of its recognition on the international stage, and the promotion of its international reputation as a responsible world power. Thus at the 26th United Nations General Assembly in 1971, among the 23 countries that submitted the proposal to the General Assembly to restore all legitimate rights of China, 11 countries had been recipients of CMTs, and among the 76 countries that voted for the proposal, most were developing countries. In many ways, the cause for this diplomatic success could be traced to the contributions made by China's foreign aid, including CHAFC. Needless to say, it is also with this goal in mind that China had provided aid to many developing countries in the world, at a time when China's own economic strength was weak and living standards were lower.

This self-interested aspect of CHAFC is underlined by the statement made by a CMT representative when she was accepting the Award of Public Affairs at the '2008 You Bring Charm to the World Award Ceremony': 'We fully understood that we were not only health workers but diplomatic envoys to improve the friendship of all the countries worldwide' (IFENG, 2009).

Sovereignty and global governance

The notion of sovereignty, meaning having supreme and independent authority over a territory, is both a cornerstone of kingdoms and nation-states and a signature of modern political systems and international relations. Respect for sovereignty means, among other things, freedom from external control. However, in a globalizing world, the traditional notion of sovereignty is being challenged. In the field of global health, infectious diseases can spread, sometimes very rapidly, across national boundaries. The recent outbreaks, notably SARS, H1N5, and H1N1, have led to increased calls for the establishment of some level of global health governance.

Its fundamental foreign policy principle being non-interventionist, China's consistent emphasis on independent sovereignty and no strings attached in aid policy has made it steadfastly refuse to criticize or to involve itself in the internal affairs of the recipient countries. As a result, China has tended to attract, disproportionately, those countries that have been denied aid by other (Western) countries. There has been much international criticism of China's aid policy because of its disregard of human rights violations in the recipient countries.

China maintains that pressures brought through aid withdrawal or denial are unlikely to force the leaders of those countries to change policy, nor would aid withdrawal result in a political dynamism that leads to change. On the contrary, it could bring about a hardening of the leaders' positions, thus leading to increased suffering among the vulnerable groups that the aid is intended to target, and in health aid, this can often mean life or death. China therefore argues that a conciliatory, non-confrontational approach is most appropriate, and does not bring about negative impacts on targeted populations.

Two critical questions are raised here: the wisdom of using aid generally, and health aid in particular, as political means to engineer changes in a foreign country and respect for recipient country sovereignty.

China's most fundamental foreign policy tenet is non-interventionism. In respecting the sovereignty of other nations, it similarly desires and expects its sovereignty to be honored. China has strongly defended its sovereignty, even in matters of global health. The 2003 SARS outbreak, however, forced many within the central government to rethink their position. Key informant interviews indicate that central government health policy makers have now realized that China's insistence on sovereignty is in conflict with the demands of global health governance. Even conservative policy makers now realize that traditional strategies of prevention (i.e. doing everything to keep it inside or outside the border) will not stop a highly infectious disease from moving from one country to another. Many have now accepted that China will have to relinquish some degree of sovereignty to enhance global health governance (Interviews D, E, G and H).

While there have been instances where international pressure has led China to take a particular course of action that would not have been possible before (i.e. China's active cooperation with the WHO on H1N1), the extent to which China is ready to compromise on its sovereignty stance and engage actively in global health governance remains a question. The changes at present are still limited, largely due to the consistently cautious attitude of Chinese leaders to issues of national sovereignty as a fundamental principle that governs international relations (Interview D). It is also possible that vested bureaucratic interests remain hostile to change. International pressures for China to be more transparent and more in line with global norms and standards in health matters are unlikely to fully achieve their aim without the strong support and collaboration from party and government officials at all levels (especially the grass-roots level).

Mirroring its concern with its own sovereignty, China is, by and large, still rather reluctant to explicitly attach political conditions to its foreign aid, including health aid, and it has continued to take a non-interventionist approach to recipient countries' domestic affairs. On the other hand, as a rising power with rising expectations and influence, China may well have to rethink its position on its own sovereignty and that of other countries in matters of public health (Interviews F and G).

Multilateralism and bilateralism

Our review of the history of CHAFC indicates a slow but clear shift in emphasis from bilateral to multilateral health aid, including contributions to such international agencies as the WHO, UNICEF, UNFPA, ICRC and the Global Fund. China's contributions to these agencies are still rather limited, compared with those from developed countries such as Japan (Table 3.8). Nevertheless, the level of China's contributions compares favorably with similarly large developing countries such as India.

While the weight of China's aid to date has been on bilateral approaches, contributions to multilateral and international agencies have been increasing, reflecting a more global perspective of the country in its dealings of foreign aid. The level of a country's contribution to international agencies and the weight of this contribution in its total foreign aid can be a measure of a country's commitment to the establishment and/or improvement of a global protocol and governance. Compared with narrow bilateral aid where explicit national interests may be involved (and often pursued), contributions to international agencies are unlikely to give the donor a specific advantage, other than to increase its say in those agencies' decision making, which may or may not help to serve any specific national interests of the donor.

This changing pattern of aid is understandable given that, before 1971, China was barred from joining the United Nations, and the isolationist policies of the Western nations towards China gave it little opportunity to act on the international stage, other than through bilateral relationships (it did once join the Socialist Block led by the Soviet Union but even that relationship ended in the early 1960s). The real opportunity for China to act on the world stage through international organizations and agencies emerged only after the early 1970s.

In health, China's involvement with international agencies goes beyond making financial contributions. It has been an active member of the WHO, in particular since the SARS outbreak in the 2003. As seen earlier, over 60 Chinese health research institutions are now WHO-collaborating institutions, working with and supporting WHO on various issues of health. And one of its nationals, Dr Margaret Chan, has become the head of the organization, in part thanks to the support of China as a WHO member state.

Currently, a widely shared view among Chinese health policy makers and academic scholars is that global health governance is the direction of future health development for all countries, and the use of global action is the way to improve population health in all countries of the world. China should and could play a major role in this field (Interviews D, G and H).

Within such a multilateral framework, bilateral aid also has obtained a new meaning and significance. Bilateral aid may play an important part in the construction of an effective global health governance system. Rather than as a means of diplomacy, bilateral aid may contribute to strengthening the health systems of the recipient countries, drawing on the experiences and strengths of the donor countries. All of this should contribute to the building of an effective global health system.

Regional cooperation

Until recently, China's foreign aid strategy has been bilateralism within the framework of South–South cooperation. However, it has moved decidedly from being over-reliant on bilateralism to more active participations in regional cooperation. In the view of some Chinese commentators, global health governance could actually be better facilitated by and built on regional cooperation (Interviews B, C and G). Countries from the same region would benefit from forming regional associations that both regulate regional relations and represent member countries in negotiations with other countries, or other associations of countries, to advance their common interests. Representations through such regional associations can better facilitate real dialogue between countries, save time in negotiations and reduce the transaction costs involved. Wider use of such regional associations might be the first step to building up a truly functioning global health governance system. From this viewpoint, China's active involvement in regional cooperation should be seen as making a positive contribution to global health governance.

The China–Africa health cooperation discussed above is only one type of regional cooperation. Another important example of regional cooperation that China takes part in is the Greater Mekong Sub-region. Begun in 2005, the Greater Mekong Sub-region cooperation involves the border provinces of Yunnan and Guangxi of China, and the neighboring countries of Laos, Myanmar and Vietnam. It is meant to promote cooperation for purposes of, among others, disease control, including malaria, AIDS and TB prevention. Recent years have also seen increased health cooperation between China and ASEAN countries (10+1 and 10+3). The biannual ministerial conference between China and ASEAN, the China–ASEAN Investment Cooperation Fund, and the China–ASEAN Fund for Public Health are testimony to the substantial steps China has taken in regional health cooperation with South East Asia. Similarly, the ministerial conference between China, Japan and the Republic of Korea on health is yet another example of regional cooperation, in this instance among the three North East Asian countries with a view to improving regional health coordination. Likewise, the Shanghai Cooperation Organization has instituted mechanisms of health cooperation covering health emergency response, cross-border infectious disease prevention and control, disaster health relief, etc.

As one interviewee suggests, China's current engagement in regional health cooperation (with Asian and African countries mainly, but also with countries of other regions) can be seen as China taking a major step onto the stage of regional and global health governance (Interview B). Such cooperation has not only involved China sending its health care workers to other countries, but also China inviting many health experts and leaders from other countries and international organizations to China to discuss various health issues, including the use of better ethical standards and transparency of clinical trials.

Aid system and capacity-building

The 'aid system' of a country means the entire array of institutions, protocols and processes that support the decision making, implementation and evaluation of a country's assistance to foreign countries. As described earlier, China's health aid system has evolved. What began as a response to a request from the Government of Algeria expanded over the subsequent 20 years into flow of health aid to foreign countries, especially African countries. During that time, the system that now governs and manages China's aid to foreign countries developed, but only as the culmination of various ad hoc decisions and arrangements. Throughout the period one thing was clear: health aid, as any other aid, must serve the country's foreign policy and obey its general principles.

As described earlier, expressions of need for health aid would first come from various foreign governments. These requests would then be submitted to the Chinese embassy in the countries concerned, and be directly handled by the ECO of the embassy, whose superordinate ministry in Beijing was the now defunct Ministry of Foreign Trade and Economic Cooperation (MOFTEC). It was only when that ministry merged with MOC that foreign aid, quite by historical accident, became part of the portfolio of the MOC. One downside of this is that aid policies and implementation too often became fragmented and lack coordination. Aid policy, at times, appeared to lack vision and strategy. If China is to further project itself internationally, as it undoubtedly will with its rising economic power, there appears to be a strong case for it to institute an independent central agency taking important decisions on strategy and vision, and overseeing all matters of aid. The existence of an independent agency would also help its aid programs to be seen to transcend China's immediate commercial interests, and address larger issues of a global nature, including global health governance. Additionally, it could help China's aid system to become more transparent and accessible not only to recipients, but also to non-state actors, whose potential has yet to be tapped.

Thus far, China's health aid, as other aid, has almost entirely been dependent on the government; the role of civil society has almost entirely been missing. However, the expanding private sector and NGOs can potentially engage in health aid as well. In the past decade, a number of Chinese NGOs played an active role in the emergency rescue operations, for example after the Indian Ocean tsunami in 2004, and more recently after Haiti was hit by a severe earthquake. Lately, private hospitals have begun to participate in CHAFC with the permission of the government (Interview B).

Currently, many policy makers and academics in China hold the view that there is no conflict between the state and non-state actors in the arena of health aid and global health governance. These two groups of actors could complement each other. Indeed, in the case of humanitarian assistance, the aid from NGOs rather than the state might actually be easier for recipients to accept (Interview H), and a wide international network of NGOs will have an advantage in identifying problems, including early warnings, technical support, and resource mobilization (Interviews G and H). However, before civil society can widely participate in public affairs in China itself, the scope and ability of non-state participants to engage in foreign health aid are likely to be limited.

Many Chinese policy makers and academics express the view that an effective global health governance system should be built up on the base of interactions among nation-states, civil society (including NGOs) and international organizations (such as the WHO), rather than between nation-states only. One hopes that civil society and NGOs could soon play a significant role within China's own health system, and this should help China to contribute, to an even greater extent, to the building of an effective global health governance system (Interviews F and H).

Conclusion

This chapter has reviewed CHAFC from the perspective of global health governance. Through literature review, historical records analysis and analysis of in-depth interviews with policy makers and scholars, this research has attempted to identify key characteristics of CHAFC, and its role, if any, in contributing to global health governance.

We have seen that CHAFC first began as responses to the need of recipient countries, rather than acting on some prior, proactive program aimed to gain a strategic national interest (although it eventually did so). Furthermore the system that governed and managed it arose from some ad hoc arrangements, rather than from any well-thought-out plan. CHAFC's emphasis was toward bilateralism, although multilateralism has also increasingly received attention. Regional cooperation has been emphasized in recent years and has now become a major vehicle of health aid. Concerns about sovereignty have led China to continue to insist on a non-interventionist stance, though it has made significant concessions on matters of global health following the SARS outbreak in 2003.

While CHAFC has not been entirely altruistic, and China itself has emphasized mutual benefit, it has undoubtedly brought benefits to the population of recipient countries. Its bilateralism need not conflict with the demands of GHG, and its emphasis on regional cooperation could also contribute to the development of GHG. In spite of its general concerns with sovereignty, China has endorsed the basic principles of GHG, and has made concessions on its sovereignty to accommodate these principles. As the Asia century progresses, it will be unthinkable to have an effective GHG system without the active involvement and participation of China.

Notes

1 China began its reform and opening-up in 1978, a process which covered a wide range of policies aimed to reform the then planned economy and integrate China more closely into the world economy and community.

2 Tikki in his comments on an early draft of this paper points out: 'as an Indonesian Chinese, I have a personal view on this. In the late 1950's to the late 1960s, there was real concern in SE Asia as to China's true motives, especially in some of the SE Asian countries. The Indonesian Communist Party (strongly linked to Peking) staged a *coup d'état* attempt in 1965 so many were suspicious of China during that period of history.'

3 For a long time countries such as Vietnam, the Democratic People's Republic of Korea and Albania had been the largest recipients of CHAFC.

4 According to available data, in the three years 1967, 1972 and 1973, for example, the ratio of foreign aid to China's total state financial expenditure reached as high as 4.5, 6.7 and 7.2 per cent respectively, exceeding even the same ratio for the richest and most developed countries, then and now (www.china.com.cn/news/60years/2009-08/28/content_18422630.htm).

5 China's aid to Iraq, Afghanistan and South East Asian countries has, for example, been for this purpose.

6 See www.china.com.cn/news/60years/2009-08/28/content_18422630.htm.

7 Why the MOC, not another ministry such as MOFA or MOH, became the ministry in charge of CHAFC is a matter of historical happenstance. For a long time, the now defunct Ministry of Foreign Trade, later the Ministry of Foreign Economic Relations and Trade was in charge of all foreign aid matters of China, and, needless to say, also CHAFC. That ministry was then abolished and was merged with the then Ministry of Commerce, to form the present-day MOC. With this merger the portfolio of foreign aid, including CHAFC, went over to MOC.

8 This process is very similar to that of Japan's ODA. In China, the process is designed in this way largely due to the consideration that the aid should, first of all, be based on the needs of the recipient countries. However, it does beg the question of the capacity of recipient countries to put forth appropriate and high-quality proposals truly reflecting their needs.

9 A significant feature of CHAFC is the direct delivery of health care in a recipient country, in contrast with health aid provided by some countries, for example Japan, with emphasis on other forms of aid, including significant support for health-related research.

10 Including one non-municipality city.

11 This was the case in all of the countries mentioned with the exception of Somalia.

12 This number totals more than 38 due to some projects providing more than one type of aid.

13 In Chinese, this is called 'Chuan-Bang-Dai', which means to educate local health workers during service delivery, to help the local health workers to solve the problems during the work, and to teach the local workers to be more skillful.

14 In 1975, the CMT from Hubei Province in Algeria designed and taught the first full-time training course on Chinese acupuncture. Chinese doctors laid out the teaching plans, compiled the teaching materials and translated these materials into French. In total, 25 Algerian practitioners completed this training course over two years. The area of training gradually expanded over time. The CMT in Cameroon held four training courses in acupuncture, obstetrics and gynecology, pediatrics and other topics. The CMT from Ningxia Province in Benin gave the local workers training courses including epidural anesthesia, toxic dysentery in children, normal childbirth, diagnosis and treatment of anemia, liver function tests, etc. Their teaching materials became a major reference for local doctors subsequently (Li, 2009: 36–37).

15 Nine agreements were signed between China and six Asian countries (Armenia, Brunei, Georgia, Malaysia, North Korea and Turkmenistan), five between China and four European countries (Macedonia, Romania, Russia and Slovenia), and two more between China and two Central and South American countries (Costa Rica and Argentina).

16 In the course of writing up this report, however, reliable sources have indicated that the MOC may release the related data soon. Until then, however, it will not be possible to establish a detailed picture of the financing flows in question.

17 The exchange rate is a current one, 1US$ equals 6.8RMB.

18 While it is not entirely clear if these funds come fully from the central government budget, as the source does not make it clear, we nevertheless reckon that they do.

19 Zhejiang province's work on CMT deployment began in 1968. It is now responsible for the CMT deployment to three countries: Mali, Central Africa and Namibia. To the year 2008, Zhejiang Province has deployed 40 CMTs with 915 medical workers in total. The teams have treated 11.7 million outpatients and 470 thousand inpatients.

4 India and global health governance

Past, present and future

Aravinda Meera Guntupalli and Karthik Nachiappan

Introduction

Few scholars have explored India's Official Development Assistance (ODA) paradigm and practices. Almost no one has analyzed India's development assistance for health (DAH). This paper examines India's ODA in the health sector by examining India's total DAH, the channels and modes through which it is deployed, areas where it is being channeled and the motives underpinning them. Through this, it attempts to draw some inferences and implications of India's DAH, and what this portends for global health governance.

Indian health assistance is and was historically channeled through technical and financial vehicles, primarily and predominantly through the bilateral arm. From independence until the early 1990s, India's development and health assistance was directed largely within South Asia on moral and idealist grounds. But India's development and health assistance approach is evolving as the country liberalizes and its economic and geopolitical importance grows. Strategic and geo-economic interests now greatly influence India's development agenda and policies, and will continue to do so in the foreseeable future.

India's role in DAH and global health governance (GHG) will depend on how it balances its role as a recipient and giver of aid, how it addresses the institutional deficiencies within its ODA apparatus and whether it chooses to remain a regional health player or is prepared to elevate its intentions and actions to the global level.

India's accord with official development assistance

India is simultaneously a burgeoning strategic donor and a dependent aid recipient. India's economy is now the third-largest in the world by purchasing power parity at US$4.469 trillion, and ninth-largest by nominal GDP at US$1.846 trillion (International Monetary Fund, 2011). It has grown at an average of 7 percent since 1997, and is expected to continue at that pace in the next few years (Stuenkel, 2010). India's growing financial reserves are being increasingly deployed through aid; recent estimates indicate that India expended US$500 million to US$1 billion per year on ODA (Stuenkel, 2010: 44). Despite record growth rates over the past two decades, India's internal development challenges stagger. Over half of the country's labor force works in the agricultural sector, and the majority of them live in poverty. Life expectancy in India is 64 years, compared to 74 years in China. The maternal mortality rate is 230 per 100,000 live births, mortality rate for children under 5 is 66 per 1,000 births and the adult literacy rate is 74 percent (Sen, 2011).

India has been an active donor for many years. As a provider of assistance, India's efforts are coeval with its emergence as an independent nation-state and aid recipient. In the early years, its efforts were primarily directed towards immediate neighbors, whose stability was (and remains) important to India (Rowlands, 2008: 6). In the 1950s, Delhi began providing development assistance to Nepal, a practice that has endured to date (Ayyar, 2010). Bhutan has been a major recipient of India's aid for decades; India is now Bhutan's largest trade partner and donor. One of India's goals with its development assistance is to promote peace, amity and stability within a region known as one of the world's hotspots, home to an array of conflicts between and within states (Government of India, 2009b).

Since 1964, India has deployed its human capital to train foreign professionals through the Indian Technical and Cooperation (ITEC) program, which now extends to approximately 154 countries (Ayyar, 2010). India has also displayed a strong commitment towards participating in training programs of the Commonwealth Secretariat, Asian Development Bank and World Bank, as well as other multilateral organizations. In addition, it has been an important source of United Nations peacekeepers for decades (Price, 2005: 12). In the 1980s, India sent extensive aid to Vietnam and Bangladesh, though this trend ebbed in the 1990s (Stuenkel, 2010: 38). Collectively, the Ministry of External Affairs estimates that India has provided roughly US$2 billion of development assistance since 1964 through the ITEC (Price, 2005: 12).

Until the 1980s, India's development efforts were based on Nehruvian ideals: moralism, human freedom and dignity (Sagar, 2009: 804). Under Nehru's stewardship, this rubric manifested through policies that enhanced the agency, independence and self-determination of countries across the developing world, many of whom had just exited odious colonial experiences. Amid a tense and volatile geopolitical climate characterized by unbridled superpower rivalry, Nehru forcefully advocated that developing countries steer clear of the disastrous implications of power politics through sustained and vigorous national development agendas, a view realized through non-alignment (Nehru, 1961: 27). Another corollary was the desire to act in a principled manner on the global stage, shaping and leading coalitions to ensure that the interests of the developing world were not scuttled (Sagar, 2009: 803). This Nehruvian impulse continues when India engages on behalf of the developing world in major global forums, especially with respect to issues such as climate change and environmental degradation.

As India liberalized in the early 1990s its foreign policy and diplomacy evolved, and so did its ODA. Economic growth and prosperity translated to a greater willingness to pursue strategic economic and geopolitical priorities. Moreover, future growth hinges on the government's role and capacity in securing global market access for Indian companies and products, securing energy resources to meet rocketing demand, and procuring raw materials for industrial production (Jobelius, 2007). These exigencies have influenced India's economic diplomacy and attendant ODA policies over the past two decades.

In terms of concrete assistance, greater attention is being proffered to Africa and Afghanistan. Africa has ascended the Indian policy agenda since 2003, after the announcement of a debt relief package under the fiscal budget that wrote off all the official dues of the Highly Indebted Poor Countries (HIPCs) in Africa – Mozambique, Tanzania, Zambia, Guyana, Nicaragua, Ghana and Uganda (Price, 2005: 9). Also, under the auspices of the 'India Development Initiative', Delhi created a new lending instrument through which it drew reserves from global capital markets to lend to less credit-worthy African countries. Another part of the African agenda is financial assistance through letters of credit (LoC) worth US$500 million from EXIM Bank, US$200 million LoC through the New Partnership for Africa's Development (NEPAD), and US$550 million LoC from the Focus Africa Programme (Stuenkel, 2010: 40). Following the 2008 India–Africa summit between 14 African heads of state and Prime Minister Manmohan Singh, both parties also agreed to sign an India–Africa Framework for Cooperation, in addition to Delhi's commitment to provide an additional US$5.4 billion credit line and grants worth US$500 million over the next five years (Price, 2011: 11).

India's motives in Africa are largely economic. Its development endeavors work to enhance market access for Indian companies and their products, especially products that are not competitive in Western markets (Stuenkel, 2010: 40). In addition, it is fair to add that Delhi's overtures can be attributed to a more noble impulse: to build sustainable capacity in infrastructure and human capital across African nations such that they can be counted upon to be effective stewards of their own development in the near future, instead of constantly relying on Western intervention (Stuenkel, 2010: 41).

Since 2002, India has become a critical stakeholder in the reconstruction of Afghanistan. To date, it has provided roughly US$650 million for civilian reconstruction programs, and an additional US$500 million was approved in May 2011 (Jobelius, 2007: 9; Cunningham, 2011). India's motives are largely strategic; Delhi has given considerable amounts of development assistance to prevent Afghanistan from tilting further towards Pakistan and engender an unfriendly regime (Stuenkel, 2010: 34).

Inferring from these recent trends, it is evident that strategic and instrumental reasons suffuse India's economic diplomacy and extant development agenda. Nehruvian ideals have less bearing now on foreign and development policy and a more pragmatic realpolitik impulse reigns (Stuenkel, 2010: 43). Policy makers are focused on advancing core national interests and employ different tools at their disposal to do so. Bilateralism is de rigeur. As India gains more power, it is exhibiting a clear preference towards bilateral channels to advance its interests, especially for development assistance. The Ministry of External Affairs (MEA) clearly states that India's role as a donor is 'demand-driven' and 'response-oriented' to address the needs of developing countries. India has always maintained that aid should be provided only after receiving consent, positioning itself as a country that strongly adheres to principles of sovereignty and non-interference as a donor (Government Of India, 2009b).

Philosophically, *liberals* and *strategists* appear to have acquired the upper hand within the Indian foreign policy apparatus. On the strategic side, proponents call for Delhi to eschew statecraft that is couched in high idealism and instead engage in the concerted pursuit of policies that will result in registering 'tangible, not abstract, gains for the country' (Karnad, 1994: 67). The strategic community's realization of force as the ultimate determinant of power in world politics impels them to champion development of India's economic and military capabilities, and shape policies to facilitate that goal (Sagar, 2009: 811). Liberals, on the other hand, want Delhi to do its utmost to advance India's development needs through greater economic interdependence. Cooperation is exalted. Economic diplomacy trumps all else. Building and deepening economic linkages to ensure access to markets and resources is the key, liberals propound, towards realizing India's promise (Bajpai, 2002: 254).

Finally, before moving to consider India's DAH practices, it is necessary to present an estimate of India's entire ODA. Data on India's ODA is sparse and not well accounted for because India is not a member of OECD-DAC, nor does it have a centralized agency or a lexicon within that can deftly aggregate requisite data (Ayyar, 2010). Current estimates, however, range from US$450 million in 2006 (Ayyar, 2010) to US$610 million (Stuenkel, 2010) to US$1 billion for the same year (Rowlands, 2008). Problems of definition, delineation and comprehensiveness continue to plague the enumeration of India's aid.

India and global development assistance for health

Incumbent under the ongoing revolutions in global health has been the rise of emerging power donors, such as India, and their burgeoning emphasis on global health initiatives. These donors have entered the fray as global health donors, disbursing aid bilaterally, regionally and globally to tackle prevailing and emergent health challenges. Within this emerging donor contingent, India is playing a greater role vis-à-vis development assistance for health. Below, we present an empirical overview of India's global health financing patterns, focusing on their preferred channels and modes of health assistance, and geographic preferences.

India's global DAH contributions

As discussed above, it is difficult to create an accurate estimate of India's ODA, and similarly, securing an accurate estimate of India's global health financing is equally challenging. India, like China, lacks concrete data detailing its global DAH contributions. However, one estimate by Devi Sridhar in 2008 pegs India's foreign health aid at US$226 million in 2007–08 (McCoy *et al*., 2009: 409).

Complementing the bilateral health assistance, India has also upped its financial contributions to multilateral channels, mainly the WHO, UNICEF, International

Red Cross and the Global Fund to Fight AIDS, Tuberculosis and Malaria (GFATM).

WHO

India's contribution to the WHO totalled US$7 million between 2004 and 2009. In the year 2008–09, India's contributions have declined, amounting to nearly US$2 million (Table 4.1).

The International Red Cross

With respect to the International Red Cross society, India's contributions have been meager. India provided US$30,000 between 2004 and 2007, with no contributions in 2006 and 2007. However, India increased its contribution to US$2.5 million in 2008 and to US$2.8 million in 2009 (Table 4.2).

UNICEF

Despite being a major recipient of aid for child health related programs, India's contributions to the UNICEF have been consistently increasing over the period from 2000 to 2009. Based on the UNICEF annual report, India contributed US$4 million in 2009 with roughly US$1.5 million given by the government and the rest from the private sector (Table 4.3).

Table 4.1 India's contribution to the WHO

Year	*Amount in US$*
2008–09	1,170,429
2006–07	3,760,020
2004–05	3,247,180

Source: WHO Annual report (2005, 2006, 2007b).

Table 4.2 India's contribution to the International Red Cross

Year	*Amount in CHF (Swiss francs)*	*Amount in US$*
2009	3,085,298	2,776,768
2008	2,734,431	2,460,988
2007	–	–
2006	–	–
2005	16,404	14,764
2004	17,633	15,870

Source: Annual report of the International Red Cross (2005, 2005, 2006, 2007, 2008)

Table 4.3 India's contributions to UNICEF

Year	*Public sector*		*Private*		*Total (US$)*
	Government	*Other sources*	*Regular*	*Other*	
2009	1,533,816			2,413,241	3,947,057
2008	886,160	1,913,968		1,534,122	4,334,251
2007	938,220	2,976,088		1,378,917	5,293,225
2006	844,444	1,852,428	1,049	805,688	3,501,512
2005	900,121	2,181,433		79,177	3,160,732
2004	1,370,510	692,537			2,063,047
2003	–	–	–	–	–
2002	643,250	548,687	10	417,653	1,609,600
2001	649,140		6,730	2,183	644,593
2000	959,710	308,174		356,143	1,007,679
1999	718,270		125,410	105	843,575

Source: UNICEF annual report (2001, 2002, 2003, 2004, 2005, 2006, 2007)

Global Fund to fight AIDS, Tuberculosis and Malaria (GFATM)

India's contributions to the GFATM pale in comparison to the financing it has received from the multilateral institution. India's contributions to the GFATM remained nearly constant between 2006 and 2009. In 2010, India increased its contribution by US$3 million. However, the role of India as a recipient is significantly larger than its role as a donor. The total approved grant amount from the GFATM to India 2010 is US$1.1 billion, with close to US$700 million already disbursed. To date, it has pledged and given US$11 million to GFATM (Global Fund to fight AIDS, Tuberculosis and Malaria, 2010) (Table 4.4).

Financing by mode of health assistance

Substantial portions of DAH disbursed by India are in the form of in-kind services. India's preferred mode of assistance on overseas health projects is

Table 4.4 India's contribution to the Global Fund in US Dollars

Year	*Amount contributed*
2010	3,000,000
2009	2,000,000
2008	2,000,000
2007	2,000,000
2006	2,000,000
2005	–
2004	–
2003	–
2002	–

Source: Global Fund to Fight AIDS, TB and Malaria (2010).

bilateral technical and financial assistance (Ayyar, 2010). Programmatic data from the Indian Ministry of External Affairs indicates a heavy concentration of DAH being directed for the construction of hospitals and clinics, deputation of medical and paramedical experts, as well as the development of water sanitation, agricultural processing projects, etc. (Government of India, 2009b). India also channels assistance through the provision of LoCs to developing countries through the EXIM Bank for financing imports of Indian expertise, technology, projects and goods, which are also used for health system and infrastructure development (Ayyar, 2010).

Financing by regional focus

The largest share of ODA for health globally goes to sub-Saharan Africa, followed by Asia (merging the East Asia-Pacific and South Asia) with Latin America following thereafter. India's preferences, however, deviate from prevailing patterns. India directs a predominant share of its ODA and incumbent health assistance to the South Asian region – Afghanistan, Bhutan, Bangladesh, Nepal, Sri Lanka, the Maldives and Myanmar (Government of India, 2007). As Table 4.5 indicates, India's ODA allocations have largely been focused within the South Asian region, with Africa and parts of Central Asia following in the picture.

Furthermore, India's DAH to its South Asian neighbors has been primarily in the form of technical and economic cooperation. In Bhutan, India focuses on project assistance, mainly in the areas of infrastructure development in healthcare (Government of India, 2009b). Aid to Nepal is similar; MEA data reveal a major portion of financing directed towards the construction of small-scale health infrastructure projects, including the construction of hospitals. In addition, India has also provided close to 300 educational scholarships to train Nepali students in areas of scientific expertise in India (Government of India, 2009b). India's DAH to Sri Lanka also manifests in the form of technical and infrastructure cooperation.

Table 4.5 Allocation of aid from India (million USD)

Country or program	*2007–08*	*2008–09**
Bhutan	175.3	210.4
Bangladesh	14.4	3.5
Nepal	24.0	30.9
Sri Lanka	6.7	7.5
Maldives	4.7	3.9
Myanmar	4.8	12.4
Other developing countries	43.2	39.0
African countries	12.0	17.7
Central Asia	4.8	6.2
Afghanistan	104.1	98.2

* These figures are based on the proposed budget in rupees.
Source: Government of India (2009b).

Small-scale health projects including the construction and upgrade of hospitals has occurred in Trincomalee and Dinckoya (Government of India, 2009b). Notwithstanding recent commitments by the Manmohan Singh government that total an additional US$500 million, India's health assistance in Kabul has primarily been in the form of health facility construction, development of small-scale projects in health and sanitation, rural development and agriculture and higher education scholarships for Afghani students (Government of India, 2009b).

India has also concurrently maintained a marginal influence across the African continent since 1964 through its two flagship training programmes – ITEC and the Special Commonwealth Assistance for Africa Programme (SCAAP), both of which invest in human resource capacity-building for those engaged in social and economic development projects (Government of India, 2011). Recent Indian MEA budget outlays (2010–11) to Africa reveal an increase in the transfer of funds to facilitate technological development in healthcare across the continent (Government of India, 2010). The scope of this approach has considerably widened given India's expertise in information technology; a pan-African e-network is being developed to link Indian universities and hospitals to 5 regional universities, 5 specialty hospitals, 53 regular hospitals and educational institutions in Africa (Ayyar, 2010).

Recent agreements formalized under the India–Brazil–South Africa (IBSA) Tripartite Framework present another South–South forum for India to share its experiences, comparative advantages and finances in the area of public health (India Brazil South Africa Dialogue Forum, 2011). Finally in 2011, the Indian government offered US$5 billion to several African countries in development assistance, including health-related projects. The tranche will be transferred through a series of lines of credits for infrastructure projects, regional integration, human capital and skills development (Maasho, 2011).

Institutional management of ODA and DAH in India

In India, the international development policy and health assistance portfolios fall under the purview of MEA. The MEA is also principally responsible for bilateral development assistance (Price, 2011: vii). It functions as the coordinating unit for conceiving development policy and advises other ministries on fulfilling their respective development mandates (Jobelius, 2007: 7). MEA's official tasks vis-à-vis development and health assistance include offering technical and project assistance to developing countries, consultancy services through project formulation and implementation, provision of foreign students in Indian educational institutions and other kinds of humanitarian assistance as and when they occur (Ayyar, 2010). The MEA also takes direct charge of coordinating development aid packages for countries in South Asia and Afghanistan (Joebelius, 2007: 7).

The Ministry of Finance (MOF) chips in to fulfill the attendant financial tasks involved and receives advice from the MEA on the eventual shape of bilateral assistance packages (Stuenkel, 2010: 39). Under the MOF, the Department of Economic Affairs (DEA) functions as the coordinating unit, especially with respect to coordinating development policy for countries outside South Asia (Jobelius, 2007: 7). In addition to the MEA, MOF and DEA the EXIM Bank, an entity attached to the DEA, assumes the role in financing budget support and loans for developing countries through the provision of a LoC (Ayyar, 2010). The payment and settlement of development loans and assistance is administered and managed by Indian embassies and consuls in their respective territories (Joebelius, 2007: 7).

Technical assistance constitutes a critical focus of Indian development assistance. MEA's two technical arms – ITEC and SCAAP – administer technical assistance for foreign development professionals seconded from their home countries (Government of India, 2011). Notwithstanding the deputation of Indian experts abroad, ITEC offers extensive training programs for nominees of ITEC partner countries across the developing world. Training is broken down in two segments: civilian and military. Under civilian training, over 40 Indian institutions offer a range of courses for foreign professionals and practitioners in areas such as information technology, parliamentary studies, rural development, mass communication and planning and administration (Ayyar, 2010). ITEC has also been involved in health and development programs in Afghanistan, Maldives, Sri Lanka and Vietnam, primarily through the construction of hospitals. Aid for disaster relief has also been given through ITEC (Government of India, 2009b).

Civil society's role appears to be confined to aid delivery. Eduardo Gomez discerns robust NGO activity, especially in the prevention of HIV/AIDS, in partnerships with global entities like the WHO, World Bank, Gates and Clinton Foundations, etc. (Gomez, 2009: 10). Gomez also identifies a clear want of non-governmental presence in the ODA and DAH policy process. Especially while tackling HIV/AIDS, NGOs could play a decisive role in improving the role and operative capacity of the National AIDS Control Organisation, the nodal organization responsible for the formulation and implementation of programs for the prevention and control of HIV/AIDS (Gomez, 2009: 11; NACO, 2011).

The Ministry of Health and Family Welfare (MOHFW) appears to play virtually no role in determining global health assistance (Government of India, 2009a). However, the MOHFW does play a role within the IBSA Forum. In the IBSA framework, under a joint memorandum of understanding on health signed in 2009, the three countries agreed to 'promote and develop cooperation in health and medical sciences, based on equality, mutual benefits and in accordance with the laws and regulations in each country' (IBSA, 2009). To lead and facilitate this endeavor from the Indian front, Delhi appointed the Ministry of Health and Family Welfare. It is responsible for implementing the actions agreed upon by the working group on health cooperation, which will manifest through the exchange, dissemination and sharing of health and medical information, professionals, technology and innovations (IBSA, 2009).

This institutional apparatus is poised to change with the announcement of the India Agency of Partnership in Development in July 2011 – a proposed centralized foreign aid institution designed to streamline India's burgeoning aid commitments, curb delays, reduce operation costs and ensure India's aid agenda and attendant programs are driven by developmental considerations. The institution is also expected to better harmonize India's role as a critical aid recipient and donor. As of now, the agency has been entrusted to oversee US$11.3 billion over the next five to seven years (Patel, 2011).

India, development assistance for health and global health governance

Can India contribute substantively to global health governance through its development assistance for health? What do their DAH practices signify? These are, no doubt, critical queries that emerge after discussing the Indian government's global health assistance footprint. Indeed, the amounts, types and modes of DAH being disbursed by the Indian government does indicate that Delhi is and will play a role as a global health donor in the near future, complementing its role as an aid recipient. However, acute development and public health challenges at home, coupled with a weak and inadequate institutional apparatus to manage development assistance, will restrain their ability to contribute substantively to GHG through foreign health aid.

Donor–recipient balance

Domestically, it is worth considering the state of India's public health system. Doing so enables us to place Delhi's foreign health financing patterns in perspective and provide a more complete picture of their global health aid practices and what can be expected of them vis-à-vis global health governance.

India's public health capacity is feeble. WHO statistics reveal that India expended 4.2 percent of the government spending on domestic healthcare in 2009 (WHO, 2011). Until 2005–2006, government health spending in India had been declining. Rising fiscal burdens on the state in the 1980s and 1990s forced Delhi to pare its health expenditures. After three decades of declining healthcare spending, however, India has increased total government spending on health by roughly 1–2 percent of GDP. Since 2006, government spending has risen on healthcare (Mahal and Yip, 2008: 926). But current spending patterns are not adequate to address menacing public health threats. Non-communicable diseases such as diabetes, cancer and heart disease are rampant; they caused 60 percent of Indian deaths in 2005 (Mahal, Karan and Engelgau, 2010). The National Family Health Survey-3 report (International Institute for Population Sciences and ORC Macro, 2006) showed that under-nutrition is predominant among women confined to a low standard of living, while one in two women aged 15–49 suffer from chronic energy deficiency. Also, the report shows that India is facing a double burden of over-nutrition and under-nutrition. India also faces a daunting challenge on the infectious disease front, which represents close to 30 percent of the national disease burden (John *et al.*, 2011: 254). UNAIDS also contends that India has the third largest number of individuals with HIV/AIDS after South Africa and Nigeria (UNAIDS, 2010). Tuberculosis is also resurging across the country, with two million new cases surfacing in 2009 and a disturbing presence of multi-resistant strains of the pathogen (John *et al.*, 2011: 255).

This problematic state of affairs will force India to continue as a thriving recipient for the foreseeable future, complicating its ability to lead concurrently with global health initiatives. As GFATM statistics reveal, India has paid US$26 million to date in assistance to the Fund (The Global Fund, 2011). However, it currently possesses approved grant amounts that total US$2 billion, with disbursals that collectively stand at over half a billion US$ each (The Global Fund, 2011b). The Gates Foundation has pledged US$338 million to India to combat HIV/AIDS. The World Bank has boosted its HIV funding to India by US$250 million in 2007 (Gomez, 2009: 10–11). Such heavy use of global health resources also distorts the process through which funds are allocated to tackle pervasive global health threats, siphons funding away from low-income countries, especially those in Africa that are decimated by these diseases, and places immense fiscal pressures on entities like the GFATM, which is struggling to renew investments (Chow, 2010).

Material contributor to global health

Perusing India's DAH practices, one can discern a trend towards investing in assistance that is material in nature. Across South Asia and Africa, the sheer numbers of projects that focus on health systems, hospital construction, training of development foreign professionals through the ITEC and other initiatives have a tangible impact on their aid recipients. Delhi has displayed a penchant to focus more on assistance that is practical in orientation, largely in the form of small-scale development projects, training and capacity-building programs, and infrastructural development, whose impact remains long after project completion. India is choosing to leverage and channel its inherent comparative and competitive advantage in capacity-building, information and communications technology, and infrastructure in conceiving and structuring development and global health assistance initiatives.

Thus, they are playing a beneficial functional role in building the sovereign public health capacities of beleaguered developing countries, which do complement the litany of 'soft' initiatives being developed and implemented by Western countries, private foundations, civil society organizations and other global health actors. As such, there is tremendous value added from India's development trajectory, challenging extant notions that claim emerging donors are impeding global development efforts through their independent aid agendas.

Institutional inadequacies

Institutionally, India's apparatus is clearly wanting and deficits reign. India lacks a clear and comprehensive aid lexicon that could help to track and estimate the funds it allocates and disburses. Notwithstanding the recent announcement of a centralized aid agency, India's ODA and DAH processes are principally driven by agencies that have limited knowledge of development or health issues. Policy formulation in India is concentrated in the Ministry of External Affairs, which solicits assistance from other functionally specialized entities like the Ministry of Finance, Department of Economic Affairs and the EXIM Bank. Also compounding the problem is the absence of the Ministry of Health and Welfare in the aid policy process. Non-governmental organizations are also missing.

Such a structure prevents health concerns from entering and influencing the assistance policies that Delhi formulates. Institutional barriers also complicate the harmonizing of national development and public health agendas with the global health paradigm. This is reflected in the technical and financial outlook of their international development and health assistance packages that only require calibration with Delhi's governing philosophies and agendas. It also fundamentally prevents the establishment of a conceptual link with the governing episteme of the GHG paradigm that stresses the interdependencies of global health. If India is and can be expected to discharge a global health role, institutional reform is merited to ensure that India's development assistance for health is in lockstep with larger global health assistance trends.

In addition, the implications of India's ongoing tryst with novel institutional modalities like the IBSA forum are unclear. The IBSA's *raison d'être* is to mobilize expertise, experiences and resources of emerging market-oriented democracies to bear upon and address salient development challenges. It also constitutes a clear and emergent attempt to institutionalize South–South cooperation in order to challenge and counter prevailing models of development cooperation that are more hierarchical in nature (Stuenkel, 2010: 41). But as emerging countries, like India, engage exclusively with each other in these avenues, they are also refraining from making extensive policy commitments in areas of cooperation, which does arguably suggest that these emergent fora constitute avenues of metaphorical, not actual, importance.

Regional hegemon

A broad look at India's DAH patterns demonstrates the significance that Delhi attaches to regional interests and concerns. Regional stability constitutes a major national interest. Since the 1950s, India has deployed its largesse to maintain and advance regional peace and prosperity. As Oliver Stuenkel describes, 'India embraces its transition from aid recipient to donor more wholeheartedly in the regional context, where it clearly seeks to define its role as regional hegemon and donor' (Stuenkel, 2010: 43).

However, this regional focus also constricts India's global ambitions. In the global context, India does not necessarily feel a part of the multilateral system of donors, as it might lead to greater calls for more leadership and greater financial contributions. India's penchant to exclusively invest on bilateral, not multilateral, channels of assistance affirms their regional preferences. Relying on institutions that govern foreign and strategic considerations to determine development policy also suggests that regional interests will trump global objectives. Thus, it might be time for global health actors and institutions to revisit the global expectations being foisted on India and, perhaps, explore whether and how India's regional health expertise and experiences should be further leveraged.

Conclusion

India has been a donor since it attained independence. Over the first few decades, its development and health assistance was directed within South Asia to enable countries to achieve their development needs through technical assistance, largely influenced by Nehruvian ideals of non-alignment, self-sufficiency and autonomy. These fundamentals still hold sway and South Asia continues to feature large in India's current development outlook. As India liberalized in the 1990s, however, its priorities and values began to evolve. Economic and strategic priorities are trumping ideals and moral discourses and India's overtures to Africa and Central Asia are a direct outcome of this shift. Health assistance continues to be channeled through technical means but the objectives underpinning aid are also extra-developmental, to either unlock market access for Indian enterprises and products or secure geopolitical leverage.

In terms of development assistance for health, India prefers to channel it bilaterally through technical and financial means. Its multilateral assistance pales in comparison to its bilateral assistance. Technical assistance vis-à-vis health typically manifests through the construction of hospitals and clinics, deputation of medical and paramedical experts, and the development of water sanitation, agricultural processing projects, etc. (Government of India, 2009b). India also deploys assistance financially, through the provision of letters of credit to developing countries for financing the import of Indian expertise, technology, projects and goods, which are subsequently used for health system and infrastructure development.

Institutionally, four national entities are responsible for the provision of ODA and health assistance – the Ministry of External Affairs, Ministry of Finance and its Department of Economic Affairs, and the EXIM Bank. The Ministry of Health and Welfare and non-governmental organizations do not have a place in the development of India's global health policy. As a result, economic and strategic considerations dominate the determination of health and development assistance. However, India has also commenced cooperating with Brazil and South Africa on public health issues through the IBSA framework, which does include and involve the Ministry of Health and Welfare. Though the Ministry of External Affairs, Delhi finalizes the aid allocation decisions, and state governments occasionally influence the aid process. For instance, the state of Tamil Nadu has requested the Ministry of External Affairs to provide aid to Sri Lanka through the International Red Cross in 2008 and 2009 (Meier and Murthy, 2011).

Inferring from India's DAH patterns, it is evident that it chooses to operate as a material operator and contributor, directing assistance predominantly to areas it finds strategically attractive. On the one hand, this practice does complement the global health initiatives of Western actors that are 'softer' and fungible in nature.

On the other hand, it prevents India from developing its global health ambitions and contributing to innovations within GHG. This disconnect is exacerbated by a lax ODA apparatus that is littered with myriad deficits.

Finally, it is necessary to situate, connect and reconcile India's role as a donor character with its role as an active and robust aid recipient to better understand its global health role and potential. Acute developmental and health challenges will likely inhibit India's capacity to play a substantive role in GHG since they rely on the largesse and know-how of a litany of global health actors without commensurately contributing in return. If the government feels compelled to allocate greater resources to public health causes, India could better internalize lessons of health cooperation and interdependence, which could then inform and shape its global health assistance policies and benefit global health governance as a whole.

Part 2

Asian contributions to collective action instruments to address global health challenges

5 The International Health Regulations (2005)

Asia's contribution to a global health governance framework

Adam Kamradt-Scott, Kelley Lee and Jingying Xu

Introduction

On 15 July 2007, the International Health Regulations 2005 (IHR, 2005) officially entered into force following a 12-year process to update the only intergovernmental legal framework specifically designed to limit the global spread of infectious diseases, while minimizing disruption to international traffic and trade. Although the decision to fundamentally rethink and update the IHR was made as early as 1995, the greater part of diplomatic negotiations were completed at three meetings held by the Intergovernmental Working Group on Revision of the International Health Regulations (IGWG) between November 2004 and May 2005. The proposed text that emerged from the IGWG meetings was then submitted to the World Health Assembly (WHA) in May 2005, where it was adopted by member states. This began an 18-month grace period that concluded in July 2007, when the IHR became binding on all member states of the World Health Organization (WHO).

Under the terms of the new Regulations, all governments had until July 2012 to develop certain 'core capacities' to detect, assess, notify and respond to 'public health emergencies of international concern' (PHEIC). In this chapter, we analyse the contribution that selected Asian countries made to the IHR revision process, and specifically the IGWG. In addition to examining these contributions, we will examine how these governments are currently progressing in implementing the revised IHR. We conclude with a discussion of the challenges faced by many lower- and middle-income countries (LMICs) in ensuring the necessary technical infrastructure is in place to meet IHR 2005 requirements.

This chapter is based on a review of primary and secondary literature, and over 25 semi-structured interviews with government officials, representatives of non-government organizations (NGOs), as well as leading academics based throughout China, South Korea, Japan, Thailand and Taiwan.

Background to the revision process

The WHA first adopted the International Sanitary Regulations (ISR) in 1951. Reflecting the interests of the largely European-focused agreements drawn up during the International Sanitary Conferences of the late nineteenth century, the ISR initially pertained to six reportable diseases. When the ISR were renamed the 'International Health Regulations' in 1969, their scope was reduced to four diseases and, in 1981, following confirmation that smallpox had been eradicated, to cholera, plague and yellow fever.

By the mid-1990s, as a result of this progressive narrowing of scope, the IHR were seen to be increasingly irrelevant to the broader international control of disease outbreaks. The public health community, faced with several new and resurgent diseases including HIV/AIDS, ebola haemorrhagic fever (EHF), West Nile virus, variant Creutzfeld–Jakob disease, polio and tuberculosis to name a few (World Health Organization, 1996), found the framework outdated and dysfunctional. In addition, some governments had become reluctant to report outbreaks of disease subject to the IHR, often choosing instead to use inventive means to avoid notifying the WHO, due to the risk of punitive measures being imposed by other countries. The risk of adverse effects on trade and other economic activity has been acknowledged as a problem for the ISR since their adoption in 1951 (Minze *et al.*, 1998). Thus, as an effective legal framework designed to 'ensure maximum security against the international spread of diseases with a minimum interference with world traffic' (World Health Organization, 1983), the IHR were no longer seen as fit for purpose.

A number of developments during the 1990s created a new incentive within the international community to revise the IHR. First, there were several serious infectious disease outbreaks. These notably included the reappearance of cholera in Latin America in 1991 a decade after it had been eradicated from the continent, an outbreak of plague in the Indian city of Surat in 1994 that caused losses of over US$2 billion to the Indian economy, and an outbreak of EHF in Zaire in 1995. These latter two outbreaks, which occurred very close to the annual WHA meeting where the IHR were to be discussed, provided ample evidence that both the IHR, and the WHO's outbreak policies and procedures, needed urgent attention.

Compounding concerns over naturally occurring disease outbreaks was the discovery in 1991 of substantial stockpiles of biological and chemical weapons during the first Gulf War, which raised the spectre that outbreaks could be caused deliberately (Tucker, 1999). This was followed in 1992 by the disconcerting Russian admission that an offensive biological weapons program had been maintained throughout the Cold War. Aside from the risk of such weapons falling into hostile hands, there were also fears that the scientists who had worked on developing these weapons might be recruited to work for terrorist organizations. The Aum Shinrikyo terrorist attack on a Tokyo subway in March 1995 appeared to confirm that such fears might in fact be well founded. Consequently, as member states assembled at the WHA in May 1995, a new consensus emerged to revise the outdated IHR and strengthen the WHO's disease outbreak alert and response capabilities.

Thus, a clear accord emerged at the 48th WHA that both the existing IHR, and the WHO's disease outbreak response strategies, required extensive revision. Adopting two resolutions to that effect – WHA48.7 *Revision and Updating of the International Health Regulations* and WHA48.13 *Communicable Disease Prevention and Control: New, Emerging, and Re-emerging Infectious Diseases* – the WHA requested that the Director-General immediately initiate a program to evaluate and update the IHR legislative framework. To inform this process, the Secretariat was also charged with developing and testing new and effective disease eradication policies and procedures. These new policies and procedures were to be used as a basis to revise the IHR, and improve the Organization's ability to protect and assist its member states (World Health Organization, 1995a, b).

Between 1995 and 2003, progress in revising the IHR was painstakingly slow. Several factors, notably the failure of trials testing the proposed syndromic reporting method, the internal reform process following the appointment of Gro Harlem Brundtland as Director-General, the failure of the Biological Weapons Convention negotiations post-11 September 2001, and the launch of the Global Outbreak Alert and Response Network (GOARN), contributed to the delays. It was not until the 2003 Severe Acute Respiratory Syndrome (SARS) outbreak, and the renewed threat of an H5N1 avian influenza pandemic in 2004 (following the Hong Kong outbreaks of the late 1990s), that sufficient momentum built to bring the IHR revision process to conclusion.

The SARS outbreak served as the perfect catalyst to bring the revision process to a close, engendering a sense of urgency and spurring the international community into action. For the WHO Secretariat and member states, SARS also provided a timely opportunity to assess the organization's new communicable disease outbreak strategies. The disease's rapid international spread enabled the Secretariat to field test, for example, a number of the protocols that were being proposed for inclusion in the revised IHR. As a consequence, the Organization released a report as early as May 2003 outlining the 'lessons learned' from the SARS outbreak, indicating how the WHO's response to the disease would be incorporated into the revised IHR framework (World Health Organization, 2003a, b). Likewise, as reflected in the text of WHA resolution on SARS, member states believed that the outbreak had given 'concrete expression' of the need to revise the IHR and develop disease-eradication procedures that all governments could agree upon (World Health Organization, 2007d). To that effect, the Assembly authorized the creation of an IGWG to finalize the process, and a series of regional consultations were held to allow member states to contribute their views on the draft framework ahead of the formal intergovernmental summit. The first IGWG meeting was conducted in November 2004, and drew together approximately two-thirds of the WHO's member states to debate and negotiate a new framework. While considerable progress was made, it took a further two sessions of the IGWG in February and May 2005 to conclude the revision process. The final draft text of the IHR was then submitted to and approved by the 58th WHA in May 2005.

The contribution of Asian countries to revising the IHR

In light of these meetings, all WHO member states were provided with formal opportunities to contribute to the IHR revision process. The two most prominent forums were the regional consultation meetings held in the lead up to the formal IGWG meeting, and the IGWG itself. Following the distribution of an early draft of the proposed IHR text in early 2004, only two of the Asian countries identified in this chapter – the Republic of Korea and Japan – submitted comments to the WHO Western Pacific Regional Office (WPRO) suggesting specific amendments. Similarly, although attendance at the regional consultations hosted by the WHO in WPRO and the South East Asian Regional Office (SEARO) was relatively high (World Health Organization, 2004a, b), a number of Asian delegates appeared to lack a firm understanding of the IHR and the proposals under consideration. As one official noted:

> We didn't have regional meetings in the lead-up to or during the IHR negotiations other than the formal meeting arranged by WPRO in Manila. Even at that regional consultation in April 2004 it was clear that many countries didn't exactly know what the IHR meant and they hadn't caught the full implications of what the negotiations were about.[1]

Each country surveyed in this study did assemble teams that were tasked with examining the draft legislation, to propose amendments and to inform negotiating positions. In each case, however, these groups comprised between three and five individuals, and were only created between late 2003 and early 2004 just ahead of the regional consultations. This meant that teams were not always fully briefed and/or had been only given very general guidance. As one informant noted in relation to their country's IHR negotiation team,

> We were given a very, very broad mandate from the government when we entered the negotiations, so we had a large amount of flexibility. The only guidance or direction we were given was that our first priority was the health of our nation's population, second was the health of the all the region, and third, the rest of the world. That was the extent of the mandate we were given.[2]

The structure of the teams also reportedly varied considerably with differing levels of expertise and experience in public health, international law, and/or foreign affairs and diplomacy. Some teams even lacked legal expertise as they entered the formal IGWG talks, as one respondent later recalled:

> At that time our negotiation team comprised the Director of the Infectious Disease Control Division, some of his colleagues, and myself. Unfortunately the expert on international law could not attend the meeting and I just remember that throughout the negotiations there were so many legal issues that came up, and it was very difficult for us to understand the differences at times between distinctions such as 'should' and 'shall'. We were conscious that other teams had their international lawyers with them, so we went to speak to representatives from the United States and other countries to get their help.[3]

Another factor that appears to have affected the extent to which teams were able to contribute to the negotiations was language skills. As one respondent noted,

> One of the biggest difficulties we faced was language. It was interesting to observe that the Chinese often insisted on speaking in Mandarin throughout every meeting, even though all the Chinese delegates spoke perfect English. It seemed to be a point of pride for them as no other country could understand Chinese. We then always had to wait for the translation into English, and then sometimes we didn't always understand it as English isn't our mother tongue.[4]

As a consequence, it appears that at least some delegations viewed the IHR negotiations as beyond their ability to influence. As one official summarized,

> We didn't feel the need to get heavily involved in some parts of the negotiations because it was clear that they were between the United States and some European countries on one side, and Iran and some other countries on the other. So we just watched what was going on and kept out of the way.[5]

Such observations may potentially explain why the size of negotiating teams fluctuated so markedly over time and between countries. As Table 5.1 shows, whereas some countries (notably China, Bangladesh, Malaysia and Myanmar) increased their representation at each successive meeting, other countries reduced the

Table 5.1 Asian Country Participation in the IHR Intergovernmental Working Group Meetings by number of delegates

Country	*Nov. 2004*	*Feb. 2005*	*May 2005*
Bangladesh	3	3	5
Brunei Darussalam	4	2	4
Cambodia	1	2	2
China	12	15	17
India	3	3	3
Indonesia	9	5	6
Japan	9	7	7
Lao People's Democratic Republic	1	–	1
Malaysia	3	4	6
Maldives	–	1	1
Mongolia	1	1	2
Myanmar	1	2	5
Nepal	–	–	–
Philippines	3	3	4
Republic of Korea	5	2	4
Singapore	5	4	4
Sri Lanka	1	–	1
Thailand	3	1	2
Timor-Leste	–	–	–
Vietnam	1	–	1

Source: Compiled from World Health Organization (2004) *List of participants*. Document: A/IHR/IGWG/DIV/3_Rev.1; World Health Organization (2005) *Provisional list of participants*. Document: A/IHR/IGWG/2/DIV/3; and World Health Organization (2005) *List of participants*. Document: A/IHR/IGWG/2/DIV/3_Rev.2.

number of their representatives (Indonesia, Japan, Singapore and Thailand), while still others (Lao People's Democratic Republic, Maldives, Sri Lanka and Vietnam) sent representatives only intermittently. Of the countries identified in Table 5.1, only Timor-Leste and Nepal failed to send any delegates at all. Various factors may account for the size and fluctuation of the negotiation teams (e.g. domestic political considerations such as elections, internal instability and financial costs associated with sending delegations to Geneva, etc.). It is reasonable to assume, however, that those countries that increased their representation believed the IHR negotiations warranted increased attention, expanding the size of their delegation accordingly. China, for instance, progressively increased its number of delegates from 12 to 17. By comparison, the United States (US) government, which as noted above proved to be another highly influential actor in the negotiations, maintained its representation at 12 delegates throughout all 3 IGWG meetings. Only limited conclusions can be drawn from such data. Increasing the relative size of negotiating teams can enable governments, however, to take advantage of processes such as concurrent breakout sessions where controversial matters are debated, or 'corridor' negotiations where representatives from various countries meet informally to advance certain agendas and debate proposed amendments.

The influence of state sovereignty on Asian contributions to the IHR negotiations

One of the more widely debated issues throughout the formal negotiations pertained to how the revised IHR potentially infringed upon state sovereignty. As early as the April 2004 WPRO regional consultation, for example, the Secretariat observed,

> International law, by its very nature, impinges on country sovereignty. Some participants consider the proposed IHR needs to be modified to shift the balance more towards the rights of Member States. As well as the question of team deployment, some participants wish to retain the right to impose measures in excess of those recommended by WHO, where there is an appropriate rationale. Most participants feel that the issue of charging for patient services should be left to their own discretion, especially with regards to medical examination, vaccination and prophylaxis.[6]

As the talks progressed, additional examples were raised. A core motivation for revising the IHR was to encourage greater openness and transparency, and ensure more rapid notification of events. To that end, it had been proposed that countries should immediately report outbreaks of specific diseases such as polio, new strains of influenza, smallpox and SARS that were listed in Annex 2 of the draft legislation. For some countries though, this proposal equated to an infringement of state sovereignty on the basis that they may be compelled to reveal information that may adversely harm their national interests. The Chinese delegation was amongst those countries that argued strongly against the inclusion of any formal list and against identifying SARS in particular. As one informant later recalled,

> SARS had been a big embarrassment for the Chinese Government. They basically had been caught out trying to engage in a cover-up over the number of cases they had. The WHO Director-General, Dr Brundtland, then publicly criticized the Chinese authorities. That had never been done before by a Director-General. I am still not entirely sure why they objected so strongly to having SARS included in the list of reportable diseases. They gave a list of reasons in the negotiations such as that it would be a further burden on developing countries and so on, but I personally suspect that they saw it as a matter of national pride. They did not want to end up in a situation where they would be again embarrassed by SARS.[7]

The Chinese government's proposal did not have widespread support though, even amongst its more immediate neighbours, as a key respondent later noted,

> We were not happy with the degree of transparency China demonstrated in the SARS incident, so we didn't agree with China's attempts to exclude SARS from the list of reportable diseases.[8]

It was also in the context of concerns regarding SARS that the issue of Taiwan's status was raised. In 2003, the Taiwanese government's attempts to obtain technical assistance from the WHO to control its outbreak of SARS, and the rejection that subsequently ensued, became headline news around the world. In late 2003, the Taiwanese administration formed a 'special task force' to review the draft IHR and provide comments on how the framework could be improved. They also sent a special representative to Geneva to attend the IGWG meetings. Intriguingly, although the special representative was physically prevented from entering the building to meet with government officials,[9] Taiwan's status was raised on a number of occasions, with delegates voicing either their support or opposition for special recognition of the disputed territory. One of the more vocal opponents was China, which maintained that any move to recognize Taiwan independently from China equated to an infringement of their sovereignty. As a result, Taiwan's requests for special recognition were repeatedly denied.

The Taiwanese government was evidently aware of the sensitivity surrounding their attempts to become further involved in the negotiations, but they were uncomfortable with approaching neighbouring countries for support. As one Taiwanese respondent noted,

> Asian countries considered this to be very sensitive. The Chinese government was particularly aware of the fact that Taiwan was an issue. We were also aware and understood the sensitivity, so we intentionally didn't solicit support from Asian countries. We had some contact from the United States through our representative in Geneva, and we spoke with several friendly

> countries who understood our situation, but we didn't approach any Asian countries.[10]

As such, despite the fact that it was widely recognized that all geographical areas were at risk of disease outbreaks, and that if these outbreaks were not rapidly contained they could potentially develop into PHEICs, governments were clearly divided over whether Taiwan warranted special recognition.

A third example of where Asian sovereignty concerns visibly entered the negotiations pertained to the issue of investigative teams. Under the terms of the GOARN operational framework the WHO was authorized to send investigative teams to verify an outbreak (World Health Organization, 2000a). Throughout the IHR negotiations, however, this authority began to be openly challenged with Asian countries amongst those that opposed such measures. As one government representative noted, for instance:

> During our discussions, we did raise the issue of on-the-spot investigations and supported the idea that the WHO should be able to make them mandatory. This obviously went against the notion of national sovereignty, but we felt that sovereignty should give way in this instance to what is in the better interests of human beings.[11]

By way of contrast, other Asian countries, such as China, vehemently opposed the notion that investigative teams could enter a country uninvited, claiming such actions amounted to an infringement of their sovereignty. Ultimately, the latter view gained the majority of support, and under Article 10 of the revised IHR the WHO is now required to obtain the consent of governments prior to sending investigative teams.

Institutional diversity and Asian governments' approach to the IHR negotiations

Of the countries surveyed for this study, it would appear that Asian governments approached the IHR negotiations in a state-centric and nationally focused, rather than multilateral-orientated manner, declining to form alliances or partnerships, or even seek advice from other actors (both state and non-state) in developing or negotiating policy positions. Asian governments did not, for example, pursue input from NGOs or seek to form partnerships with other actors prior to the regional consultations and the IGWG negotiations. In a move designed to further restrict the input of non-state actors, the majority of Asian governments voted with other delegations to exclude all organizations in official relations with the WHO at the commencement of the November 2004 IGWG meeting on the basis that they were deemed 'intergovernmental' meetings. This occurred despite the fact that these organizations had previously been invited to attend and contribute to the discussions. It was not until the February 2005 round of talks and a series of interventions by the WHO Secretariat that NGOs were permitted to re-engage in the process.

This pattern of engagement appears to have been in stark contrast to the approach taken by countries in other regions. Indeed, Asian governments appear to have sidestepped forming regional or coordinated positions on the IHR. As one official noted,

> There were the regional consultations ahead of the intergovernmental working group but I don't recall that we really discussed things with other countries. We attended the meetings, and we listened to what other countries raised and we raised a couple of things ourselves, but we didn't form any partnerships or make any deals.[12]

Even in the period leading up to the formal IGWG talks, whereas several groups of countries such as the Andean Group (Peru, Bolivia, Venezuela, Colombia, Chile and Ecuador) and the Mercosur Group (Chile, Brazil, Argentina, Uruguay and Paraguay) had met as early as 2002 to develop a coordinated position on the draft text, no equivalent meetings were held by Asian countries (World Health Organization, 2010d). Asian governments also declined to raise the IHR negotiations in other state-based regional forums, such as ASEAN and APEC, selecting instead to approach the negotiations individually. In this regard, Asian countries not only maintained a very state-centric approach to the negotiations, shunning the opportunity to engage with non-state actors such as NGOs and the private sector, but they also approached the negotiations virtually in complete isolation from each other. Thus, there is little evidence to suggest that a sense of collective solidarity emerged amongst those Asian countries attending the IGWG. As described by one respondent,

> Usually in negotiations countries don't fight alone. Usually a country will seek out other friendly countries to work together with. Africa, for example, now tends to unite as one. The European Union usually unites as one. Even the Commonwealth countries headed by the UK usually have informal meetings during these important negotiations. But here in the East Asia region we have difficulties with this. That actually lessens the Asian voice.[13]

The consequence of this approach was that Asian countries might have failed to capitalize on an opportunity to strengthen their diplomatic influence by adopting alternative negotiating methods, such as regionally based partnerships or non-state actors.

Asian conceptions of the IHR

For the most part, much of the IHR revision process was framed in the language and context of 'global health security' (World Health Organization, 2007e). Among Asian countries, however, it does not appear that this discourse resonated strongly. For example, several Asian delegations expressed their objections towards the inclusion of terrorism and/or terrorist-related activities within the scope of the IHR. As one respondent observed,

> One of the main issues for us throughout the formal negotiations was the definition of 'disease' in the IHR. North America and Europe really wanted to include terrorism and terrorist events, but our government objected to this notion. There was no need to include this.[14]

Asian countries were not alone in their objections to this proposal and, with support from the WHO Eastern Mediterranean and African regions, a compromise deal was struck on the definition of 'disease' that avoided explicitly mentioning terrorism and terrorist-related activities (Kamradt-Scott, 2012).

Since 2005, the health security discourse has become more nuanced in recognition of the wide-ranging socio-economic, cultural and political consequences arising from disease outbreaks and/or pandemics. In turn, governments have been encouraged to comprehensively prepare all sectors of society to defend against this threat, in what has become known as 'whole-of-government', 'whole-of-society', or 'multisectoral' preparedness (Horvarth *et al.*, 2006). Some Asian governments, such as China, declare they have embraced such an approach:

> The Government used to be very fragmented about these sorts of things, about how to respond to infectious disease outbreaks. For example, our department for entry and exit inspection and quarantine used to regulate only those functions at the borders, while the health department used to be responsible for only local hospital issues and epidemic prevention. The departments used to communicate with each other, but not very well. The emergence of the IHR and several recent outbreaks though has given us a real opportunity to get things working better. Now when an epidemic occurs, it is recognized that it is not something that can be resolved by a single department. The Government has recognized that it needs to unify and activate the whole society so we have established new joint prevention and control mechanisms.[15]

Whereas other governments appear to be still struggling with ensuring better coordination:

> One of the big challenges for the IHR, and for the WHO, is something that is happening within our government. Because it has traditionally been the Ministry of Health that has had responsibility for working with the WHO on matters, we have found that the other ministries don't feel the need to pay attention to things like the IHR. So when the Ministry of Health has gone to the other ministries to talk with them about how we need to implement the IHR, they say they don't want to be bothered with it. In their view, it is a health matter and therefore it is up to the Ministry of Health to deal with. This is a big challenge for us at the moment.[16]

Noting these challenges though, at least amongst the participants surveyed for this study, there was a strong consensus that the revised IHR was a useful tool for encouraging greater intra- and inter-state collaboration in controlling disease outbreaks. In this sense, it would appear that Asian governments are very comfortable with a framework that emphasizes a state-centric, rules-based approach that identifies a strong role for government in preventing and controlling disease outbreaks.

Asian countries' progress in implementing the IHR

Following the conclusion of the revision process, the response by Asian governments in how they view the IHR appears to be somewhat mixed. Some countries, such as China, claim to attach considerable importance to the Regulations and have undertaken massive reforms of their health system as a result. For instance, as one Chinese official has recalled,

> Since the IHR has entered into force, the general direction of our country in relation to pandemic surveillance and containment has changed considerably. The Government has learned the lessons of SARS and attaches great importance to this issue. It is very clear now that if an event occurs at the local level it must be reported immediately to the next higher level, right up to the Ministry of Health. So the first area where we have seen an improvement has been in enhancing the reporting mechanisms, and the second is the level of importance leaders now attach to this. In China, attention by leaders is very important and the more attention they pay, the more measures will be adhered to.[17]

Other administrations, however, appear to have given the Regulations less attention. Korea and Taiwan, for example, have passed new domestic laws to ensure their compliance, but general awareness and political commitment to the IHR currently appears to be low. As one respondent observed,

> Many officers in our organization don't know about the IHR. At a guess I would say that there are about ten officers in total in this building that know about the IHR. The high-ranking officers definitely know of the framework and its implementation, but the employees working in other divisions or departments have probably never heard of it. It's a shame but that is the reality. It is at least a relief that the high-ranking officers think it is important.[18]

In Japan, it appears that the attention afforded to the IHR varies across government departments, as one respondent noted:

> Within our department, we see the Regulations as a treaty that we have to comply with under international law. But most of the government sees the IHR as just an agreement. This has meant at times that when the WHO has

> suggested we create a committee to oversee implementation of the IHR or to assess our national core capacity requirements, some view it more as just a suggestion that they don't have to pay as much attention to. Other ministries just don't think of it as an issue.[19]

In what is perhaps further evidence of either low prioritization or a lack of capacity, many Asian countries have failed to nominate representatives to the IHR Roster of Experts. This roster is particularly important because members are drawn from the IHR Roster of Experts to sit on an advisory committee (known as the Emergency Committee) that has responsibility for advising the WHO Director-General on whether to declare a PHEIC. Therefore the roster is central to the revised IHR decision-making processes, and in ensuring greater accountability and transparency. By mid-2008, the SEARO region, which comprises 11 member states, had nominated only 8 individuals (World Health Organization, 2009d). To prompt further interest, the regional office issued a call for nominations (World Health Organization, 2008a), and governments were again encouraged to nominate representatives at the Third Regional Meeting of IHR National Focal Points held in Bangladesh in February 2010 (World Health Organization, 2010f). As of 1 March 2010, the Director-General had nominated over 200 experts to the IHR Roster, including 54 individuals nominated by member states (World Health Organization, 2010c). As shown in Table 5.2, although Asia constitutes the bulk of the world's population, currently only 34 out of 200 (17 per cent) 'experts' are presently from Asian countries.

While enthusiasm may be lacking in some areas, Asian governments have increased the extent to which they are working collectively on issues surrounding the emergence and spread of infectious diseases. Many of the new links are based on informal networks between public health and scientific colleagues who share information on a regular basis via e-mail, telephone, or the Internet. Many of these professional networks have not been documented, and have emerged distinct from more formalized intergovernmental processes. At the same time, a number of governments have sanctioned their public health officials to engage in more formal technical assistance programs. As one individual recalled,

> In 2005, we hosted a meeting for countries in the WPRO region on the International Health Regulations. We had just gone through the process of amending our own domestic laws to be compliant with the IHR, and we offered those countries that attended the meeting to help them do the same. I've participated in a number of other meetings as well, with the Pacific Island countries, and with New Zealand, to see how we can make some progress.[20]

Giving even further weight to these initiatives, a new inter-ministerial forum has been established among the Health Ministers of China, Japan and Korea. This annual meeting, known as the Tripartite Health Ministers' Meeting, was first convened in 2007, and is held to discuss such issues as disease outbreak prevention and control, and food safety (Relax News, 2009).

Table 5.2 Asian representation on the IHR roster of experts at April 2010

Country	*WPRO*	*SEARO*	*Number*
Bangladesh		x	1
Brunei Darussalam	x		–
Cambodia	x		–
China	x		7
India		x	5
Indonesia		x	1
Japan	x		4
Lao People's Democratic Republic	x		–
Malaysia	x		2
Maldives		x	–
Mongolia	x		–
Myanmar		x	–
Nepal		x	1
Philippines	x		2
Republic of Korea	x		1
Singapore	x		5
Sri Lanka		x	1
Thailand		x	3
Timor-Leste		x	–
Vietnam	x		1

Source: World Health Organization (2010) *IHR roster of experts*. Accessible http://intranet.who.int/ihre/default.asp (accessed 24 April 2010). Thanks to Dr Tikki Pang, WHO Director of Research Policy and Cooperation, for providing this information.

Moreover, while Asian governments joined with other countries to sideline non-state actors from the IGWG negotiations, some Asian countries appear willing to explore alternative, innovative arrangements for implementing the IHR. As one WHO official noted, for instance,

> The first thing is you have to make sure the government sector has the foundation to control things. Once that is achieved then you can start including other partners. We are exploring some possibilities of engaging the services of the Red Cross in countries like Laos and Vietnam, and we are also encouraging various NGOs like CARE to come in and do part of the surveillance work. But at the moment these organizations can only really be involved in data collection activities. They can't evaluate the data, nor is it their responsibility. We have noticed in trials that NGOs involved in the surveillance system 'Event-based Surveillance System' have produced very good results. But there is still a question of sustainability, and we're not sure if this can be expanded or if it will just be an exceptional case.[21]

Equally important to note is that much of the recent emphasis and activity on disease surveillance and outbreak control has not necessarily been entirely attributable to the IHR. As one respondent commented,

> In the first four to five years after the completion of the IHR negotiations, there has been a much closer and more frequent exchange of information among Asian countries, especially China, Korea and Japan. These three countries have established new networks, and they have been increasingly working through ASEAN, even though they're outside the ASEAN network. But my understanding is that it is not directly coming from the fact that the IHR have now been updated. Rather, the more important factor in driving all this work has been pandemic influenza preparedness. Everybody was worried that the next pandemic would come from this region, so we all need to prepare, and that is what has been behind the close communication that has developed.[22]

Indeed, much of the impetus for these activities appears to be self-interest as opposed to camaraderie or altruism. As one Korean official succinctly noted,

> We maintain constant contact with our Chinese and Japanese associates. We share our information and surveillance data, and in the future we'd like to communicate more with our colleagues in South East Asia because obviously that's where most of the emerging infectious diseases come from.[23]

Furthermore, although there is some indication that countries have begun to work more collaboratively on these issues, such as implementing bilateral exchange programs between scientific and/or public health personnel, it is just as apparent that not every government is willing or able to assist. As one official observed, for instance,

> No, we are not helping other countries because obviously other countries, other more industrialized countries like the US, are helping them. This means that we don't have the chance to help. And I hate to say it but we don't have the capacity to look out for other countries. We share information with our immediate neighbours, but that's about all . . . Some countries do lack sufficient disease surveillance systems, but it's not something that we can do anything about.[24]

The notable exception has been Japan, which has devoted a large proportion of its official development assistance (ODA) to global health (see Chapter 2 this volume). As one respondent summarized,

> The health sector is one of the most important sectors of Japan's development program. It has invested a lot of resources into health, not only in terms of financial contributions but also human capital. You could even say that it is uniquely important to the Japanese government's development policy. And even from the very beginning of Japan's official development assistance in the 1950s, Asia has remained the most important focus. Admittedly, some countries have developed themselves to the point where they now don't

> receive direct Japanese assistance – countries such as China or Malaysia – but certainly the less developed countries of the region are a primary focus.[25]

In the context of Taiwan, in 2009, the Chinese Government gave its permission for the Taiwanese authorities to have special observer status at the WHA. Alongside this decision, Taiwan was granted permission to liaise with the WHO Secretariat regarding disease outbreaks. Significantly, however, the Taiwanese authorities remain only permitted to liaise with the WHO headquarters in Geneva and not, for example, directly with the WHO regional office or programmes. As one Taiwanese official noted,

> We have been given the name of one person in Geneva that we can speak to if we have a disease outbreak, but it is only that person. We are not allowed to contact the Western Pacific Regional Office, and we receive no communication from them. We send surveillance data and information about any disease events we have to our neighbouring countries like Japan and so on, but we never get any reports or communication back.[26]

In this regard, there is some evidence to suggest that, at least in the case of China, concerns to protect national sovereignty remain an issue and, indeed, there may be growing recognition of the complementarity of national interests and collective action. At the same time, however, it became clear in interviews with Taiwanese officials that how long this special status will last is unclear. As one Taiwanese interviewee summarized,

> The IHR is genuinely more a matter of technical cooperation so we are hopeful that our ability to cooperate in this area will continue. But on the wider issue of our status as an observer to the Health Assembly it is a little less clear. Last year, for example, we wanted to participate in the FCTC (Framework Convention on Tobacco Control) negotiations on illicit trade in tobacco. We asked if we could join, but we got no response. My personal view is that China wants to keep this card close to its chest, so they can decide when to play it. I suspect that if there is something that happens that doesn't please China, next time they'll play a different card and we won't be able to be an observer again.[27]

Conclusions

While limited in scope, this analysis has found that the majority of Asian governments had limited engagement with the negotiation process to revise and update the International Health Regulations. It is argued that Asian governments thereby lost a very valuable opportunity to influence what is arguably one of the most important pieces of legislation affecting global health in the twenty-first century. However, during the implementation process, there is evidence to suggest that some Asian governments have begun to pay more heed to enhancing the region's capacity to combat infectious diseases, with some even trialling public–private partnerships to enhance disease surveillance capacity. Several governments have now also implemented programs to exchange information and enhance the region's capacity via the exchange of technical personnel. New forums, such as the tripartite meeting of health ministers between China, Korea and Japan, have additionally served to raise overall awareness of the need for greater cooperation in tackling infectious diseases. While the bulk of this work may be attributed to other factors, such as the 2003 SARS outbreak and the threat of pandemic influenza rather than the revised IHR per se, there are clear indications of a greater awareness among government officials of the need to work collaboratively to prevent disease outbreaks. At the same time, however, a number of Asian governments continue to approach implementation of the revised IHR as a matter for the state, and, in many cases, a single government department's responsibility. In other words, compliance with the IHR is largely seen as an area of national responsibility as opposed to a region-wide collective problem. Consequently, as much as there is evidence to suggest a greater willingness for cooperation has emerged, there are also indications that existing power dynamics and Asian conceptions of sovereignty have not really altered in any meaningful way.

Notes

1 Interview, 23 February 2010.
2 Interview, 23 February 2010.
3 Interview, 25 February 2010.
4 Interview, 23 February 2010.
5 Interview, 23 February 2010.
6 World Health Organisation (2004a: ii).
7 Interview, 10 March 2010.
8 Interview, 26 February 2010.
9 Interview, 1 March 2010.
10 Interview, 2 March 2010.
11 Interview, 2 March 2010.
12 Interview, 22 February 2010.
13 Interview, 26 February 2010.
14 Interview, 25 February 2010.
15 Interview, 5 March 2010.
16 Interview, 25 February 2010.
17 Interview, 5 March 2010.
18 Interview, 22 February 2010.
19 Interview, 25 February 2010.
20 Interview, 23 February 2010.
21 Interview, 20 November 2009.
22 Interview, 26 February 2010.
23 Interview, 22 February 2010.
24 Interview, 22 February 2010.
25 Interview, 24 February 2010.
26 Interview, 1 March 2010.
27 Interview, 2 March 2010.

6 The global health governance of pandemic influenza

A snapshot of Asia's contribution

Adam Kamradt-Scott and Sungwon Yoon

Introduction

While rare, influenza pandemics are a regular feature of human existence. In the last century alone the world's population was subjected to three such events in 1918, 1957 and 1968, respectively. In April 2009, the World Health Organization (WHO) declared that another influenza pandemic was underway following the spread of a novel H1N1 virus strain. Fortunately, the first pandemic of the twenty-first century was shown to be comparatively mild and short-lived; but reflecting the conventional response of governments to such threats, the event nonetheless resulted in billions of dollars being spent on procuring vaccines and antiviral medications. These acquisitions were based on advice from the WHO, which has been at the core of international pandemic influenza governance arrangements for over 60 years. Since 2007 however, several Asian leaders – a number of whose populations are considered at greatest risk from the H5N1 avian influenza virus – have openly challenged the existing regime on the basis that it favours those countries that can afford to procure vaccines, namely Western developed states.[1] This questioning, and Indonesia's actions in withholding influenza virus samples, has contested the legitimacy of existing pandemic influenza governance structures.

This chapter analyzes the contributions made to the global governance framework surrounding pandemic influenza by Asian countries, intergovernmental and non-governmental actors. By drawing on a wide variety of published and unpublished literature and interview material from over 30 key informants, the chapter explores the progress four Asian countries, Indonesia, China, Thailand and Vietnam, have made towards strengthening their own health systems and participating in international efforts to prevent and mitigate the effects of pandemic influenza. In addition, the chapter explores the contribution that state-based actors, such as the Association of South East Asian Nations (ASEAN) and the Asia-Pacific Economic Cooperation (APEC), and other non-state actors (i.e. non-governmental organizations, charitable foundations, the corporate sector) have made in responding to the threat. In so doing, the chapter also explores the controversy surrounding existing policy responses (i.e. virus-sharing and access to pharmaceuticals), identifying the key actors and agents that have actively promoted particular governance arrangements.

Background

The framework for the existing global influenza governance system was established more than 60 years ago, coinciding with the creation of the WHO. The Interim Commission of the WHO officially endorsed the creation of the World Influenza Program in September 1947, following a request by a respected group of virologists earlier that year (Hampson, 1997). Recalling the impact of the 1918 Spanish Flu pandemic that killed an estimated 50 million people worldwide, the objective of the WHO program was threefold: (i) to plan against the reoccurrence of future influenza pandemics, (ii) to develop control methods to limit the impact when a pandemic did appear, and (iii) to limit, as much as possible, the economic consequences of influenza epidemics and pandemics. As part of this broader program, in 1947 the Interim Commission also authorized the creation of the World Influenza Centre (WIC) to be based in London. The primary objective of the WIC was to collect and distribute information, conduct and coordinate laboratory work on the virus and train new laboratory workers to undertake the necessary scientific work. Later, in 1952, the WHO formed the Expert Committee on Influenza to provide technical advice and general oversight for the Organization's program of work (Payne, 1953: 763).

The cornerstone of the contemporary global influenza governance system is the Global Influenza Surveillance Network (GISN), which was established in 1948. Throughout the years, GISN has served as the primary vehicle for the international distribution of influenza-related information and viruses for scientific and research purposes. The network operates by receiving influenza virus samples from participating countries via their National Influenza Centres (NICs). NICs then forward these samples to one of six WHO Collaborating Centres (WHO CCs) where the virus samples are analyzed to identify which strains of the virus are currently circulating. Augmenting GISN's work is FluNet, an Internet-based program operated by the WHO that links together the NICs and WHO CCs in a virtual worldwide network to ensure the rapid exchange of global surveillance data. The data generated by these research systems is then passed to pharmaceutical companies, which use the data to inform the development of seasonal influenza vaccines and, in the event that a new strain of the virus emerges, a new pandemic-specific vaccine. Given that GISN, which has now been renamed the Global Influenza and Surveillance system (GISRS), also currently incorporates some 140 institutions throughout 110 countries, the network has considerable global reach (World Health Organisation, 2012).

In 2007, both GISN and the WHO came under heavy criticism from several low- and/or middle-income countries (LMICs) over the network's virus-sharing practices. Claiming a breakdown of 'mutual trust', Indonesia's health minister, Dr Siti Fadilah Supari, announced that her country would no longer share H5N1 influenza virus samples with GISN. At the core of Indonesia's concerns was the WHO's practice of passing the virus samples GISN received from affected countries to pharmaceutical companies who then used the samples to develop new vaccines, which they then patented and sold for profit. Like most pharmaceuticals, however, production capacity is limited (Lee and Fidler, 2007) and residents in high-income countries who can afford to pay higher prices purchase the majority of vaccines (Garrett and Fidler, 2007). While this system has operated for decades, following the re-emergence and progressive international spread of the H5N1 avian influenza virus from late 2003 onwards, the issue of equitable access to influenza vaccines gained new prominence as concerns of a new impending pandemic grew (Fidler, 2008). Indonesia, as one of the countries that has been most severely affected by H5N1, questioned why their samples were being used (without their permission) to make vaccines that Indonesia's citizens would not be able to access. Claiming several previous breaches of trust, in January 2007 Indonesia announced that it would no longer be sharing its viruses with GISN after it was revealed that an Australian company had developed a new vaccine from an Indonesian H5N1 sample (Sedyaningsih *et al.*, 2008).

Indonesia's announcement to withhold samples sparked widespread alarm amongst the international community, in large part because of fears that a H5N1 'Bird Flu' pandemic was imminent (Fidler, 2008). Invoking the Convention on Biological Diversity (CBD), Indonesia claimed that the samples were their sovereign property and that it was under no legal obligation to share the viruses with the international community. For many LMICs that confronted the same challenges of unaffordable and/or inaccessible vaccines, Indonesia's actions were seen as courageous and by 2008, Health Minister Supari claimed that as many as 112 countries supported her country's stance (Schnirring, 2008).

In an attempt to resolve the impasse that had developed and address LMICs' concerns, the WHO announced in 2007 the creation of a global stockpile of pandemic vaccines that all countries would have the ability to access based on demonstrated need (Chan, 2007). In addition, a series of meetings were held throughout 2007 between WHO and Indonesian officials to address their specific concerns ahead of an intergovernmental meeting that sought to negotiate a way through the diplomatic quagmire (Fedson and Dunnill, 2007). Representatives from 109 countries attended the Intergovernmental Meeting on Pandemic Influenza Preparedness, alongside representatives from various international and NGOs to discuss sharing of influenza viruses and access to vaccines and other benefits ('the IGM'). Given that the outcome of the negotiations was also likely to have a bearing on pharmaceutical companies, a delegation from the International Federation of Pharmaceutical Manufacturers and Associations was also invited to attend (World Health Organisation, 2007c). Despite several rounds of talks being held between late 2007 and 2010, negotiations broke down over the nature and extent of benefits that LMICs should receive from participating in the WHO Influenza Program. As such, no consensus was achieved on how the system could be made more equitable and accessible.

Asia's contribution to pandemic influenza governance

The 2003 Severe Acute Respiratory Syndrome (SARS) outbreak proved a global wake-up call for strengthening disease surveillance for many countries around the world. In Asia, this outbreak has been credited with inspiring several regional-based disease surveillance initiatives and programs (Kamradt-Scott, 2009). However, since the re-emergence and progressive global spread of the H5N1 influenza virus from late 2003 onwards, Asian countries have been placed at the forefront of international efforts to address the threat from communicable diseases, and considerable financial and political capital has been expended in an attempt to bolster surveillance and response capacities throughout the region. The United Nations group, which includes the WHO, the United Nations System Influenza Coordination (UNSIC), the United Nations Development Program (UNDP), and the Food and Agriculture Organization (FAO), combined with other actors such as the Organization for Animal Health (OIE) and several key donor countries (including the United States, Australia and Japan), have actively contributed to various programs and initiatives aimed at strengthening health systems and fostering regional collaboration. In September 2005, the WHO officially endorsed the Asia-Pacific Strategy for Emerging Diseases (APSED), which was jointly developed by the WHO Western Pacific Regional Office (WPRO) and the South-East Asia Office of the WHO (SEARO) with considerable financial support from Australia and Canada (WPRO, 2005; AusAID, 2007; CIDA, 2010). This strategy, which formed the basis of much of the region's activities, has since been revised, and an updated version of APSED was approved in October 2010 (WPRO, 2010). Likewise, in 2006, the Japanese Government contributed US$135 million to the creation of a stockpile of personal protective equipment (PPE) and antiviral medications (ASEAN, 2007), currently stored in Singapore for the explicit use of ASEAN countries in the event of an outbreak (MOFA, 2007). Moreover, both ASEAN and APEC have established pandemic influenza technical working groups to facilitate greater regional cooperation; and several regional surveillance networks, such as the Mekong Basin Disease Surveillance (MBDS), the Southeast Asian Influenza Research Network (SEA ICRN), and the Emerging Infectious Network (APEC EINet), have been created to enhance the region's surveillance and response capabilities (MDBS, 2010). In terms of global governance efforts to mitigate the impact of pandemic influenza, Asian countries could be equally viewed as both the 'governed' and the 'governors', in that several countries have functioned as major donors supporting and leading pandemic influenza initiatives, while a number of other countries throughout the region have been the recipients of this and additional international aid.

The influence of state sovereignty on pandemic influenza governance throughout Asia

As in other areas of public life, state sovereignty appears to have had a tremendous impact on international cooperation efforts to improve health. In 1954, in response to tensions over disputed territory, China, India and Burma agreed on a set of principles to guide diplomatic relations. These principles, which became known as the Five Principles of Peaceful Coexistence, emphasized the need to maintain mutual respect for territorial integrity and sovereignty, mutual non-aggression, mutual non-interference in internal affairs, equality and mutual benefit and peaceful coexistence (Kim *et al.*, 2009). Over the following decades, the Five Principles increasingly began to be reflected in numerous regional technical cooperation agreements including, for example, becoming the 'fundamental' principles of ASEAN when the organization was created in 1967 (ASEAN, 2010). Thus, as Kim and colleagues have observed,

> Curiously, even though the ideas in the Five Principles did not originate in Asia, Asian countries have embraced them and given them Asian texture. Vigilance about sovereignty, non-interference, political equality, and the creation of mutual economic benefit are recognized as characteristic of Asian diplomatic practices.
>
> (Kim, Fidler and Ganguly 2009)

It was not particularly surprising, therefore, to discover that respect for territorial integrity, sovereignty, non-interference, and mutual respect characterizes much of Asian governments' cooperation in pandemic influenza preparedness. A good example of this relates to Indonesia's former decision to withhold virus samples from the WHO. Although this action was identified to have potential implications for the region as a whole, there appeared to be a genuine reluctance to address the issue in formal diplomatic contexts, such as APEC and ASEAN. As one informant noted,

> The case of Indonesia's refusal to share viruses was not raised in ASEAN nor is it likely to be raised. The only issues that are raised are those that they are likely to get consensus on. Indonesia's refusal to share virus samples is widely perceived to be a 'national' issue even though it is recognized to have obvious transborder and regional implications.[2]

And another interviewee noted in relation to APEC,

> Those sorts of issues won't go anywhere in that sort of forum as no-one wants to be seen to be interfering in the domestic affairs of another member country just in case another issue comes up that might involve their country being criticized.[3]

Indeed, sensitivity to criticism throughout the region is high, and arguably related to concerns that such actions equate to interference in domestic affairs. These concerns also appear to be quite pervasive, as evidenced by the fact that some interviewees were reluctant to identify their own views on Indonesia's actions even when directly questioned.

> I don't know which one view is correct. Just because that is the way governments and organizations have done things in the past does not mean it should continue in that way. It is really difficult to tell. I think maybe it is not fair.[4]

At the same time, there was anecdotal evidence to suggest that the reluctance to criticize other Asian countries may be based more on the recognition that it could harm relations, and that this would negatively impact upon technical cooperation efforts. As one key informant stated,

> In this area we have to work together. Many of Asia's countries are borderless – you can cross the border into Cambodia and Laos very easily. This is a problem for disease control if we cannot then talk with Laos or Cambodia.[5]

Yet while there may be a reluctance to be perceived as interfering in the domestic affairs of neighbouring countries, political commitment to tackling infectious diseases (and particularly pandemic influenza) is high. In fact, domestic political engagement has improved considerably post-SARS, and in contrast to many Western countries, often engages decision makers at the highest level of government – in Thailand and Vietnam, for instance, both the national pandemic influenza crisis committees are chaired by their respective Deputy Prime Ministers, and involve ministers (or their senior representatives) from multiple government departments.

Institutional diversity and pandemic influenza governance throughout Asia

Throughout the countries examined in this chapter, the majority of pandemic influenza-related work has remained centralized within governments, and usually at the national level. Non-state actors have not played a major role in pandemic influenza preparedness and response matters. Certainly this is an approach that is consistent with the majority of countries around the world, and, in this regard, Asian countries appear to be adhering very closely to a conventional, government-centric approach. In fact, where external actors are involved, they are usually inter-state in nature, such as international or regional intergovernmental organizations like the Asian Development Bank (ADB) or government aid agencies, such as the United States' USAID, Australia's AusAID, or Japan's JICA. There are a few notable exceptions. For example, in Thailand a small number of NGOs support the Thai health authorities in their work, such as the Influenza Foundation and the Thai Health Promotion Foundation.[6] However, even noting these few isolated cases, one Thai official observed that

> There are not many NGOs that work with us in this area. In Thailand there are NGOs that are engaged in work with HIV/AIDS, TB and other infectious diseases, but not so much on influenza issues. This is mostly the responsibility of public hospitals. There is some private sector involvement, but it is mostly a public hospital issue.[7]

This theme was repeated in several countries examined. In Vietnam, for instance, it was found that the Red Cross played a minor role in funding local initiatives at the provincial level to enhance communication around health messages for personal hygiene, but no further evidence of participation was identified.[8] Similarly, as one Chinese respondent observed,

> China is very different from Western countries. We do not have a lot of private sector involvement in public health. There are some institutions or foundations like the Red Cross that provide some assistance when things like earthquakes occur, but not in pandemic influenza issues.[9]

Other non-state actors engaged in pandemic influenza-related work were occasionally identified, but upon closer investigation they were revealed to be proxies for governments. A good example here is ABT Associates, which is a private company that has previously had a limited role in enhancing disease surveillance for H5N1 avian influenza throughout several countries in the region (ABT Associates, 2006). The funding for ABT Associates' work has been provided by USAID, and therefore could be considered an extension of that government's efforts to enhance regional preparedness as opposed to a civil society or business-inspired initiative.

The most notable exception to this overall trend can be found in Indonesia, where the century-old faith-based organization Muhammadiyah is playing a key role in enhancing community awareness around pandemic influenza, including assisting in technical activities, such as disease surveillance and containment. In his work, Paul Forster identified decentralization of government functions as one of the reasons why Muhammadiyah has assumed such a critical role in these activities (Forster, 2009), a finding that was further substantiated by the interviews conducted for this chapter. As one Indonesian interviewee noted,

> There are many parts to the process and a number of government departments that are involved. In Indonesia you have the central government and the local government authorities, and the implementation for this kind of issue was designated as the responsibility of local authorities.[10]

Specifically in relation to Muhammadiyah, a key informant observed,

> We are aware that in Indonesia pandemic influenza is very much associated with poverty. It is the poor, the backyard chicken farmers who suffer the most from this. As an organization, Muhammadiyah has a comparative advantage at the community level as it is an extensive organization that is already running community education programs, health programs, welfare programs, training in income generating activities, and Islamic counselling services. Pandemic influenza is considered just another type of disaster and so it was a natural extension of the organization's existing work.[11]

In this sense, unlike other Asian countries that followed a more conventional 'top-down' managerial style with clearly delineated command and control structures, the Indonesian government has adopted a more 'hands off' approach, preferring instead to set the overall policy direction and delegate much of the day-to-day implementation of programs to a third party.

At the regional level, just as the national level, intergovernmental organizations such as ASEAN and APEC do appear to have played a key role in enhancing pandemic influenza preparedness and response. Since the organization was established in August 1967, ASEAN has periodically hosted high-level meetings between health ministers. In the wake of the 2003 SARS outbreak, these meetings have become much more frequent, with ministers meeting on an annual basis or once every two years to discuss health security-related issues. Several declarations and statements of cooperation have been produced on a variety of topics ranging from cooperation on H5N1 avian influenza prevention and preparedness, cooperation in health emergencies and regional production of vaccines and antiviral medications (ASEAN, 2010c). Similarly, in late 2003, APEC established the Health Task Force (HTF), which met initially on an ad hoc basis to discuss 'health-related threats to economies' trade and security' (APEC, 2008). Pandemic-related matters were a key feature of these discussions in the wake of SARS; and, recognizing the ongoing importance of cooperation in this area, in 2007, the HTF became the APEC Health Working Group. In 2009, the Group's annual program of work explicitly identified enhancing avian and human pandemic influenza preparedness and response capacity as its top priority (APEC Health Working Group, 2009).

However, at least in terms of the interview material gathered for this chapter, there also appears to be some dissatisfaction with these regional organizations. As one government official noted, 'There is no genuine collaboration between ASEAN. It is just rhetoric. There is no sense of partnership.'[12]

Similarly, another key informant was more circumspect in their comments, but agreed,

> Yes, ASEAN is extremely weak but it is not a criticism per se. You have to remember that ASEAN was effectively established to be an anti-communism forum, but that is obviously not as big a threat as it once was. As such, there are no strong incentives for these countries to really work together anymore.[13]

Several reasons were cited for why organizations like ASEAN and APEC continued to underperform. One of the more commonly identified causes was a residual lack of trust between Asian governments toward each other. One official, for example, noted

> Singapore is outstandingly bad in terms of collaboration. They don't have the ASEAN perspective. It is the only rich country within ASEAN, and yet when we have an initiative that we need funded they simply say 'no'. They take and they never give.[14]

Likewise, the Japanese government's announcement in 2005 that it would fund the creation of a stockpile of antiviral medications and PPE for ASEAN countries to access was viewed with some scepticism:

> Japan donated the funds via JICA [Japan International Cooperation Agency] but no-one knows how it will be mobilized during the first phase even of the H1N1 pandemic. I don't know. Ultimately it was funded by Japan for the security of Japan.[15]

More broadly, a lack of trust also appears to have contributed to undermining regional efforts to establish a new framework for whole-of-government pandemic preparedness. As one key informant relayed,

> A specific example I could share with you relates to the issue of multisectoral preparedness – a group of countries were supposed to be doing an assessment in every country which they had agreed they would then pilot in Indonesia. Firstly though, it took a lot of time to get buy-in on what should be the indicators and how was the assessment going to be done. Then when they did do the pilot momentum was lost as individual countries said, 'Well, we don't really need that team of consultants from other member states to come into our country. We can do a self-assessment.'[16]

Culture was yet another reason given for countries' preference for individualized approaches, as opposed to working through collective action bodies. One informant from China observed,

> Compared to Europe or North America, Asian countries have a very different culture which does not easily translate into collective action. For instance, they [Asian countries] often say to each other 'that's your population, nothing to do with any other country'.[17]

Cultural differences were also identified as existing as one of the primary obstacles to improving collaboration. It was suggested, for instance,

> Improving technical collaboration between Asian countries is one issue. But all these countries have different cultural backgrounds, and culture influences our way of thinking in so many ways, including how we respond to these sorts of challenges. It is really difficult to overcome.[18]

At the same time, it is apparent that there are large divides between the economies of the region, and this may also account for the disjuncture in working collectively. As one informant summarized,

> I think there are many different contexts in this region. For the more developed countries like Japan and Korea, they can survive by themselves because they have enough medical resources and access to vaccines and such. With the exception of Singapore, the picture is very different in Southeast Asia. Thailand, Laos and Cambodia need a lot of technical and financial support. In Laos, for example, there are just a few hospitals. The health

system in Cambodia is mostly based on the support it receives from external donors.[19]

Pandemic influenza governance 'gaps' and success stories in Asia

As the above analysis has demonstrated, considerable enthusiasm exists to enhance pandemic influenza preparedness and response capabilities throughout the region. At the same time, the majority of Asian governments appear to be more inclined towards building national capacities (thereby contributing to regional preparedness) as opposed to investing directly in regional initiatives. While this may yet be further evidence of the influence of the Five Principles (particularly in terms of mutual respect for state sovereignty and territorial integrity), it was observed that Asian governments emphasize independence over regionalism. Chinese officials, for example, expressed a reticence for working through regional bodies stating that, in their view, China's greatest contribution to the international community (and the region as a whole) would be to manage their own country's disease outbreaks and epidemics in the first instance.

> If China is able to control the pandemic well, then, because we have such a big population, it helps out the entire world. One in three people throughout the world is Chinese, so I think if China manages itself okay, then that is a big contribution to global pandemic preparedness.[20]

Another responded, 'I think that given China has one-fifth of the world's population, if we manage our response to these disease outbreaks well, then I think that is a really big achievement.'[21]

Giving further weight to the argument that Asian governments prefer individualistic as opposed to multilateral approaches, each country has actively pursued bilateral arrangements, and continues to do so. Indeed, every country examined in this chapter has signed either one or more bilateral agreements with neighbouring countries aimed at enhancing their respective pandemic influenza preparedness and response capabilities. Vietnam, for instance, signed formal agreements to exchange information and facilitate greater technical cooperation in pandemic preparedness with Laos PDR in December 2001, Cambodia in March 2006, and China in 2003 and a further agreement in 2008.[22] One Vietnamese official characterized this sentiment by stating,

> I think bilateral cooperation is better because we can discuss directly how we can get support in terms of technical and financial issues, directly between this country and that country, or this country with that organization, and so on.[23]

Establishing formal bilateral arrangements is certainly consistent with how other countries around the world have sought to improve pandemic influenza preparedness. It is also the case that other regions, such as North America, have adopted region-specific strategic frameworks for avian and pandemic influenza cooperation and response similar to APSED (Security and Prosperity Partnership for North America, 2007), and yet still pursue bilateral arrangements with specific countries independent of each other. As also identified above, the lack of NGO participation throughout pandemic influenza preparedness in Asia is not peculiar to that region. In this regard, the general approach taken by Asian governments appears to be in line with how other countries are currently approaching pandemic influenza preparedness.

Equally, a number of Asian governments appear to be struggling with many of the same challenges that other countries currently confront. This is perhaps no more evident than in the field of multisectoral preparedness. In recent years, the idea for greater multisectoral collaboration has found form in the UN's 'One World, One Health' agenda that emphasizes closer collaboration between the animal and human health sectors, particularly in disease surveillance (UNSIC, 2008). Presently, however, there appears to be a reticence amongst some countries in the region to pursue this approach, as one informant noted,

> The 'One World, One Health' was pushed by international agencies here, but it wasn't put under that heading. There's not really anything at country-level yet here, or pretty much anywhere, that I've heard about. We may start to see it emerge in the next year or so in some countries, but my sense is that countries are saying to each other 'let's wait and see if it's really going to get up globally', or 'let's wait to prove that it can be done' before they're prepared to move towards implementing it.[24]

For other countries in the region, it would appear that overall progress has been made, but challenges still remain. One Chinese official noted,

> Disease surveillance and response are all under the Ministry of Health and that works very well. But when more than one ministry start to get involved, that is where the system gets weaker and things don't happen very easily unless there is engagement by officials at the highest level. Things have gotten better from where they were in the sense that things now go through the State Council and that tends to pull everyone together, but if the top brass aren't involved then problems can emerge.[25]

In yet other countries where there is a desire for greater multisectoral coordination, existing governance arrangements and practices have been (and are) inhibiting coordination. For example, although a national pandemic influenza taskforce was previously established in Indonesia that draws together representatives from various government departments, multisectoral collaboration remains an issue, in part, due to the fact that decision making within the Indonesian government is divided into specific 'clusters'.[26]

In this regard, the lack of progress in implementing both the 'One World, One Health' agenda and achieving greater multisectoral coordination is generally consistent with existing global trends, in that few countries have made significant progress in these areas (UNSIC 2008). At the same time, a small number of Asian countries appear to be bucking this trend. Vietnam, for example, is one country that have made significant progress, as one external observer has noted,

> We don't see a turf war here with Vietnam because you've got a relatively strong, confident and thoughtful Government led by the Party, and you often get the best of the international agencies here. I'm not saying the international agencies are perfect, but there has been very good cooperation here between human–animal health area.[27]

Thailand is also reported to have experienced similar successes, with at least one official noting,

> We have made quite a lot of progress in establishing multisector cooperation, especially between the public health sector and the animal health sector in relation to H5N1. And that was just the start of broader multisector cooperation. In the first phase of the response to H5N1 there were two authorities mainly working together – the Ministry of Public Health and the Ministry of Agriculture via the Department of Livestock and Development. But in the process we have been able to organize a systematic multisectoral system, and in my view this has been the hallmark of our success in recent years with preventing further H5N1 transmissions.[28]

Thus, while many countries have and continue to struggle with achieving greater multisectoral coordination, some countries in Asia may potentially offer a template for others to follow, particularly in terms of how they are structured.

Discussion

There is undoubtedly a new willingness on behalf of some Asian countries to challenge the status quo around existing health governance arrangements – what Lawrence Gostin has previously described as the 'entrenched power structures' of global health governance whereby 'Economically and politically powerful countries, principally in Europe and North America, have had a disproportionate influence on the global health agenda' (Gostin, 2005). Thailand's decision to issue compulsory licenses for antiretroviral medications (Ford *et al.*, 2007), and Indonesia's decision to withhold sharing virus samples with the WHO's GISN are two good examples of this new trend. It would appear, however, that even if a new paradigm is emerging, it is, first, at a very early, embryonic stage, and secondly, it is currently a very frail consensus. It can be observed from the material gathered for this chapter, for instance, that despite a high level of political commitment to tackling communicable diseases such as pandemic influenza, and considerable technical initiatives to enhance the region's disease surveillance and response capabilities, mistrust pervades contemporary diplomatic relations. While cultural differences and a strong adherence to the Five Principles of Peaceful Coexistence may also have served the region well in the past, it remains unclear whether these now are inhibiting greater regional cooperation and understanding.

Added to this, a number of Asian governments seem to be determined to follow their own path, irrespective of the implications it may have for the wider region. Aside from Indonesia's aforementioned former stance on virus-sharing, another example was identified in the context of Vietnam, where the government persisted with a nationwide campaign to vaccinate all poultry despite warnings that the approach was unsustainable in the long term. It became apparent in interviews, however, that the program is now under serious threat of closure due to high costs and the labour-intensive nature of its operations.[29] If the program is stopped, it raises the risk that new, resistant strains of the H5N1 virus may emerge to threaten the region.

Equally, even though this chapter has only explored the activities of four countries, there is no denying that Asian countries have made a valuable contribution to pandemic influenza governance, both within their region and more broadly. According to one official, for example, it was Thailand that originally proposed the creation of the regional stockpile of antiviral medications and PPE that is currently based in Singapore. It was observed,

> At the height of the avian influenza outbreaks, we tried to promote this vision of stockpiling resources, such as antiviral medications and protective equipment. That idea was then taken up by ASEAN, and ASEAN created the stockpile with donations from Japan and some other donors. Originally we had suggested that every country that had already developed a national stockpile of antivirals should donate about 5 per cent of their stock to put into a regional stockpile that could be accessed by any member country in the event of an outbreak. When we proposed it initially though, it wasn't so well accepted, I think because of the fact that Asian countries just don't have these types of budgets to be able to do this sort of thing. When Japan heard about the idea though, they loved it and allocated the money for it to be established.[30]

In addition to this, Thailand was also reportedly instrumental in advancing the idea of creating multiple rapid response teams (RRTs) that could be immediately deployed in the event of an outbreak to assist in containing it and preventing the disease from spreading. As one interviewee noted,

> One of the proposals we put forward was training on disease outbreak and containment. The US use the term rapid response, but in Thailand we call it surveillance and rapid response team. But the idea is effectively the same: to have, in every district, a team that can be moved in to investigate and contain the outbreak. That is one we tried to introduce as well, and the CDC [US Center for Disease Control and Prevention] have taken this idea and produced a training package, and now if you visit another country you will see each country has their own RRTs.[31]

Vietnam's contribution, by way of contrast, is often considered a 'model' that other countries both within the region and internationally should potentially emulate. As one informant noted,

> I think they can assume the mantle of being the health policy leaders among ministries. Especially in relation to influenza it has gone pretty well because the Ministry of Health and Ministry of Agriculture have collaborated in a way that's been robust and fairly effective. Everybody recognizes there is room for improvement. But I think the government deserves really good marks for that type of inter-ministerial collaboration, not just in influenza, but they've managed to take this approach in all sectors and all health issues . . . As such, Vietnam is often held up as a sort of poster child.[32]

Even Indonesia's actions in refusing to share H5N1 virus samples, while widely condemned by many high-income countries, has nevertheless had a fundamental impact upon the GHG of pandemic influenza, prompting an extensive review of the existing system and processes. Given the level of in-principle support these actions have garnered throughout the majority of low- and middle-income countries, and the fact that even policy makers from several high-income countries have acknowledged the rationale behind Indonesia's actions, it is difficult to conclude that the actions have been entirely negative.

Similarly, although it may not necessarily be described as a 'concrete' contribution, China has had a marked impact on the global governance of influenza by the mere fact of its population size and geopolitical status. Indeed, it is generally agreed that China's ongoing participation in international efforts to control the spread of infectious diseases such as H5N1, as well as their domestic capacity to conduct surveillance and implement control measures, is critical to successfully mitigating the threat.

Finally, in the wake of the global controversy regarding virus samples and access to vaccines, at least three of the countries surveyed in this chapter have recently commenced infrastructure programs aimed at ensuring sufficient domestic production capacity for influenza vaccines to cover their entire populations. These initiatives are being supported by a variety of sponsors, including other Asian countries,[33] and while the initiatives undoubtedly speak to the tendency for Asian countries to emphasize sovereign capacity over multilateral reliance, they nevertheless will prove beneficial in enhancing global production capacity overall, thereby benefitting the entire international community.

Conclusion

In summary, while it must be acknowledged that this study was limited in scope, it is apparent that Asian countries have made a varied but considerable contribution to the global health governance structures and processes surrounding pandemic influenza. Several Asian countries have, for example, sought to take a key leadership role within the region, donating significant financial or in-kind technical assistance. Even those countries that lack the equivalent capacity have contributed in other ways, such as looking to enhance national surveillance and response capacities and actively working to improve multisectoral collaboration. At the same time, the extent of economic disparity throughout the region, combined with the lack of trust between countries, the inclination to elevate national interests and state sovereignty above collective interests, and the lack of faith in regional bodies (such as ASEAN and APEC) has meant that progress has been notably restrained. In this regard, several key challenges to effective collaboration in pandemic influenza health governance remain, and more work is and will continue to be required in the foreseeable future to encourage health system strengthening and political commitment to tackling this disease.

Notes

1 The term 'international regime' as used here is based on Stephen Krasner's 1983 definition of the same that defines international regimes as 'implicit or explicit principles, norms, rules, and decision-making procedures around which actors' expectations converge in a given area of international relations'. See Hansenclever *et al.* (1997).
2 Interview, 3 November 2009.
3 Interview, 22 November 2009.
4 Interview, 4 December 2009.
5 Interview, 4 November 2009.
6 See Influenza Foundation (Thailand) (2010). See also Thai Health Promotion Foundation (2010).
7 Interview, 4 November 2009.
8 Interview, 6 November 2009.
9 Interview, 10 December 2009.
10 Interview, 13 November 2009.
11 Interview, 13 November 2009.
12 Interview, 3 November 2009.
13 Interview, 16 November 2009.
14 Interview, 3 November 2009.
15 Interview, 3 November 2009.
16 Interview, 6 November 2009.
17 Interview, 10 December 2009.
18 Interview, 10 December 2009.
19 Interview, 4 November 2009.
20 Interview, 4 December 2009.
21 Interview, 5 December 2009.
22 Interview, 6 November 2009.
23 Interview, 6 November 2009.
24 Interview, 5 November 2009.
25 Interview, 5 December 2009.
26 Interview, 13 November 2009.
27 Interview, 5 November 2009.
28 Interview, 4 November 2009.
29 Interviews, 5–6 November 2009.
30 Interview, 4 November 2009.
31 Interview, 4 November 2009.
32 Interview, 6 November 2009.
33 Interviews, 3–18 November 2009.

7 The Framework Convention on Tobacco Control

Contributions by five Asian countries

Kelley Lee and Wayne Kao

Introduction

The signing of the Framework Convention on Tobacco Control (FCTC) in May 2003, led by the World Health Organization (WHO), was heralded as a major achievement within the public health community. The treaty's stated objective, 'to protect present and future generations from the devastating health, social, environmental and economic consequences of tobacco consumption and exposure to tobacco smoke', was accompanied by wide-ranging commitments of what States Parties must do at a minimum to prevent and reduce the more than five million deaths annually from tobacco use.

In addition to catalysing support for advancing tobacco control worldwide, the FCTC offers insights for understanding the contribution of five Asian countries to global health governance (GHG). The region has much to gain from stronger tobacco control: Asia holds three of the five-largest tobacco-using countries in the world (China, India and Indonesia) and is expected to suffer the majority of the 8.3 million projected tobacco-related deaths by 2030 (Mathers and Loncar, 2006). Tobacco control has received varying levels of priority among Asian countries, and the FCTC offered an opportunity to raise the issue's public policy profile. The negotiation of a strong and effective international treaty offered potentially key support for addressing this public health challenge.

Asia also has a large and thriving tobacco industry comprised of both domestic and transnational tobacco companies (TTCs) seeking to expand markets worldwide. Given an increasingly globalised industry, such issues as smuggling, trade and tobacco and cross-border advertising require effective collective action across countries. In this context, how Asian countries have contributed to the negotiation and implementation of the FCTC offers insights into Asia's role in global tobacco control, as well as the region's broader contributions to GHG.

Based on documentary sources[1] supplemented by key informant interviews, this chapter analyses the contributions of Japan, China, Indonesia, India, and Thailand to the FCTC process. The chapter finds that, despite the significant public health burden from tobacco-related death and disease in the region, there was varying support for the negotiation of comprehensive and binding measures under the FCTC in Asia. Since the signing of the treaty this has given way, to some extent, to a shift towards stronger measures, suggesting that the FCTC process catalysed increased policy support for tobacco control in many Asian countries. However, the chapter concludes that the ongoing struggle to implement the measures eventually adopted suggests that tobacco control remains defined in Asia by the prioritisation of perceived national interests, rather than a commitment to collective action in a global health context.

Spoilers and leaders: Asian contributions to the FCTC

While the challenges encountered by the public health community during the FCTC process have been widely acknowledged (Ulrich *et al.*, 2004) there has been limited political analysis of the FCTC, and even less of Asian contributions to the negotiations. The former includes an analysis of the FCTC as part of emerging GHG by Collin *et al.* (2002), with particular attention to the role of CSOs. The critical role of CSOs, notably centred around the Framework Convention Alliance (FCA), has been a particular focus (Mamudu and Glantz, 2009; Lenchucha *et al.*, 2010). Beyond CSOs, Mamudu et al. reveal how the industry's Project Cerberus sought to undermine the FCTC process focused on advocating for a global voluntary regulatory regime (Mamudu *et al.*, 2008). The latter focuses on the implications of the FCTC for tobacco control in specific countries (Lando *et al.*, 2005; Lee *et al.*, 2010). The following sections analyse the contributions of five Asian countries to the FCTC process.

Japan

For almost 90 years, the tobacco industry in Japan was a state monopoly and, since privatisation in 1985, the government has remained a major shareholder. Today, Japan Tobacco International (JTI) is the third largest tobacco company in the world. It was subject to relatively few public health regulations before 2004, and previous analyses have suggested that the industry has acted strategically to undermine the adoption of stronger tobacco control regulation. For example, JTI joined Philip Morris (PM) in supporting the 'Courtesy of Choice' initiative that advocates ventilated smoking areas in public places instead of public smoking bans (Aguinaga Bialous *et al.*, 2006). The government has also been relatively liberal on the presence of tobacco advertising on television (Lambert *et al.*, 2004). Overall, observers and public health advocates argue that Japan 'has not kept pace with the rest of the global community', given a fundamental conflict of interest within the government between public health and economic goals (Asukai *et al.*, 2005).

Japan's contribution to the FCTC process, led by the Ministry of Finance given its responsibility over the government's controlling interest in JTI, can be understood in this context. Japanese opposition to the FCTC was expressed early during WHO public hearings where JTI representative Axel Gietz claimed advertising bans and tax increases did not work, called instead for 'sensible and meaningful tobacco control regulations' (Price, 2000). This often used term by TTCs meant non-binding recommendations and guidelines that member states would be invited to comply with voluntarily, as circumstances permitted. Assunta and Chapman describe how the Japanese government was a negative influence by pressing for optional and qualifying language:

> With regard to Article 13 on regulating cross-border advertising, Japan doubted the need for a protocol. Elaboration of guidelines should take precedence . . . He favoured guidelines in the form of non-binding recommendations containing examples of worldwide best practices on specific measures.
>
> (World Health Organisation, 2007b)

Given the desire by WHO to enable as many countries as possible to accede to the treaty, negotiators sought to agree 'the lowest acceptable common denominator in clause development' (Assunta and Chapman, 2006).

Japan's position during negotiations on the adoption of such measures as 'light' and 'mild' labelling, health warnings and bans on vending machines were, according to reports, influenced by a 'fear that implementing such policies in the country where 340 billion cigarettes were sold last year would be devastating to tax revenues and tobacco farmers' (Asahi News Service, 2000). This was also evident in the Japanese delegation's opposition at the First Conference of the Parties (COP1) meeting in 2006 to a request by developing countries for increased resources to support the implementation of the FCTC. Despite being one of the world's largest donors of health development aid (see Chapter 2 this volume), Japan argued that 'contributions should be entirely voluntary':

> Dr KASHIWAGI (Japan) stated that the review had shown that there were already sufficient resources in donor countries to assist developing countries in tobacco control activities: the task was to raise awareness so that those resources could be effectively tapped.
>
> (World Health Organisation, 2006)

In seeking to protect domestic economic interests by diluting the language of the treaty and weakening commitment to its implementation, Japan was largely seen as a 'spoiler'. This elicited strong criticism by CSOs which 'named and shamed' the Japanese delegation during the INBs:

> During the FCTC negotiations international and local media applied pressure on Japan to re-examine its stance on tobacco control . . . Outside Japan, international NGOs participating in the FCTC negotiation played a part in keeping pressure on the Japanese government by meting out public shame such as the awarding of 'Dirty Ashtray Awards' (of which Japan received the most) over its weak negotiating positions. In March 2002, at INB4, Japan was labelled by an NGO as one of the 'axis of evil'.
>
> (Assunta and Chapman, 2006)

For Japanese negotiators, however, this criticism came as an unpleasant surprise: officials were 'shocked to be blamed and to be framed as such' (Assunta and

Chapman, 2006). For public health advocates, such as the Anti Smoking Parliamentarian League, this international criticism created 'political leverage' for a domestic policy debate on tobacco control. As well as ratifying the FCTC on 8 June 2004, Japan revised the Health Promotion Law in 2003, and strengthened legal measures in support of tobacco control. As claimed at COP1 (2006):

> [W]e are taking measures domestically and internationally . . . Japan is not only concerned about the health of its own people; in the international arena Japan has been providing financial and technical support to the Tobacco-Free Initiative. In our official development assistance . . . Tobacco-related measures requested by partner countries are an important element and it goes without saying that we will continue to support WHO in this field.
>
> (World Health Organisation, 2006)

Tobacco control advocates, however, are less sanguine about the progress made to date:

> Japan is making efforts to follow the FCTC, but it is insufficient and present anti-tobacco measures seem to have only a little impact on decreasing smoking rates. More effective measures should be developed for reducing smoking rates and for making a smoke-free society.
>
> (Satomura *et al.*, 2008)

Internationally, Japan's participation in negotiation of a FCTC protocol on illicit trade in tobacco products also suggests that the country continues to be reluctant to commit to a strong and binding agreement. Japan has continued to insert optional language based on arguments regarding the creation of binding instruments and the primacy of national authorities:

> Japan would not support the imposition under the protocol of a uniform obligation on States Parties to create new categories of crime or to introduce a special international cooperation mechanism solely for tobacco products. Anti-counterfeiting measures for tobacco products should give careful consideration to existing international agreements and domestic legislation. The protocol should be a multilateral instrument that many States could accept. Too many specific obligations might reduce the level of acceptance and, consequently, the number of signatories. The protocol should be elaborated on the basis of diverse legal systems and social and cultural backgrounds and allow for a degree of discretion and flexibility.
>
> (World Health Organisation, 2008c)

China

China is the largest producer and consumer of tobacco in the world. Tobacco production is controlled by a state monopoly, the China National Tobacco Corporation

(CNTC), and regulated by the State Tobacco Monopoly Administration (STMA). The industry supplies 9–11 percent of government revenues through taxation and has thus been nurtured as a valued economic sector. As described by Jiang Cheng Kang (Director of the STMA and General Manager of CNTC), '[T]he tobacco industry of China . . . represents the fundamental interests of the overwhelming majority of the Chinese people . . . The state tobacco monopoly is . . . the most practical and most powerful measure for tobacco control' (Jiang, 2006).

China's participation in the FCTC negotiations, therefore, was strongly influenced by industry interests. Perceiving the treaty as a threat, the STMA formed a working group consisting of its research arm, as well as the Yunnan Tobacco Science Research Institute, and Ministry of Foreign Affairs. Funded and staffed by the STMA and CNTC, the working group's aim was 'promoting its own countermeasures against the WHO FCTC and developing strategies for the tobacco industry in China to mitigate the impact of the FCTC' (STMA Working Group, 2006). The Working Group's report, submitted to the Chinese INB delegation, proposed 128 countermeasures to the proposed treaty's text. The report claimed approximately 51 were included by the Chinese delegation in documentation prepared for the negotiations (Nerc, 2004).

As well as advising on text negotiations (Zhou and Cheng, 2006), members of the STMA Working Group also served on the Chinese FCTC delegation. Indeed, unlike most delegations which were led by senior public health officials, the Chinese delegation was led by the Commission of National Development and Reform (CNDR) under which the STMA is located. This inclusion of industry interests was heavily criticised by other delegations and CSOs, leading to calls for INBs to be 'closed' to tobacco companies. The Chinese government opposed these proposals in 'the spirit of inclusiveness and openness' (World Health Organisation, 2006).

> Mr GOU Haibo (China) wondered how the wish to ensure maximum transparency and inclusiveness by making public meetings the norm could be reconciled with Article 5.3 of the Framework Convention, which specifically excluded representatives of the tobacco industry. Subsidiary bodies, the type and number of which could not be foreseen, should be able to decide for themselves whether their meetings should be public or restricted.
>
> (World Health Organisation, 2006)

The presence of industry representation on the Chinese delegation, and incorporation of industry-led countermeasures in its negotiating position, shaped the country's contribution to the FCTC process.

First, China supported the need for the treaty to be 'broad, comprehensive and inclusive', allowing flexibility especially for developing countries that should receive 'financial and technical support' for 'losses' incurred in implementing the agreement (World Health Organisation, 2000b, c, d). The impact on China's 22 million tobacco farmers was of particular concern:

> Dr ZHAO Baidong . . . drew attention to . . . agricultural diversification and alternative crops to tobacco. The Conference should provide financial and technical support for the study group. Tobacco was often grown in less-developed regions where practical problems could slow down crop diversification.
>
> (World Health Organisation, 2006)

China thus opposed ending government subsidies for leaf production as 'detrimental to the development of the tobacco industry' (STMA Working Group, 2006). The draft article aimed to mitigate this concern by promoting viable alternative activities to tobacco farmers. However, the STMA proposed that this be omitted given 'mass employment in the tobacco economy, and that promoting alternative activities would be difficult and impossible to achieve' (STMA Working Group, 2006).

Secondly, the Chinese delegation firmly resisted economic measures, such as taxation and price controls (Article 6), to reduce tobacco use. For example, China opposed the 'allocation of a part of the revenues from tobacco taxes to tobacco control programs' (World Health Organisation, 2002b) on the basis that 'national policy does not have to be internationalized, need to respect national sovereignty' (STMA Working Group, 2006). China also opposed restrictions on tax-free and duty-free tobacco sales (World Health Organisation, 2000b, c, d). In the final text, wording was softened to 'prohibiting or restricting, as appropriate, sales to and/or importations by international travellers of tax- and duty-free tobacco products' (World Health Organisation, 2003c). On Article 19 (Liability), which was strongly supported by European countries as an 'important means of rectifying damage caused by tobacco use', China was among the countries which opposed its inclusion. While not excluded from the final text, the phrase 'where necessary' was added to weaken its impact: 'For the purpose of tobacco control, the Parties shall consider taking legislative action or promoting their existing laws, where necessary to deal with criminal and civil liability including compensation where appropriate' (Cheng, 2006).

Thirdly, China opposed strengthening regulation that had 'a direct effect on the tobacco business', such as restrictions on marketing and advertising, health warnings, packaging and labelling (Zhou, 2004). The delegation argued, for example, that 'the radical languages used by EU, Canada and other countries' on warning labels were inappropriate to Chinese culture, as was restricted use of 'red and other traditional, festive colours'.

> [T]he form of print warning on cigarettes must accommodate the value orientation of traditional culture of our nation and consumer psychology of the mass. The print format of package labelling must fit the orientation of traditional values and psychology of mass consumers.
>
> (STMA Working Group, 2004)

This argument against the globalisation of tobacco control measures continued beyond the negotiations to the Third Conference of Parties (COP) in 2008. As Malone writes,

> The Chinese delegation argued forcefully and passionately during discussion of guidelines for implementing the Article 11: Packaging and labelling of tobacco products, that their country could not possibly institute graphic warnings on cigarette packs because those packs featured revered cultural icons. To cover them with graphic warnings, they explained, would convey a terrible disrespect.
>
> (Malone, 2010)

Given the above, evidence of an apparent government shift favouring the strengthening of tobacco control policy in China is notable. In part, this can be attributed to the FCTC process which drew unprecedented attention in China to startling data on the scale of the predicted population health impact of tobacco use. Following the conclusion of negotiations, attention shifted to encouraging China to ratify the agreement:

> WHO also convened two national awareness-raising and capacity-building workshops for China from 30 May to 3 June 2005 and for Nigeria from 31 October to 1 November 2005. The workshops aimed to support national processes to become Contracting Parties and to create the conditions for implementing the Convention.
>
> (World Health Organisation, 2006)

Faced with a predicted rise in tobacco-related deaths, from one to three million by 2030 (including one-third of young men) (Niu *et al.*, 1998), China somewhat unexpectedly ratified the FCTC in 2006. International support for tobacco control activities began to be received, and broadly based meetings in China were held on such issues as tobacco economics and taxation (World Health Organisation, 2008). As described by Yang Gonghuan (Director of the National Office of Tobacco Control):

> Before 2006, attempts at tobacco control were mainly research by health experts and basic health education. Since China joined the WHO Framework Convention on Tobacco Control (WHO FCTC), the Government, media, research institutions and the public have acknowledged the need for tobacco control. The Ministry of Health has published an annual tobacco control report and there have been campaigns to increase tobacco tax and warnings added to packaging.
>
> (World Health Organisation, 2010a)

As described by Jiang Yuan (Deputy Director of National Tobacco Control Office, Chinese CDC), the FCTC process also galvanised a nascent tobacco control movement, which gained political impetus (World Health Organisation, 2010a).

Interestingly, it has been the issue of public smoking bans (Article 8 on protection from exposure to tobacco smoke) that has received the most public attention in China in relation to the implementation of the FCTC. While WHO documents suggest the STMA did not explicitly oppose such restrictions, industry documents suggest BAT sought to undermine the scope of public smoking bans (Muggli *et al.*, 2008). The 2008 Beijing Olympic Games provoked unprecedented Chinese debate about smoke-free places:

> China, with its 350 million smokers, was particularly concerned about the implementation of Article 8 on protection from passive smoking. Guidelines to prohibit the use of tobacco in public places must be prepared and applied before the 2008 Olympic Games in order to give China a smoke-free public environment, thereby reducing the effects of passive smoking.
>
> (World Health Organisation, 2006)

After several years of limited restrictions in selected municipalities and venues, 17 pro-public health delegates proposed national legislation on a smoking ban at the Eleventh National Peoples Congress in 2010. While unsuccessful, the government agreed to explore the issue as potential legislation (Jin, 2012).

The nascent state of tobacco control in China, following ratification of the FCTC, offers insights into the relationship between national and global health governance. China entered negotiations with a strong belief that national interests were best served by protecting the tobacco industry. Economic development remained of primary concern, and the FCTC was framed as a potential hindrance to a thriving sector. Participation in the negotiations led Chinese officials to gain a fuller understanding of the looming population health impacts of tobacco use in China and, significantly, the serious implications this would have on China's adult male population. In other words, large-scale death and disease from tobacco use was increasingly seen as a threat to national interests, and national and global health governance began to be more closely aligned.

Beyond tobacco control, China's engagement with the FCTC can also be understood as part of the country's growing profile in international relations. As the world's largest producer and consumer of tobacco products, according to Jiang Yuan, China is eager to be respected as a responsible stakeholder committed to working with other countries. Like Hong Kong, Singapore and South Korea, Jiang Yuan believes China could contribute positively to global tobacco control in spite of a strong domestic tobacco industry. AS the Chinese Ministry of Foreign Affairs stated in 2001, 'The Chinese delegation (to the FCTC negotiations) not only safeguards China's rights and interests as a big power of production and consumption of tobacco in the world but also establishes its image as a responsible big power' (quoted in Jin, 2012: 12).

> As a nation of courtesy and propriety, and as a big tobacco country, to actively support WHO in the enactment of the FCTC would create an image of being supportive of tobacco control, protecting public health and being a responsible country. And in the process of promoting human civilization, to fully fulfill China's positive influence over the process of the FCTC is helpful in raising

> the international status of our nation, and beneficial in creating a tall and big image for our country.
>
> (Cheng *et al.*, 2001)

Fulfilling this aspiration, however, will require continued attention to powerful vested interests that retain considerable influence over public policy in China. The FCTC's ratification, according to STMA Director Jiang, has not necessarily reflected diminishing influence by the industry:

> On Jan 9th, 2006, the FCTC went into force in China . . . the research achievement scored by the Working Group will be of far-reaching influence on the development, improvement and practical application of theories on the tobacco economy and for tobacco control.

Indeed, the countermeasures proposed by the STMA Working Group continue to shape implementation:

> At the Durban session of the WHO FCTC in November 2008, I was one of the Ministry of Health's representatives on China's delegation, which was led by the Ministry of Industry and Information Technology. But as the director of the State Tobacco Monopoly Administration also sits on the party committee of the ministry, it was like having the Administration lead the delegation. The attitude towards tobacco control shown by the delegation was terrible. One speaker argued that Chinese tobacco packaging featured mountains, rivers and monuments, and placing 'ugly' pictures besides such scenes would 'humiliate the Chinese people'. But I don't think these behaviours represent the essential attitude of China's government . . . The delegation's behaviour at the Durban session was merely a manifesto of the opposition from vested interest groups.
>
> (Cheng *et al.*, 2001)

Indonesia

Indonesia has been another challenging environment for tobacco control, given an economically powerful domestic tobacco industry. The tobacco sector is the second-largest employer after the government, and the country is the world's seventh-largest tobacco producer and fifth-largest tobacco consumer (Healthbridge, 2007). In 2005 Philip Morris bought Sampoerna, one of Indonesia's tobacco giants, as part of its goal to remain the world's largest TTC. Other TTCs actively seek market access (Lawrence and Collin, 2004; *Smokers News*, 2009). It is estimated that 80 million Indonesians smoke (62 percent of adult males), with clove cigarettes dominating the market. The industry is closely aligned with the government (Reynolds, 1999), which has been reluctant to regulate a thriving business (*Jakarta Post*, 2009). Five key ministries – Finance, Agriculture, Industry, Trade, and Manpower and Transmigration – oppose the FCTC as harmful to the tobacco industry. As David Stanford (Indonesia Consumers Foundation) states, 'from the tobacco company's perspective Indonesia is a paradise' (Thompson, 2009).

FCTC documents suggest that unlike other South East Asian countries, Indonesia was not an active contributor to the negotiations. As reported by the NGO HealthBridge,

> Most of the countries located in WHO's South East Asian Region (SEAR) have demonstrated a strong commitment to the WHO Framework Convention on Tobacco Control (FCTC). Indonesia, however, is an exception—there is much apathy on the part of the Government to accede to the FCTC and implement tobacco control policies.
>
> (Cheng *et al.*, 2001)

This observation is supported by Wasis Sumartono (National Institute of Health, Ministry of Health) who believes 'so far the impact of the FCTC is very small':[2]

> Singapore is the best example of a country where control of tobacco supply and demand are undertaken simultaneously, very similar to suggestions in the FCTC. Bangladesh has encouraged crop substitution for tobacco farmers and supervised farmers to grow healthier produce. Brunei Darussalam, a country that has declared war on smoking, says tobacco is 'harmful' and that 'smoking is against Islamic teaching'. The views of Singapore, Thailand, Brunei, Bangladesh, India and Japan are probably united. But views in Indonesia are still being left far behind these leading countries in tobacco control.
>
> (Thompson, 2009)

During negotiations, this was reflected in the delegation's support for a broad, non-specific approach:

> [T]he convention should be flexible so that as many countries as possible could participate, even if that meant removing specific obligations. The convention should focus on broad, comprehensive and inclusive principles, reflecting the political wills of different governments, and should help to protect developing countries in particular from the international trade in tobacco, while developed countries that exported tobacco products should be held accountable.
>
> (World Health Organisation, 2006)

Indonesia has yet to sign and ratify the FCTC as of September 2010, with former Minister of Health, Farid Anfasa Moeloek, even downplaying the FCTC's importance: 'Indonesia has no reason to ratify the FCTC, because tobacco is already covered by the Law on Health' (Asia Pulse Data, 2009). Outside of government, there has been limited tobacco control advocacy. The Indonesian Tobacco Control Network, led by Alex Papilaya, coordinates advocacy activities, including public information campaigns. Yet activities are limited in scope and progress remains slow. Even where tobacco control measures have been adopted, their implementation has been ineffective. Barber and Ahsan, for example, report that the new tobacco excise system has hindered tobacco control because price increases (Indonesia has the cheapest prices in the world) were not passed on to consumers (Barber and Ahsan, 2009). In this context, public health advocates look to WHO and other countries in the region for support:

> The WHO, they have a role in warning a country like Indonesia about the importance of smoking epidemic control and prevention. Singapore, Australia, Brunei Darussalam, Japan, Bangladesh, Thailand and India play important role models for Indonesia about what kind of tobacco control strategies have been proven to be effective.
>
> (Thompson, 2009)

Thus, while Indonesia's tobacco industry has been entwined in domestic politics in similar ways to Japan and China, to date there is little evidence of public engagement of tobacco control issues. Indonesian participation in the FCTC process has been notable in its absence for such a major tobacco-producing and consuming country (Achadi *et al.*, 2005). Ongoing tensions between WHO and the Indonesian government over virus-sharing may further hinder engagement by the government with strengthening global health governance.

India

India has been a strong supporter of the FCTC process, taking a leadership role throughout (Samet and Wipfli, 2009). The country chaired four regional consultations during the inter-session periods between the second and sixth rounds of the Intergovernmental Negotiating Body (INB), and 'catalysed consensus development and consolidated strong and unified regional positions on the draft text of the FCTC' (Reddy and Gupta, 2004). This role carried over into the INB where India was unanimously elected as the coordinator of WHO South-East Asia Regional Office (SEARO) member states, 'principle negotiator, on their behalf, on the advertising issue', as well as the Group of 77, with China serving as the principle negotiating team on issues related to financial resources. India is described as working closely with WHO throughout to promote the FCTC process. For instance, an International Consultation on Tobacco Control in Developing Countries, convened by the WHO and held in New Delhi in January 2000, served as a 'curtain raiser' for the negotiations. India also co-hosted the International Conference on Global Tobacco Control Law at the same time, the first multisectoral meeting to facilitate legislation on advertisement and promotion (SEARO, 2000).

According to Monika Arora (Director of HRIDAY, New Delhi), efforts were exerted simultaneously at the domestic and global policy levels, leading to a 'parallel culmination of the FCTC and Indian Tobacco Control Act' in 2003. Arora described India's success as mutually reinforcing: 'The strong provisions of the tobacco control bills approved by the Indian cabinet for introduction in Parliament enabled India's strong advocacy for a strong FCTC.' Correspondingly, Parliament was in favour of strong domestic legislation due to India's 'lead role in the FCTC negotiations'. This mutuality was also recognised by Indian delegates in negotiating specific treaty provisions:

> Dr REDDY (India) said that it would be difficult to proceed until the actions required at national level had been identified. The weaker the national interpretations of Article 13, the greater the risk for global cross-border advertising. Any future guidelines should not be limited to cross-border issues but must encompass domestic provisions.
>
> (World Health Organization, 2007a)

India's leadership role during the FCTC negotiations was widely acclaimed by the NGO community, with the FCA awarding India four Orchid Awards. Lead negotiator Srinath Reddy was given a WHO award for outstanding contributions to tobacco control, and the Ministry of Health was presented with a prestigious Luther Terry Award in 2006.

Notably, India's support for domestic and global tobacco control was achieved despite being the second-largest producer of tobacco in the world after China. However, chewing tobacco and *bidi*s (small, hand-rolled cigarettes) represent 86 percent of the market (cigarettes are 14 percent), and India has only 0.7 percent share of the US$30 billion global tobacco trade. Thus, India signed the FCTC on 10 September 2003 and became the eighth country to ratify the agreement on 5 February 2004. During INB-5, India proposed an export tax on manufactured tobacco products that would be used to finance tobacco control activities:

> Mr CHOWDHURY (India) considered that it was necessary to establish a global fund financed by an export tax on manufactured tobacco products. Such a tax would discourage tobacco exports which, in a way, exported disease. The funds could be used to provide support to developing countries to introduce income-generating activities to replace tobacco growing and processing. Those countries were faced with the gigantic task of shifting human resources into other means of gainful employment and would be unable to carry out any serious tobacco control measures unless a safety net of that nature were provided.
>
> (World Health Organisation, 2006)

During COP meetings to discuss implementation of the FCTC, the Indian delegation remained supportive of measures to build capacity in the developing world:

> Mr TRIVEDI (India) . . . Practical achievement of the Convention's objectives depended on the financial mechanisms put forward for those countries most in need. A dedicated fund was a good idea and merited more work. The activities of the Secretariat must be more measured and predictable, and, at the

> same time, the commitment of the Parties to the objectives must be demonstrated. Needs assessments should identify available funds, total requirements, potential achievements in the short term and longer-term priorities.
>
> (World Health Organisation, 2006)

> Mr TRIVEDI (India) agreed with Norway that working methods should be streamlined to build capacity at country level, and with Kenya that much had been promised that was yet to be delivered. He agreed with the Islamic Republic of Iran that a review of funding was needed. Every year, at the Health Assembly, Member States agreed that strengthened capacity was needed, but results took time. The issue of basic needs assessment recurred because it addressed the larger issue of capacity to meet collateral budget requirements. A working group and a dedicated fund would introduce more predictability. Donor funds, which were voluntary, could dry up if the donor considered the 'performance' of a country to be inadequate, unless such funds formed part of a core budget.
>
> (World Health Organisation, 2006)

> Mr TRIVEDI (India) said that, in considering any such reduction, the Health Assembly should maintain core competencies and equity between countries. The predominance in recent years of extrabudgetary funding in WHO's programme budget had created a dichotomy between the commitment of Member States to WHO's work and the financial resources they were prepared to provide.
>
> (World Health Organisation, 2006)

The commitment of the Ministry of Health and Family Welfare to implementing the agreement is described in John's assessment of 'best practice' in fulfilling FCTC obligations (John, 2008). Similarly, Reddy, Arora and Yadav (2008) compare the FCTC with Indian tobacco control legislation. Finally, the hosting of the World Conference on Tobacco or Health in 2009 in Mumbai confirmed the ministry's ongoing commitment to strong global tobacco control. Domestically, the battles over health warnings, increased taxes, youth marketing, public smoking bans and other measures have remained fierce (Shimkhada and Peabody, 2003; Jandoo and Mehrotra, 2008; Asian News International, 2008). As Gupta (2006) writes, 'there are a few successes but much remains to be done'.

Thailand

Thailand has been seen as one of the leading lights in global and domestic tobacco control within the developing world since the late 1980s. It is one of the few developing countries with national institutions specifically responsible for tobacco control. The National Committee for the Control of Tobacco Use, which was established in 1989 to conduct governmental tobacco control activities, leads Thailand's efforts. President of the Thailand Health Promotion Institute and former Permanent Secretary in the Ministry of Public Health, as well as Thai representative to the negotiations and President of the COP Hatai Chitanondh states:

> Since 1992, Thailand has enacted two strong tobacco-control laws: one to control tobacco products and another to protect non-smokers' health. The laws include the prohibition of smoking in public places and workplaces; a total ban on all forms of advertising, sponsorship and promotions, such as free sampling and exchanges; a ban on advertising trademark diversification products; the prohibition of tobacco sales to minors, including by vending machines; pictorial health warnings on cigarette packages; and the requirement to disclose the ingredients and emission products in each brand of tobacco product. Recently, we managed to totally ban point-of-sale displays at all 500,000 retail outlets. This is the biggest distribution network in the world. This year, we will have a ban on misleading descriptors, prohibition of the sale of packs with less than 20 sticks and flavoured cigarettes, and also mandate low ignition propensity in products.
>
> (World Health Organisation, 2006)

From the earliest stages of the FCTC process, Thailand has been an active supporter of a strong treaty. Thailand (like India) saw the treaty as essential for achieving domestic policy goals.[3] As Bung-on Ritthiphakdee (ASH Thailand) stated,

> The FCTC is needed since tobacco is a global problem . . . It's impossible for any single country to cope with the tobacco problem because it is a transnational problem. Thailand would welcome protocols on the effective eradication of tobacco smuggling, a global ban on tobacco advertising and sponsorship, the elimination of duty-free sales of tobacco products, the harmonization of taxes on tobacco products at international level, the exemption of tobacco products from reduced taxation under regional free-trade agreements, the mandatory testing and reporting of toxic constituents, and the establishment of a mechanism for information-sharing.
>
> (JTI Weekly News Report, 2000)

To support the FCTC process, Thailand (in partnership with WHO) hosted several major meetings to facilitate negotiations including, the second Intersessional Meeting for Member States in ASEAN, which was held in Bangkok in 2002, and chaired by Thailand (World Health Organisation, 2002a). Between INBs, Thailand also played a lead role in several working groups including the Working Group on Health and Education Issues (after the first INB) (Smith, 2000). To support implementation of the FCTC, Thailand hosted the second COP in 2007, and was conscious of the significance of having developing countries play this role:

> Because Thailand is the host country of this session of the Conference of the Parties, Thailand supports South Africa as the future host country because

> South Africa is a developing country just like Thailand, and because Thailand has proved that a developing country can host a big conference like this one.
>
> (World Health Organisation, 2008d)

At this meeting, Dr Chitanondh was elected COP President in recognition of his leadership role throughout the FCTC process:

> Dr Hatai (Chitanondh) has the personal commitment and, backed by the institutional support of the Thai Government, he has done wonders in the world of tobacco control. He just mentioned that he is not a career diplomat, but being a career diplomat and having served in a few missions, I know the importance of leadership. All ambassadors are not necessarily leaders. I say this in my personal capacity as an experienced Foreign Service officer. All we need in tobacco control is leadership. And Dr Hatai has amply demonstrated his ability to lead the tobacco-control efforts.
>
> (Smith, 2000)

Thailand demonstrated particular leadership in relation to specific FCTC's provisions on trade and health issues. The country's team was able to lead effectively based on its past experience facing down pressure by the US Trade Representative to open its domestic tobacco market (World Health Organisation, 2006). Described as 'perhaps the central issue of the negotiations', Thailand took the firm view that health should take precedent over trade policy: 'If the Framework Convention does not explicitly state that its public health provisions are to take priority when they conflict with trade rules, it would allow the industry to challenge other provisions of the Convention as trade violations' (Boltz, 2002).

As described by Dr Chitanondh,

> Over the past decade Thailand had attempted to implement effective, comprehensive tobacco control measures as recommended by the World Health Assembly, but at the same time has had to fight repeated attempts by the tobacco industry to use international trade laws to weaken those measures. The proposed framework convention would therefore have to be a robust instrument of international law. It should assert the importance of good health and of comprehensive tobacco control as an integral part of health protection both nationally and internationally, and provide strong protection for national and international tobacco control regimes from the effects of international trade law. It should not be subordinate to any other international agreement, including trade agreements. While liberalized trade was an important engine of socioeconomic development, public health protection should take precedence over the interests of the tobacco industry.
>
> (World Health Organisation, 2000b, c, d)

Moreover, ASH Thailand supported the exclusion of tobacco from all trade agreements; 'tobacco products should not take advantage of free trade and be kept out of all trade agreements' (Asahi News Service, 2000). The trade issue remained a sticking point throughout the negotiations, leading to the creation of a special working group to reach a compromise. BAT documents describe the impasse:

> At the end of the negotiations, Thailand, which has had its tobacco control measures challenged by the industry as trade violations, insisted that its proposal putting health first remain under consideration. The Thai proposal states, 'In the event of a conflict between the Convention or any of its Protocols and any other international agreement, this Convention and its Protocols shall prevail.' While it appeared the Thai proposal was still alive, it remains to be seen whether it will be in the Chair's Text when it is released in July.
>
> (BAT, 2001)

Indeed, the ambiguous language of the final text did little to resolve the trade or health issues, and the issue remains a point of debate to the present day.

Relatedly, Thailand drew important attention to the broader economics of tobacco control. Prakit Vateesatokit (Secretary of ASH Thailand) argued that the 'misconception that tobacco benefits the economy should be brought out into reality to show how tobacco imposes enormous economic costs on governments, consumers and private employers' (World Health Organisation, 2001). A workshop on the economic analysis of tobacco control held at SEARO brought together economists from seven countries (including Thailand) to strengthen the evidence base on the real costs of tobacco:

> Country case studies were presented on situation analysis of prevalence, health and economics, demand analysis, and estimations of health burden and costs resulting from tobacco use. Recommendations from the meeting included using electronic means for communication between economic researchers and exploring the possibility of an international consultation involving ministries of finance and health to enhance collaboration between those sectors for tobacco control.
>
> (World Health Organisation, 2001)

Of particular concern was the need to draw attention to, and prevent the undue influence of, the tobacco industry in the FCTC process and tobacco control more widely. In Thailand, in contrast to Japan and China, as Dr Chitanondh described,

> Thailand still has a government tobacco monopoly but the monopoly never had any influence on Thailand's position on the FCTC negotiations. China's delegation included members from its national tobacco monopoly. China's stand during negotiations was not supportive of the FCTC.[4]

This concern about industry influence led the country to play a lead role in negotiating Article 5.3, Guidelines on the protection of public health policies with respect to tobacco control from commercial and other vested interests:

> Thailand was willing to act as a key facilitator for the working group on Article 5.3. India and Thailand were willing to be partners in the working group on Article 11, and India, Sri Lanka and Thailand were willing to be partners in the working group on Article 12.
>
> (Smith, 2000)

Overall, Thailand can be described as playing a lead role in the FCTC process, both within the Asian region and globally. In turn, the country has seen the FCTC as enhancing its domestic efforts: 'Although Thailand already has a "gold standard" of legislation for tobacco control, the FCTC has been boosting Thailand's performances in non-legal interventions, for example, countering the tobacco industry's strategies' (World Health Organisation, 2006).

Global tobacco control and changing perceptions of sovereignty in Asia

The traditional notion of sovereignty, focused on the exercise of supreme authority over a defined territory, was raised regularly during the FCTC process, largely by state and non-state actors opposed to a comprehensive, strong and binding treaty. First, the primacy of state sovereignty vis-à-vis the FCTC was maintained, with some member states seeking confirmation through the insertion of phrases such as 'in accordance with its national laws'. Some Asian countries used such interventions to weaken the binding nature of adopted measures. China, for example, asserted that 'price and tax measures were matters for national authorities' (World Health Organisation, 2006) and that 'Every Party should formulate and promulgate the relevant specific provisions concerning licensing arrangements in accordance with its national laws' (World Health Organisation, 2008d). As Zhao (2006) stated, 'Our governmental delegates (at INB sessions), based on confirmed negotiation principles by the Nation, acted insistently and uncompromisingly concerning issues involving sovereignty.' Regarding a protocol on illicit trade Japan similarly argued that 'since responsibilities were allocated by individual governments, the protocol should not seek to regulate the issue' (World Health Organisation, 2008c).

The alleged encroachment by the FCTC on state sovereignty was also a frequent argument put forth by the tobacco industry. BAT claimed that proposed measures 'risk undermining governments' self-determination', calling on the WHO to 'take proper account of national governments' different priorities' (World Health Organisation, 2001).

> The INB is now starting substantive negotiations for the first time. These offer governments, particularly of developing nations, an important opportunity to ensure that their sovereignty is not undermined or their domestic priorities ignored. So far, many governments' health ministers and officials have only been partly involved. The FCTC process is mainly being driven by a small number of countries with a particular 'anti-tobacco' agenda, such as

> Canada, Australia, New Zealand, Thailand and the European Union – which appears to be attempting to act without a clear mandate from its individual member states.
>
> (Zhao, 2006)

A JTI representative, speaking at the pre-negotiation public hearings, argued that a 'one size fits all' global solution to smoking was flawed, and that 'national governments were best placed to know what their country needed' (Fijii and Price, 2000). A related argument by industry was that the public health community was going beyond its mandate:

> Many proposed measures go far beyond the competence of health ministries, and of the WHO itself. There are potentially major impacts on financial, tax, economic, employment, agricultural, trade, and legal policy. We believe that key government ministries should take care to examine the WHO proposals, to ensure that balanced government views can be reflected in national negotiating positions.
>
> (Zhou and Cheng, 2006)

In the end, while the term 'sovereign' appeared only three times in the final text, the adoption of qualifying language throughout the FCTC reflected the uneasy balance eventually achieved between strong, binding measures to protect public health, and weaker, non-binding measures to protect vested economic interests. Strong emphasis was placed on national, regional and international efforts and multisectoral collaboration to implement the FCTC's universal minimum standards agreed by States Parties.

There is evidence from the FCTC process that some Asian countries may be moving beyond traditional notions of sovereignty. Recognising that the globalisation of the tobacco industry can pose a threat to sovereignty, Thailand and India have embraced the treaty as an instrument of global health governance. More broadly, the FCTC process challenges territorially defined notions of interests, highlighting how the protection and promotion of public health involves supporting and opposing interests that span national jurisdictions. Global health governance, in this context, challenges Asian countries to redefine sovereignty.

Institutional diversity in Asian tobacco control

The FCTC process has been widely recognised for the degree to which non-state actors contributed to the negotiation process. With the notable exception of tobacco industry-related interests, The Tobacco-Free Initiative (TFI) actively supported the mobilisation and participation of CSOs. This began with a grant from the UN Foundation to foster tobacco control advocacy in developing countries. Then TFI fast-tracked applications by selected NGOs for officially recognised status to enable them to attend negotiations (Collin *et al.*, 2002). As a result, non-state actors played a key role at all stages of the FCTC process, going beyond the usually circumscribed engagement by NGOs with WHO (Collin *et al.*, 2002).

In Asia, Thailand was among the strongest supporters of a Canadian proposal to allow 'national NGOs "with relevant expertise"... to apply for accreditation and attend, but without the right to vote in plenary meetings and in the main committee meetings' (BAT, 2000).

> Dr CHITANONDH (Thailand) commended the Canadian proposal but suggested refining it by explicitly excluding nongovernmental organizations that received financial or other support from tobacco companies and their acolytes, thus echoing the recommendations made by the August 2000 committee of experts on the tobacco industry's strategies designed to undermine the work of WHO... accredited nongovernmental organizations should have the right to participate in all meetings of the Negotiating Body – working groups, ad hoc bodies or any other committees – helping to craft a strong convention.
>
> (World Health Organisation, 2000b)

Canada and Thailand were subsequently appointed to coordinate enquiries from NGOs. Similarly, India supported regional consultations that would enable, inter alia, broad involvement by NGOs:

> Dr PRASAD (India), speaking on behalf of the Parties to the Convention in the WHO South-East Asia Region, suggested the addition of a phrase at the end of paragraph 7(2), calling for regional consultations [to] facilitate participation by lower-income countries, nongovernmental organizations, customs and law-enforcement officials and other stakeholders.
>
> (World Health Organisation, 2006)

While nascent in many countries, NGOs from supporting countries played prominent roles in the FCTC process. ASH Thailand played a lead role in FCA briefings on such matters as graphic warnings, illicit trade and cross-border advertising Philip Morris International (n.d.):

> Thailand. Thanpuying Sumalee Chartikavanij, President of Thai Women Watch, promised to disseminate and share information concerning the outcome of this conference to the regional network as well as her organization in Thailand and integrate it into the Beijing process. Ms Bung-On Ritthhipakdee, Project Director of Action on Smoking and Health, pledged to mobilize more media women, to enhance the beauty contest anti-tobacco strategy and to make pharmaceutical companies more active in anti-tobacco campaigning.
>
> (World Health Organisation, 1999)

The creation of the Asia Pacific Conference on Tobacco or Health (APACT), and its mobilisation of advocacy in the region, generated substantial support for tobacco control in the region. According to Dr Chitanondh, 'the Region consists of less than a dozen countries and we are a closely-knit small family. That allows us to work successfully. Member countries of the Region will forge ahead both at the regional and global levels' (World Health Organisation, 2006).

Asian conceptions of global health governance

The Asian region contained a full spectrum of positions on the FCTC, from strong industry-driven opposition, to equally strong public health-based support (i.e. India, Thailand, Singapore). As such, the region was far from uniform in its conceptions of GHG. What is notable is the shift over time during the negotiations towards regional positions based on WHO regional structures, with Thailand and India nominated respectively to speak on behalf of these groupings.

The strengthening of a regional presence at the FCTC negotiations was the result of efforts to develop and support regional governance, with efforts spanning pre-negotiations through to ongoing protocol negotiations. Beginning with regional consultations held in 1999–2000 and leading up to the opening of formal negotiations, regional working groups met between INBs, and subsequently created regional coordinators for treaty implementation. In some cases, regional positions arose from these meetings. For example, eight SEARO countries adopted the Jakarta Declaration on the FCTC in 2001. ASEAN also became a regional mechanism 'to debate matters regarding the framework convention, such as tobacco-related problems common to the members of ASEAN and possible solutions' (World Health Organisation, 2002a). Similarly, the second Intersessional Meeting held in Bangkok in 2002, attended by ten ASEAN countries and seven NGOs, reviewed the Chair's proposed text and endorsed the Bangkok Declaration on Tobacco Control as a tool for briefing their respective governments. It was also agreed that, for those items on which consensus was reached, interventions at INB-5 would be presented as ASEAN positions (JTI Weekly News Report, 2000)

Conclusions

It must be recognised that the FCTC, as a GHG instrument, supports rather than undermines Asian countries in a global political economy. With the global burden of tobacco-related disease and death shifting to the developing world, and Asia in particular, prior to the FCTC, few Asian countries had adopted effective tobacco control policies. As of September 2010, there were 171 parties to the FCTC, including Japan and China. The Asian countries' contributions to the negotiation and implementation of the FCTC show considerable diversity, often closely aligned with the political economy of the tobacco industry. The subsequent growth of the tobacco control movement in Asia, led by state and non-state actors, suggests great potential for the FCTC as a GHG instrument. The effectiveness of the FCTC ultimately depends on how it catalyses action at the national and regional levels, and how its flexibilities and qualifying language are overcome. In this respect, much work remains to be done. Incomplete data on tobacco production and consumption worldwide, weak capacity to adopt and enforce stronger regulations, and limited resources remain major challenges preventing Asia from adequately addressing this looming public health crisis.

Acknowledgements

This research was funded in part by the US National Cancer Institute, National Institutes of Health Grant Number R01 CA91021-01; and the European Research Council under the European Community's Seventh Framework Programme – Ideas Grant 230489 GHG. The authors wish to thank Jingying Xu for undertaking keyword searching of the official documentation on the FCTC and protocol negotiations, and the Legacy Tobacco Documents Library for industry documents on selected Asian countries.

Notes

1 This research used official records of the FCTC negotiations available at http://apps.who.int/gb/fctc/e/ which include the Process for the WHO Framework Convention on Tobacco Control (1999–2005) (http://apps.who.int/gb/fctc/e/E_process.html), documentation and reports of working groups, Intergovernmental Negotiating Body (INB) sessions, Conference of the Parties (COP) meetings, and INBs on a Protocol on Illicit Trade in Tobacco Products (see Appendix C). Background documents include summary records of the composition of specific bodies, and member state contributions vis-à-vis the evolving treaty text. In addition, the research analysed internal documents of the tobacco industry which are publicly available as a result of litigation. Keyword searches were carried out on the Legacy Tobacco Document Library (LTDL).

2 Interview with Wasis Sumartono, National Institute of Health, Ministry of Health, Jakarta, 17 March 2010.

3 Interview with Hatai Chitanondh, Bangkok, 20 January 2010.

4 Interview with Hatai Chitanondh, Bangkok, 20 January 2010.

Part 3

Asian participation in governing global health research and knowledge products

8 Rule-makers, rule-shapers and rule-takers

What role for Asia in the global governance of intellectual property rules and global health?

Suerie Moon and Nicole Szlezák

> Of all the issues discussed at WHO governing bodies, access to medicines consistently sparks the most heated, sometimes divisive, and potentially explosive debates.
>
> World Health Organization Director-General
> Margaret Chan, cited in Lamy, Chan and Gurry (2010)

Introduction

In an era of increasing interconnectedness and exchange, global regimes have emerged to govern actor behavior in domains that have come to be seen as transnational, such as trade, climate change, human rights and health. We define global regimes as the *formal and informal* 'principles, norms, rules, and decision making procedures' (Krasner, 1982) that govern the behavior of state and non-state actors at the global level. Such regimes signal the coming into being of a 'global' domain of public policy making – a set of rules that is no longer purely based on Westphalian principles of interaction between sovereign nation-states, but based on networked coalitions between a diverse set of players – governmental and non-governmental, private and public (Ruggie, 2004). The emergence of such regimes raises important questions for global governance. For example, how are global regimes created, amended and enforced? Who shapes and is shaped by them? How do various actors influence global rule-making, and what role do health considerations play?

The Agreement on Trade Related Aspects of Intellectual Property Rights (TRIPS), a set of formal rules on intellectual property (IP) that have profoundly impacted the field of pharmaceuticals, is a useful case for shedding light on these questions. Negotiated by member states of the General Agreement on Tariffs and Trade during the Uruguay Round of trade negotiations, TRIPS was one of the core treaties that came into force with the creation of the World Trade Organization (WTO) in 1994. By requiring all WTO Members to provide a minimum level of IP protection domestically, TRIPS was intended to harmonise IP policies across industrialised and developing[1] countries against the backdrop of economic globalisation. However, its introduction sparked a major public health controversy:

TRIPS required the introduction of patents on medicines in many developing countries, which would enable patent-holders to sell medicines at high prices that could easily exceed a country's ability to pay. Especially in the context of the HIV/AIDS pandemic, these new global trade rules sparked a vociferous response from a global network of civil society organisations (CSOs) and public health advocates. According to its critics, TRIPS imposed a global intellectual property regime on developing countries that was unsuited to meet their development needs in general, and threatened access to medicines in particular.

While the *formal* provisions of TRIPS provided developing countries with some degree of flexibility to bring their national patent policies into compliance with the treaty, the exact shape and scope of this policy space, i.e., the *informal* rules governing how the provisions could be used, were undefined and a subject of heated political contestation (Deere, 2008). For example, a powerful safeguard explicitly allowed within TRIPS is 'compulsory licensing', in which a government may authorise use of a patent without the permission of the patent-holder in order to protect the public interest. Compulsory licensing is intended to counteract the potential abuse of monopoly power by patent-holders, and is a standard feature of industrialised country patent systems. This measure could be used, for example, to authorise a generic version of an essential medicine if the patent-holder refused to supply it or to make it available at a price affordable to the local population. While TRIPS expressly permitted national governments to employ compulsory licensing and other public interest safeguards, the political space for developing countries to do so was extremely constricted in the late 1990s. National governments of developing countries found themselves in a grey zone shaped by three disparate forces: first, external pressure from industrialised countries seeking to secure worldwide protection for their intellectual property; and secondly, considerations of their own national economic and trade interests, which often included gaining access to markets and attracting investors from the industrialised countries. The combination of these factors made many governments unwilling to make use of TRIPS flexibilities. However, there was also a third factor: public health needs. Increasingly well-networked and proactive civil society organisations often pressured national governments to adopt more flexible IP policies that would make medicines more affordable.

Between 1994 and the present, there has been a remarkable transformation in the *informal* rules that govern how TRIPS is interpreted and implemented with respect to public health needs. In particular, there is greater policy space in the global IP regime for governments to take public health considerations into account in their IP policies. Asian governments and CSOs played a crucial role in this transformation. This chapter describes and analyzes how these actors shaped global IP rules, and then uses the case to explore broader implications for the role of Asia in global health governance.

The chapter is divided into four sections. The first briefly explains the origins of the global IP regime and its effects on public health. The second section covers the transformation of the global IP regime through a discussion of how Malaysia, Thailand and India (re-)defined the application of TRIPS in the public health domain. It then discusses the case of China, which provides a theoretically useful contrast to the other countries presented here. The third section discusses broader implications of the case for global health governance, along the three 'lenses' of national sovereignty and world order; conceptions and contributions from Asia; and institutional diversity. The fourth section summarises conclusions, suggests areas for future research and offers an outlook for the future.

Background: the global IP regime, public health, and Asia

When TRIPS came into force in the mid-1990s, it introduced a stringent new set of global IP rules that required developing countries to begin changing their domestic laws to provide a minimum level of IP protection, such as 20-year patent terms, across nearly all areas of technology. In practice, this meant that many developing countries had to begin granting patents on medicines for the first time.[2]

The impact of TRIPS on the affordability of medicines in developing countries became highly visible and the subject of heated political contests in the context of the growing HIV/AIDS epidemic. In the second half of the 1990s, combination antiretroviral (ARV) therapy that could effectively suppress HIV replication became available. In the industrialised countries, these drug cocktails were sold at over US$ 10,000 per patient/year (ppy). However, ARVs were largely unavailable in developing countries, many of which were undergoing far more extensive HIV/AIDS epidemics than in the industrialised countries. While generic ARVs were being sold for as little as US$ 350[3] ppy by medicines producers in India (which was not required to grant medicines patents until 2005), patents on ARVs in a number of developing countries blocked access to these lower-cost generic medicines.

Yet, by 2010, in comparison to the maximalist IP rules established in 1994, the IP regime had undergone significant changes to take public health concerns into greater account. Specifically, the policy space had considerably expanded for developing countries to take a more flexible approach to patent protection in order to ensure protection of public health. By 2010, over 60 countries had used flexibilities in IP rules to access generic medicines ('t Hoen 2009); the price of ARVs had fallen from US$10,000 to as little as US$67 ppy due to generic competition (Médecins Sans Frontières, 2010); and generics comprised 95 percent (by volume) of the global donor-funded ARV market (Waning *et al.*, 2010). Furthermore, WTO members had agreed upon an amendment to TRIPS to facilitate trade in generic versions of patented medicines (the 30 August decision), several countries had implemented patent laws with strong public health protections (most notably Brazil and India, as discussed further below), and policies to facilitate access to medicines had become commonplace across the pharmaceutical industry.

These changes were driven by a loose, globally networked coalition of several leading developing country governments, CSOs in the north and south, and a global community of legal, economic and scientific experts (Moon, 2010). Among the governments and CSOs that played an important role in re-shaping the global IP regime, a number were in Asia: Thailand, India, Indonesia[4] and Malaysia in particular.

Defining norms on trade and health – the Doha Declaration

From the outset, the effort to harmonise IP rules across countries created a rift between industrialised and developing countries. At the heart of this controversy was the question of what kind of IP system would best serve an individual country's level of development, and the extent to which developing countries would have the autonomy to adopt patent policies to meet their national needs. During the 1986–1994 Uruguay Round of trade negotiations within the Generalized Agreement on Tariffs and Trade (GATT), industrialised countries and a coalition of IP-intensive industries in the US, Europe and Japan (including pharmaceuticals, chemicals, information technology, media and other IP-intensive industries) had pushed to include IP as a trade issue (Sell, 2003). In general, developing countries had been opposed to the inclusion of IP in the Uruguay Round, since IP rights-holders were predominantly in the north. However, industrialised countries overcame their opposition with a combination of carrots (e.g. concessions on textiles and agriculture) and sticks (e.g. trade sanctions). For example, South Korea began granting product patents on pharmaceuticals in the mid-1980s after the US-based Pharmaceutical Manufacturers' Association (PMA) brought a complaint to the US Trade Representative (USTR) under Section 301 of the US Trade Act (Drahos and Braithwaite, 2002). Section 301 (later renamed Special 301) required USTR to issue an annual list of countries whose domestic IP systems did not meet US requirements, ranked in increasing order of severity from 'Watch List' to 'Priority Watch List' to 'Priority Foreign Country', which was the precursor to trade sanctions (e.g. withdrawal of benefits or increased tariffs on a country's exports to the US).

Many high-income countries had adopted flexible IP policies at various points in time as they industrialised, starting by imitating technologies developed elsewhere before developing domestic innovative capacity. Furthermore, prior to TRIPS, many countries had excluded medicines, food and agricultural technologies from patentability in order to protect social welfare. A number of high-income countries had delayed granting such patents until late in their industrialisation – for example, Spain did not begin granting medicines patents until 1992. TRIPS took these development strategies off the table by requiring developing countries to adopt the IP standards of industrialised countries. One study of 150 years of patent policy concluded that it would be problematic to 'mechanistically transfer[ing] the intellectual property practices in place in the developed world to developing countries' (Lerner, 1999).

The TRIPS regime included a number of flexibilities to give developing countries some policy space in adapting their national IP laws to meet WTO requirements. For example, TRIPS provided for a transition period, which gave national governments some leeway in deciding when to become fully TRIPS-compliant. In addition, the regime included provisions that allowed national governments to make exceptions to patent rules if they so wished; for example they could issue compulsory licenses for patented products, or allow parallel importation from countries in which they were offered at a price below the manufacturer's local price. However, the actual practice of when and how these provisions were going to be applied was unclear at the time. In fact, USTR's Section 301 effectively suggested that bilateral trade pressure could render TRIPS flexibilities essentially useless.

It was in the public health domain that TRIPS became the target of the most heated debate and contestation. In response to TRIPS in general, and to the expected increase in medicines prices in particular, a growing coalition of developing country governments, CSOs and individual experts began to challenge the new IP rules. AIDS activists advocating for broader access to treatment were a major driving force of this coalition. From the late 1990s to 2001, a number of key events took place that pushed the issue of patents and access to medicines onto the global public agenda. The rising public pressure culminated at the 2001 WTO Ministerial conference in Doha, Qatar, at which all Members agreed to the Doha Declaration on TRIPS and Public Health. The Doha Declaration stated that TRIPS

> does not and should not prevent Members from taking measures to protect public health . . . [and] can and should be interpreted and implemented in a manner supportive of WTO Members' right to protect public health and, in particular, to promote access to medicines for all.

It went on to clarify that countries had the right to make full use of TRIPS flexibilities, such as compulsory licensing (CL), and also extended the deadline for Least Developed Countries (LDCs) to implement or enforce pharmaceutical patents until at least 2016.

In the years following Doha, a number of political contests took place over the meaning, contours and degree of flexibility that would be permitted under the Doha Declaration. Malaysia, Thailand and India were key battlegrounds, as the following sections explain, and the outcome of these battles played a critical role in expanding both national and global policy space for other developing countries to make use of TRIPS flexibilities to protect public health. Such flexibilities included compulsory licensing, parallel importation, strict patentability criteria, the full use of transition periods for LDCs and a range of other measures.

Expanding policy space for health within trade rules: how Asian countries shaped the global IP regime

The Doha Declaration explicitly established the norm that, in principle, public health needs were an appropriate reason to use the flexibilities contained in TRIPS. However, fundamental questions remained open. First, could developing country governments actually make use of the flexibilities without suffering repercussions from industrialised countries in other areas? Secondly, how and when could they be used? For which types of medicines? What would qualify as a politically acceptable reason to issue a compulsory license? How extensively or often could these provisions be used in practice?

Legally, based on the text of the TRIPS Agreement and the Doha Declaration, it was clear that countries had wide latitude 'to determine the grounds upon which such [compulsory] licenses are granted' (World Trade Organization, 2001). However, politically, what counted as rule-breaking in 2001 was not very clear. The evolution of perceptions around the use of TRIPS flexibilities – which have become more widely accepted as rule-shaping rather than rule-breaking – was a key change in the access to medicines policy arena over the past decade.

The cases of Malaysia, Thailand and India shed light on how these changes came about. In each of these cases, the national government was pressed by CSOs to balance public health needs with outside pressures in the trade domain. As the following paragraphs will show, the three cases vary along two dimensions – first, the type of national intellectual property systems that governments first implemented, and at what point they implemented them. And secondly, the degree to which they used the TRIPS flexibilities, and for what types of public health needs. The two points are interrelated. Malaysia and Thailand yielded to US pressure and implemented Western-style IP systems earlier than required by TRIPS, but then issued compulsory licenses on drugs they considered essential. In contrast, India made full use of the transition period and amended its patent law to become TRIPS-compliant in 2005; rather than using compulsory licensing on a case-by-case basis, as other countries had, the Indian Parliament built a number of public interest safeguards into the 2005 Patents (Amendment) Act that systematically expanded policy space for the production of generic medicines (Kapczynski, 2009; Park and Menghaney, 2010).

Collectively, these Asian countries contributed to reshaping shared understandings regarding how TRIPS could be interpreted and implemented.[5] In contrast, China did not make use of any of the main TRIPs flexibilities with respect to medicines, despite clear public health needs; it therefore provides an exceptional and theoretically useful case to test broader propositions regarding the role of Asian countries in shaping the global IP regime.

Malaysia: establishing a precedent

Malaysia was the first developing country in Asia to issue a compulsory license on a medicine, and only the second developing country to do so worldwide (after Zimbabwe). As in Zimbabwe, the CL was issued for HIV/AIDS drugs. In the context of the global HIV/AIDS epidemic, which was increasingly being conceptualised as a global threat, Malaysia's example helped establish the principle that developing countries could make use of TRIPS flexibilities to obtain generic ARVs at lower cost to address the HIV/AIDS epidemic.

Since 2001, the Malaysian Ministry of Health (MoH) had been negotiating with pharmaceutical companies GlaxoSmithKline (GSK) and Bristol Myers Squibb (BMS) for lower prices on several HIV medicines, but without success. In 2002, Penang-based Third World Network, one of the leading international NGOs active on IP and medicines issues, began providing technical support to the MoH to begin working on a compulsory license (personal communication, Yoke Ling

Chee, 2010). Bolstered by the Doha Declaration, in November 2002, the MoH received Cabinet approval to begin importing generic versions of patented ARVs under a government use authorisation (a compulsory license for public non-commercial use) to supply the national health system (Chee, 2006). Several months later, GSK offered to drop the price of its two-drug ARV combination (zidovudine + lamivudine) by 57 percent – a significant decrease, but still costlier than the generic equivalent. The Ministry of Domestic Trade and Consumer Affairs, which had authority to grant a compulsory license under Malaysian law, was initially opposed to the compulsory license for fear of its potentially negative effect on foreign investment. However, the provision of technical expertise and mobilisation from civil society groups – including influence wielded by the Prime Minister's daughter, who was an AIDS activist – helped to shift the opinion of the government. In November 2003, the Trade Ministry agreed to issue the CL for a period of two years for three drugs patented by GSK and BMS, which had earlier warned that this decision would set an undesirable precedent and could hurt Malaysia's investment climate. Soon after, the MoH began providing ARV treatment free of charge with generic drugs imported from Cipla in India, which cost about 80 percent less than their patented counterparts. This price decrease enabled the Ministry to increase the number of patients on ARVI from 1500 to 4000 (Chee, 2006).

The Malaysian decision did indeed set a precedent and drew attention, particularly in neighbouring countries. TWN and other international NGOs, such as Médecins Sans Frontières (MSF), Knowledge Ecology International (KEI), and Oxfam, used their global networks to share details of the Malaysian experience with other developing country governments. In October 2004, Indonesia followed Malaysia's lead, and in 2006 Thailand would as well. The Malaysian CL was of particular importance because it was one of the first signals to the global community that developing countries could and would indeed make use of TRIPS flexibilities in the post-Doha era. While the language in the Doha Declaration unambiguously stated that 'each Member has the right to grant compulsory licences and the freedom to determine the grounds upon which such licences are granted' (World Trade Organization, 2001), in 2003, it was not yet clear whether countries would actually make use of this new political space. Two full years after the Doha Declaration, only two countries had, and fears still ran deep among developing country governments that use of such measures would hurt trade and investment relations. Therefore, Malaysia's precedent-setting decision and its impact on other countries qualify it as a 'rule-shaper'.

Thailand: extending the exception to chronic diseases

Thailand has played a central role in shaping global IP rules on pharmaceuticals. The Thai government first yielded to external trade pressures by implementing pharmaceutical product patents in 1992 (over a decade earlier than would be required by TRIPS), but then subsequently set a precedent in 2006–7 with the number, scope and high political profile of its compulsory licensing decisions.

Intellectual property rules have been a hotly contested issue in Thailand's foreign relations since at least the 1980s. For example, in 1988 the US-based PMA (later PhRMA) filed a Special 301 complaint on Thailand with the USTR over the country's 1979 Patent Law, which disallowed patents on food, medicines and agricultural machinery (Kirchanski, 1993). In response, the US revoked preferential access to the US market on a number of goods, denying duty-free status to US$165 million of Thai exports (Rust 1992). At the time, 20-25 percent of Thailand's exports went to the US, making it Thailand's largest export market (McDorman, 1992). Within a year of the trade sanctions, the Thai Assembly had passed a new law that granted product patents on pharmaceuticals, despite opposition from local industry, academics, NGOs, doctors associations and within government (MacLeod, 1992; McDorman, 1992). During this era, Thailand could fairly be characterised as a 'rule-taker' in the IP arena.

However, the situation began to change at the turn of the millennium, as Thai CSOs – particularly HIV/AIDS groups – began developing literacy on IP issues and building linkages with international CSOs working on IP and access to medicines. With an estimated one million people living with HIV in 1999, Thailand had been struck with the worst HIV/AIDS epidemic in Asia, but had also mounted an effective and widely admired public health response. Very few people had access to ART in the late 1990s – only 5-10 percent of people in need had access to any ARV drug at all, and only 1 percent to the three-drug combinations required to suppress HIV; triple-therapy cost about US$675/month (US$8100/year) – over five times the average office worker's salary of US$120 (Sakboon, 1999; Wilson *et al.*, 1999). The government had provided monotherapy with zidovudine (AZT, available as a generic) since 1992, dual-therapy with the addition of ddI in 1995, and in 2000, triple-therapy – but high drug costs restricted access to such treatment to only 1500-2000 patients out of several hundred thousand estimated to be in need (Revenga *et al.* 2006).

Civil society groups initially focused on the ARV didanosine (ddI), which had been invented by the US National Institutes of Health and licensed to BMS. In the late 1990s, BMS sold ddI for 178 Thai Baht (THB) (US$3.36)/day,[6] which exceeded the daily basic wage of 120 THB (US$2.26)/day (Wisartsakul, 2004). A broad coalition of Thai actors, including the Government Pharmaceutical Organization (a state-owned drug manufacturer), the academic Drug Study Group based at Chulalongkorn University, MSF, and People Living with HIV/AIDS (PLWHA) groups, formed the Working Group to Challenge the ddI Patent. The Thai Network of Positive People (TNP+) also requested that the Ministry of Public Health (MoPH) grant a compulsory license on ddI, and set up camp at the MoPH offices to draw public attention to their cause. The MoPH denied their request in early 2000, after officials from both the Health and Commerce ministries 'expressed great caution in pursuing the issue for fear of US retaliation' (Bhatiasevi and Maneerungsee, 2000).

However, the Working Group continued pursuing its challenge of the ddI patent, and in May 2001, the AIDS Access Foundation and two PLWHAs filed suit against the patent's validity at the Thai Intellectual Property court, becoming the first patient groups to contest a patent in Thailand (and possibly in any developing country). In October 2002, the court affirmed the right of patients to challenge patents as 'interested parties' – an important decision because BMS had argued that patients did not have the legal standing to contest the patent. In addition, the court found that BMS had unlawfully omitted critical information from its ddI patent application, which comprised grounds for revoking the patent. Though BMS initially appealed the decision, in December 2003, the company reached a settlement with the CSOs: BMS would withdraw its appeal in exchange for the CSOs withdrawing their suit to revoke the patent. The practical effect was the removal of the monopoly on ddI (Ford *et al.*, 2004; Wisartsakul, 2004). The overturning of the Thai patent on ddI marked a major victory for public health CSOs in Thailand, and also set an important example that civil society groups would emulate in Brazil, India and China. (CSOs in different countries often shared legal strategies, in addition to technical information, to support like-minded efforts taking place in other national contexts.) The ddI issue also built up literacy on IP issues within Thai civil society and the MoPH, which established a foundation on which Thailand's compulsory licensing decisions would build a few years later.

Thailand launched its first universal health insurance program in 2002. The newly created National Health Security Office (NHSO) had included antiretroviral therapy (ART) among its covered services, after strong civil society reaction to the initial exclusion of ART. Significantly, the high cost of ARV drugs began directly impacting the government budget. Discussions on how to address high drug prices had been ongoing within NHSO and other parts of the government for several years. According to one official present at a January 2006 intragovernmental meeting, the question arose as to why Thailand had not made use of compulsory licensing, as its fellow South East Asian countries Malaysia and Indonesia had done (Tantivess *et al.*, 2008). Precedents set in other parts of the region seemed to carry more weight than examples from Latin America or sub-Saharan Africa.

After several years of negotiations with patent-holders, in late 2006, the Thai government issued its first compulsory license on efavirenz, an ARV patented by the pharmaceutical company Merck (Ministry of Public Health [Thailand] and National Health Security Office [Thailand] 2007). The CL was one of the first decisions of Health Minister Mongkol na Songkhla, who took office after Prime Minister Thaksin Shinawatra was ousted by a military coup. Mongkol was a long-time civil servant in the health ministry and familiar with the many debates on IP and medicines prices over the years. The CL enabled the government to import generic efavirenz at half the Merck price (after Merck had offered additional discounts), which enabled the government to expand coverage with efavirenz to an additional 20,000 patients (Tantivess *et al.*, 2008).

Initial reaction to the compulsory licensing announcement was relatively muted – there was almost no coverage in the Western media, a relatively subdued public reaction from Merck, and praise from international CSOs and UNAIDS (Moon, 2010). Arguably, by 2006, a precarious norm had taken hold that compulsory licensing of HIV/AIDS medicines in developing countries was permissible.

However, the relative calm dissipated in January 2007, when the government announced CLs on two additional medicines: American firm Abbott's HIV/AIDS drug lopinavir/ritonavir (Kaletra), and French firm Sanofi's clopidogrel (Plavix), a blood-thinning agent for heart disease and hypertension. This time, the international reaction was more pronounced: the multinational pharmaceutical industry's association in Thailand publicly criticised the decision and questioned its legality; Abbott announced it was withdrawing seven medicines from Thailand; the European Commissioner for Trade, Peter Mandelson, wrote to express his concern, as did 17 Members of the US Congress; and even WHO Director General Margaret Chan seemed to question the Thai decision.

However, international support from other quarters was also strong: international CSOs, such as MSF, Oxfam, KEI and Health GAP, provided political and technical support to the government; former US President Bill Clinton defended the decision; 22 Members of the US Congress had written to USTR urging it to respect the Thai government's right to issue compulsory licenses; the European Parliament passed a resolution endorsing use of TRIPS flexibilities such as compulsory licensing; and Margaret Chan clarified her support for the decision. An international day of action to protest Abbott's unprecedented move resulted in public demonstrations at Abbott offices and research labs in the United Kingdom, France, the US (Chicago headquarters, Washington DC, New York, Austin, and Worcester, MA), India, Germany, Switzerland, Argentina, Brazil, Kenya, Singapore, New Zealand, Australia, Japan, China, Vietnam and Indonesia.

In January 2008, just before leaving office as the democratically elected government returned, Health Minister Mongkol announced compulsory licenses for four additional medicines, all cancer drugs: docetaxel, erlotinib, letrozole and imatinib (Limpananont *et al.*, 2009). When the new Health Minister, Chaiya Somsab, took over in February 2008, one of his first announcements was that he would revoke the compulsory licenses. Civil society groups reacted immediately, and within a few weeks, Chaiya had shifted his position – the compulsory licensing policy would stay. Though the initial CLs had been criticised in the Western media as illegitimate because of the military government from which they originated, the persistence of the CL policy in the new government suggested that public support for such measures was widespread. Novartis offered a donation of its blockbuster drug imatinib (Glivec), and averted the implementation of the license. The government moved ahead with the other three drugs.

The global political battle over Thailand's compulsory licensing policy was a reflection that its decisions did not impact Thailand alone. At stake were two unsettled issues: would compulsory licensing for non-AIDS medicines be politically tolerated? And how regularly could governments use compulsory licensing? It is important to point out that *legally* the answers to both questions were unambiguous; there was formal legal consensus that both TRIPS and Thai national legislation allowed for use of compulsory licensing for various public health problems. The political contest over the decision was, rather, over the *informal* rules and norms of the global IP regime, and how broadly the Doha Declaration would be interpreted. According to a pharmaceutical industry source speaking on Thailand, 'We thought we had an agreement on how the TRIPS mechanisms should be used, but obviously we have different interpretations . . . In this case, it is one government and the entire NGO community that think this is justified' (as quoted in Gerhardsen, 2007).

Indonesia issued a compulsory license on efavirenz three months after the Thai decision, and Brazil followed suit three months after. The timing of Indonesia's decision, the fact that it concerned the same drug targeted by Thailand and the close relationships between the two governments via ASEAN suggests that the Thai decision influenced that of its neighbor. Similarly, the timing of Brazil's compulsory license, and the close ties between civil society groups in Brazil and Thailand, suggest that the Thai precedent shaped the Brazilian decision. Notably, this was Brazil's first issued compulsory license, after eight years of publicly threatening to do so. Overall, Thailand's decisions expanded policy space to use TRIPS flexibilities for medicines other than ARVs, increased the political acceptability of compulsory licensing and strengthened global norms that prioritised public health over stringent IP protection. The Thai government has also influenced global norms through its active participation in global debates, for example, during the 2006–2008 Intergovernmental Working Group on Public Health, Innovation and Intellectual Property convened by the WHO. The Thai delegation was one of the most vocal advocates calling for flexibility in the application of IP rules, and for the protection of public health to remain a central concern.

The government announced in August 2010 an extension of the compulsory licenses on the two AIDS drugs until their respective patent expiry dates, 2012 for efavirenz and 2016 for lopinavir/ritonavir. It estimated that the CL policy had saved the government THB1.18 billion (US$36 million); and increased the number of patients accessing efavirenz from 4539 to 29,360, and those receiving lopinavir/ritonavir from 39 to 6200 (Treerutkuarkul, 2010).[7]

India: from exception to rule – expanding national policy space

The Indian case differs from the previous two in its more systematic approach to building a public health-friendly patent system. While Malaysia and Thailand shaped the rules that determined *exceptions* to patent protection under their own national patent laws, India designed its patent laws to reduce the need to use compulsory licensing in the first place. Consequently, while the controversies in Thailand and Malaysia were over compulsory licenses for patented drugs, India's controversies focused on the question of whether or not certain drugs were going to be granted patents in the first place.

India's generic pharmaceutical industry is one of the country's major success stories. As the 'pharmacy of the developing world', it plays a central role in the global supply of low-cost generic medicines, and is steadily increasing its share of high-income markets as well. For example, Indian-produced generics comprise over 80 percent (by volume) of the donor-funded global ARV market, and are priced consistently and considerably lower than generics produced in other countries (Waning *et al.*, 2010). The industry has its roots in the 1970 Patents

Act, which abolished product patents on medicines and reduced the term of process patents from 16 to 7 years (Sahu, 1998). In 1970, Indian firms controlled 32 percent of the domestic pharmaceutical market, while multinational firms controlled the remainder; by 2000, this ratio had been reversed (Chaudhuri, 2005).

During the Uruguay Round, India (together with Brazil) had been one of the main developing country opponents of a binding IP treaty. However, it dropped its opposition in 1989 after the US included India on the Special 301 Priority Watch List. The US elevated India to the Priority Foreign Country ranking in 1991, suspended preferential market access for some products and raised tariffs on US$80 million worth of Indian exports (Watal, 2001). However, unlike many other developing countries that underwent similar economic pressure, the Indian government did not change its patent law to meet US demands (Watal, 2001). As a result, India was able to take full advantage of the TRIPS transition period for developing countries and was not obliged to provide pharmaceutical product patents until 1 January 2005. When 2005 arrived, however, fears ran high that TRIPS would close down the 'pharmacy' and leave patients in India and around the world empty-handed.

While TRIPS meant that India could not avoid product patents on medicines altogether, its Parliament crafted a patent law that contained an unprecedented degree of flexibility intended to maintain as much policy space as possible (see Kapczynski, 2009 for a full legal analysis of the law; see Park and Menghaney, 2010 for an analysis of Section 3(d) and its application). The flexibilities in the law can be credited, at least in part, to the mobilisation of international and national CSOs, domestic industry, sympathetic Parliamentarians, international political leaders and legal experts. One clause that has drawn particular attention is Section 3(d), which sets high patentability criteria that would reduce the number of patents granted (Press Information Bureau, Ministry of Commerce and Industry, Government of India, 2005). In other words, medicines that might be patentable in other countries, such as the US or in Europe, might not be eligible for patents in India.

The first case to test Section 3(d) concerned Novartis' cancer drug imatinib mesylate (brand name Glivec), 'a miracle drug for the new century' (Strom and Fleischer-Black, 2003), used to treat chronic myeloid leukemia and other relatively rare cancers. Novartis filed a patent application for the beta-crystalline form of imatinib mesylate in 1998. In 2003, Novartis was granted a temporary market monopoly while the patent application was under examination, during which time the company sold the drug in India at US$30,000/year. When the patent application came up for examination, the application was opposed by the Cancer Patients Aid Association (a Mumbai-based CSO), represented by the Lawyers Collective HIV/AIDS Unit as legal counsel, and Indian generic firms Natco Pharma and Cipla using a procedural mechanism built into the new patent law (George *et al.*, 2009). In January 2006, the Indian patent office denied a patent on the application, arguing that the beta-crystalline form of imatinib mesylate was a polymorph of a salt of imatinib, and therefore 'only a new form of a known substance' (Office of the Controller General of Patents, Designs & Trade Marks, 2006). The patent examiner found the application did not meet the standard for inventive step nor improved efficacy set by Section 3(d) (among other grounds). This decision demonstrated that the new patent law could be implemented in a manner that would result in far fewer patents being granted in India than elsewhere.

In August 2006, Novartis challenged the patent office's decision and Section 3(d) at the Chennai High Court, on the grounds that it was unconstitutional and did not comply with TRIPS. In response, a global political mobilisation coalesced against Novartis. Protesters organised demonstrations at Novartis offices in India and Switzerland; NGOs organised international petitions demanding that Novartis drop the case; shareholders asked the CEO to drop the case at the annual meeting; high-profile individuals, including South African Archbishop Desmond Tutu, Global Fund Director Michel Kazatchkine, members from the European Parliament and the US Congress and former Swiss President Ruth Dreifuss[8] (which was particularly poignant since Novartis was a Swiss firm), did the same (Cancer Patients Aid Association *et al.*, 2007).

In August 2007, the Chennai High Court upheld the patent office rejection and the constitutionality of Section 3(d). Novartis appealed the decision on its patent application, but did not appeal regarding Section 3(d). (The Swiss government also declined to challenge the patent law's compliance with TRIPS at the WTO.) In 2009, the Intellectual Property Appellate Board (IPAB), a judicial body newly created to manage patent disputes, rejected the application, upholding the lower courts' rulings. Novartis appealed the decision: the case is expected to be heard by the Supreme Court but is still pending at the time of writing (August 2012).

In the meantime, CSOs and generic firms have successfully opposed a number of other patent applications, including those on valganciclovir, a formulation of nevirapine, and the combination of zidovudine and lamivudine – all products for the treatment of HIV infection.

The Indian Patents Act has set an important precedent, and signalled to other developing countries the possibility of new policy space. In 2008, for example, the Philippines adopted a clause identical to Section 3(d) in its 2008 Medicines Act (Hechanova, 2008); staff from India's Lawyers Collective supported efforts to adopt the legal provision in the Philippines law. In addition, similar measures may be under consideration in other parts of the region including in Bangladesh, Indonesia, Malaysia, the Maldives, Pakistan, Sri Lanka and Vietnam, according to media reports (Ollier, 2008). In addition, CSOs in Brazil have also filed oppositions on key patent applications, in collaboration with their counterparts in India. In this way, the actions of Indian civil society, companies, courts and legislature have influenced the global IP regime, and signalled India's transition from a rule-taker in the 1980s to a rule-shaper in the present era.

China: a puzzling rising power

China's approach to managing IP rules and public health concerns provides a theoretically useful contrast to the experience of the countries described above. Despite its considerable public health needs and growing power in the global system, the Chinese government did not challenge the global IP regime, nor did it take advantage of the increasing policy space in the global regime to improve access to medicines for its population. From an economic and public health perspective, China had strong incentives to challenge the TRIPS regime: a more flexible IP regime would have been favorable to many of its industries, including a significant and growing generic pharmaceutical industry, and its public health needs were considerable and increasing. China also faced a spreading HIV epidemic in the 1990s and 2000s, and the high cost of HIV medicines posed a significant barrier to the development of an effective government treatment program. What accounts for China's approach to the global IP regime?

China adopted its first patent law in 1984, and began granting product patents on pharmaceuticals for the first time in 1993 after coming under bilateral economic pressure from the US. Dissatisfied with Chinese IP policies, US businesses had succeeded in getting the country included on the Priority Watch List in USTR's 1989 Special 301 report and downgraded to the most severe category of Priority Foreign Country in 1991. USTR threatened to impose US$1.5 billion of retaliatory tariffs against Chinese exports, which ultimately led China to sign the 1992 Memorandum of Understanding on the Protection of Intellectual Property (MoU) with the US. In line with the MoU, China amended its patent law to begin granting pharmaceutical product patents in 1993, extended patent terms from 15 to 20 years, limited the scope of compulsory licensing and granted retroactive monopoly protection to pharmaceuticals patented before 1993 through the 'Administrative Protection' system. The Administrative Protection system created monopolies for over 100 newer medicines, all of which were patented by foreign nationals or companies (Gao, 1998). These legal provisions would significantly curtail the availability of effective AIDS treatment several years later when one of the most important ARVs, lamivudine, was granted administrative protection.

During this period, China could fairly be characterised as a 'rule-taker' with respect to IP. Because China was not a GATT member, it had not participated in the negotiation of the TRIPS Agreement. From 1993 to 2003, in order to alleviate US trade pressure and gain entry into the WTO, China amended its patent law several more times to adopt increasingly stringent IP measures, including a number of provisions beyond those required by the TRIPS Agreement ('TRIPS-plus' measures such as patent-registration linkage and data exclusivity).

At the same time, pressure was mounting on the government to respond to a growing HIV epidemic, which was spreading in different parts of the country due to contaminated blood-selling practices, injecting drug use and commercial sex work, among other factors. In 2003, in an abrupt policy shift following the SARS epidemic, the government began to expand its efforts to prevent and treat HIV. It launched the 'Four Frees and One Care' policy, which promised to provide ARV drugs to people in rural areas and the urban poor. As in other developing countries that had adopted pharmaceutical patents in the 1990s, several ARVs were available as generics, including zidovudine, stavudine and nevirapine. However, lamivudine, a key drug recommended by WHO for first-line treatment, was under monopoly protection by GSK. Because lamivudine was also used to treat hepatitis B (HBV), it was a particularly lucrative drug in China, which has the world's largest population of HBV carriers. GSK offered to donate lamivudine to the Four Frees and One Care program, but key conditions of the donation (such as quantities and time-limits) were kept confidential, and AIDS NGOs consistently reported lamivudine shortages throughout the country (Wang *et al.*, 2009; Zhang *et al.*, 2009). Despite persistent advocacy from national and international civil society organisations, the government did not use flexibilities in its patent law to improve access to lower-cost generic lamivudine.

The potential public health consequences of the lamivudine shortage were significant. Instead of receiving lamivudine, patients were treated with ddI-based combinations that had serious side effects; some researchers suspected the widespread use of ddI contributed to low rates of patient adherence to treatment and, as a result, high rates of resistance. A 2005 study of patients in Henan province found adherence rates of only 33.9 percent after six months of therapy (Li *et al.* 2005); these levels were far below the 95 percent adherence rate recommended to achieve effective viral suppression and minimise the risk of resistance. Low adherence rates were thought to be responsible for the high rates of resistance found in this population: 45.4 percent after three months, and 62.7 percent after six months (Zhang *et al.*, 2009). Once HIV develops resistance to first-line antiretrovirals, patients should be switched to second-line drugs; however, most of these were patented in China and considered too costly for the government treatment program. While generic lamivudine is now widely available in many developing countries, it remains under monopoly protection in China as of early 2011.

Unlike other countries in Asia, the government has not yet made use of patent law flexibilities to improve access to generic medicines, despite repeated and increasing calls from civil society to do so. In addition to advocacy around lamivudine, the CSO AIDS Care China has submitted a motion for several years in a row for compulsory licensing of ARVs and cancer drugs to the National People's Congress, China's legislative body. In 2006, PLWHA groups across the country signed a petition in support of an opposition filed by MSF against the granting of a patent on tenofovir, a key drug for both first- and second-line AIDS treatment. While the tenofovir patent was not granted in India or Brazil (in part due to public health safeguards built into each country's legal system), the patent was granted in China. In a sign of an increasingly active civil society, in 2007, Chinese CSOs demonstrated against Abbott Laboratories to express their solidarity with Thai HIV/AIDS groups after Abbott removed drugs from the Thai market following the country's compulsory licenses.

In summary, despite a clear public health need and repeated requests from an increasingly well-organised civil society, the Chinese government has neither challenged the global IP regime nor made use of the legal or political space that existed to improve access to medicines.

However, there are some signs that Chinese patent policies may be starting to shift; reversing a two-decade trend towards more stringent IP protection, in 2008 the patent law was revised to incorporate greater flexibility and public interest protections that had been weak or absent in earlier versions of the legislation. For example, the 2001 Doha Declaration has been incorporated into the law (e.g. to facilitate export of medicines produced under compulsory license), the link between competition law and patent law has been strengthened, parallel imports are allowed and measures to accelerate the introduction of generics (i.e. Bolar exceptions) have been included. In addition, in an attempt to protect its long history of traditional medicine, the law also includes for the first time a 'disclosure of origin' requirement in patent applications, when the invention draws from traditional knowledge (Cohen *et al.*, 2009; Wang *et al.*, 2009). These are important TRIPS safeguards that the WHO, legal experts and access to medicines advocates had long advised developing countries to adopt. According to the head of the patent office, revisions to the laws were intended 'to make the compulsory licensing system compatible with the need to cope with public health crises' (Yin Xintian quoted in Yan, 2010). It remains unclear whether China will make use of patent law flexibilities for public health purposes; nevertheless, the legal changes reflect an important shift in the government's thinking on how to protect public health within the IP system. These changes suggest that China may in the future shift from being a rule-taker to a rule-shaper.

Implications for global (health) governance

The previous sections explained how several Asian governments and CSOs shaped the way TRIPS is interpreted and applied with respect to public health. This section will focus on the broader implications of this case study for questions of sovereignty and world order, conceptions and contributions from Asia and institutional diversity.

Sovereignty and world order

How is the institution of sovereignty changing in an era of globalisation? The TRIPS regime as it was conceived in the mid-1990s was, arguably, the strongest challenge to classical concepts of sovereignty posed by any WTO agreement. Particularly for developing countries, it restricted the freedom to tailor national IP systems to meet national needs by mandating minimum standards based on Western laws; it also required dramatic changes to domestic laws and practices in multiple areas with impact on human well-being (e.g. health, agriculture, education, traditional knowledge). Private actors – specifically, global pharmaceutical companies – directly challenged the ability of developing country governments to set national patent policies, for example, when Novartis contested the 2005 Indian Patents Act, and when the industry opposed the Thai decision to make use of TRIPS flexibilities.

However, the global social reaction to TRIPS – particularly the mobilisation of key developing country governments in collaboration with civil society groups against the impact of TRIPS on medicines prices – suggested that sovereignty could be reasserted in the name of public health. It also demonstrated that transnational coalitions of public health actors could challenge their own and other governments, as well as international organisations. As a consequence, governments could reclaim a certain measure of sovereignty to determine their domestic patent policies within the broad confines of the global IP regime. It is important to note that governments did not win back this policy space alone, but nearly always by acting in coalitions – at national or global level – with other governments, CSOs, international organisations and experts. Thus, in a globalising system, the reassertion of sovereignty was made possible by taking a more permeable approach to the very concept of sovereignty; governments did not turn their backs on the global IP regime, but rather, challenged and re-shaped it by working in loose coalitions with other state and non-state actors. In general, a broad range of actors (multinational firms, CSOs, UN agencies and experts) influenced the extent to which developing country governments could exercise sovereignty on public health matters vis-à-vis global IP rules.

Conceptions and contributions from Asia

As detailed above, several Asian countries challenged and successfully reshaped global IP rules. In particular, Malaysia and Indonesia were among the first countries to use TRIPS flexibilities to improve access to HIV/AIDS medicines and set precedents that other countries could follow. India and Thailand further expanded the policy space to use such flexibilities for medicines beyond HIV/AIDS, and employed new strategies (patentability criteria, patient oppositions to patents on technical grounds) to broaden access to generic medicines. Notably, each of these countries was a middle-income country and an emerging market, none were least-developed countries or very small economies, thus the stakes were higher for both the pharmaceutical industry and for governments. For industry, emerging markets are expected to be the main source of global growth in the coming decade, and the interpretation of IP rules in these markets could have a significant impact on revenue. For governments of middle-income countries, many are undergoing epidemiological transitions and grappling with an increased burden from non-communicable diseases; at the same time, increased economic development can lead to growing demands for the expansion of social insurance and improved access to a broader range of medicines, with serious budget implications for governments. The Thai experience is illustrative: when the government began implementing its first universal national health insurance program in 2003, its budget was directly impacted for the first time by the effect of strict patent rules on medicines prices. However, these conditions were conducive but not sufficient. As the Chinese case illustrates, public health need and budget considerations alone are insufficient to convince a government to challenge the prevailing global IP regime. Nor was economic power a sole explanatory factor – smaller countries that depended to a significant extent on access to US and EU markets, still challenged global IP rules. The key factor seems to have been a well-organised domestic civil society that was closely networked with international CSOs, experts and international organisations;

furthermore, political space had to exist at the national level for CSOs to challenge their governments.

While several Asian countries have been influential in shaping global IP rules, there is little evidence for the existence of a general 'Asian' approach or 'Asian' conception of global IP rules. Rather, Asian countries have taken diverse positions and roles in global IP debates. Thus far, the only Asian country that could be categorised as a 'rule-maker' is Japan. Japanese trade negotiators and businesses teamed up with their US and European counterparts during the GATT Uruguay Round to negotiate the key terms of the TRIPS Agreement. However, Japan has not been as aggressive as the US or EU in pursuing TRIPS-plus measures through bilateral trade agreements or other measures. Some middle-income Asian countries, as discussed above, have become 'rule-shapers' by challenging the way TRIPS provisions are interpreted and implemented, and by making permissible certain measures that had previously been understood as off-limits. Other Asian countries have largely been rule-takers, adapting their national laws and practices largely to meet the demands of the global IP regime and/or taking advantage of the policy space opened up by other countries; China is the most notable example, but other countries such as Cambodia and Vietnam could also be characterised this way. Rather than reflecting any unified regional conception or approach to IP, the role of various Asian countries seems to have been driven more by the level of economic development and strength of civil society mobilisation (a factor linked to political regime type) than by any shared cultural or geographic background.

Institutional diversity

Asian countries have exhibited a considerable amount of institutional diversity in their approaches to meeting global demands for IP protection while protecting public health at home. The extent to which individual countries have taken advantage of the legal and political space within the TRIPS regime has varied, depending on levels of economic development, domestic industrial concerns, and – perhaps most importantly – the political mobilisation of domestic and global civil society. External economic relations or power did not determine the degree to which a country challenged prevailing global IP norms. In 2000, Thailand, India and China each sent roughly the same proportion (19–20 percent) of their exports to the US market (International Trade Centre, 2010). Thailand, with roughly one-thirteenth the GDP of China in 2006 (the year of the Thai compulsory licenses), played a much larger role in shaping the global regime.

Rather, countries with civil societies and governments that were closely networked with the global access to medicines movement, most notably, Thailand and India, developed arguably the most public health-friendly national institutions for managing IP. In addition, India's strong domestic pharmaceutical industry likely played a very influential role. In contrast, in China, until very recently there have been few signs that public health concerns have shaped domestic IP institutions. This difference can be attributed, at least in part, to three factors: first,

China has come under greater trade pressure than any other developing country to implement stringent IP rules; secondly, China's pharmaceutical industry was not as advanced or as politically mobilised as its Indian counterpart; thirdly, the political space for CSOs to advocate for more health-friendly IP institutions is restricted in China relative to other countries. Whereas in India and Thailand, CSOs (and local firms) could work through the courts, legislature and executive to shape IP policies, in China such channels for potential influence were both fewer and narrower. In addition, while CSOs (particularly those working on the HIV/AIDS response) in India and Thailand are well-organised and deeply integrated in global civil society networks, groups in China are relatively smaller, less connected to global networks, and have a more constricted political space within which to develop. Despite China's greater overall weight in the global economy, its government did not choose to challenge IP rules in the interests of public health.

These roles may shift as the global pharmaceutical market and industry evolves. Not only are China and India (along with several other Asian emerging markets) expected to contribute a disproportionate share of growth in the global pharmaceutical market (IMS Health, 2010), they are also developing increased innovative capacity to research and develop new medicines. These efforts are manifested in both home-grown research efforts of local firms, universities and government programs, as well as partnerships with the major multinational pharmaceutical firms. Between 1994 and 2009, the proportion of patent applications filed by China, Japan and South Korea under the international Patent Cooperation Treaty process grew from 7.6 percent to 29.2 percent, and South Korea and China now rank among the top five sources of international patent applications (World Intellectual Property Organization, 2010).

Institutional diversity among Asian countries is likely to continue, particularly as the two regional superpowers become both innovators and consumers of medicines, while smaller countries largely remain net-importers of IP-intensive goods. The evolution of Chinese and Indian approaches to balancing IP policy with public health needs, and the underlying drivers of each country's approach, is an important area for future research. Thailand's trajectory, and that of other smaller countries, regarding the use of TRIPS flexibilities for a broader set of medicines (beyond HIV/AIDS) will also be a critical area for scholarly analysis. The resilience of coalitions formed in earlier days between key developing countries and other concerned actors also merits ongoing scholarly attention; whether and how these coalitions change, and how these changes impact global and national IP rules is open to debate.

Conclusions and future prospects

A number of Asian countries have reshaped the global IP regime to take public health concerns into greater account. While the TRIPS regime initially seemed to pose a direct challenge to the sovereignty of many developing countries, governments and CSOs succeeded in pushing back against the strictest elements of the regime to carve out expanded domestic and global policy space to facilitate access to medicines and to protect public health. Economic interests and the level of economic development broadly shaped a country's position on the IP regime, but were not determinative; rather, whether a country was a rule-shaper or rule-taker also depended on the strength of domestic civil society groups advocating for health concerns, and the global networks of which they were a part.

Compared to low-income countries, middle-income Asian countries had both greater domestic capacity to challenge – and more to gain from reshaping – global IP rules. It is no coincidence that challenges to the regime came from emerging economies, which are currently at a stage of industrialisation better served by more flexible IP rules. Middle-income countries also had greater capacity to provide improved health security, including access to therapeutically important newer medicines for their populations, through social insurance programs. What does this imply for the future?

If the growth of Asian economies continues to outpace countries in the West or in other parts of the developing world, their political power to shape global rules may also be expected to increase. Whether such an increase is proportional to economic power or not, however, is highly debatable. Such growth suggests that Asian countries will play a larger role in shaping global IP rules in the future. As demands for health services increase, societal pressure on governments to ensure that medicines are affordable and accessible may also increase. These factors suggest that many Asian countries will continue to push for more flexible IP rules.

However, whether all developing Asian countries will do so remains unclear. Understandings of the national interest in particular countries may change as some transition from being net importers to net exporters of IP-intensive products. What do these trends imply for the global IP regime in general, and for access to medicines for poorer populations in particular? Given the multiple competing forces at play, the role of particular Asian countries in shaping global IP rules is likely to be determined in national arenas, with strong influence exerted by global actors such as firms, CSOs and intergovernmental organisations. Political contestation over how the national interest gets defined is likely to sharpen. The interests of the poorest and most vulnerable are, perhaps, most likely to be defended where they are well organised politically, have sufficient political space within which to advance their interests, and can draw on global networks for additional economic, intellectual and normative resources. This analysis suggests, then, that increasing economic growth in Asia, and the concomitant rise in the region's political power in global affairs, will not automatically lead to a more stringent or flexible global IP regime. Rather, the outcome of national debates regarding the national interest – whether defined in economic or health terms – is likely to shape how a particular state engages with the global IP regime. The normative shift of the past decade that places relatively greater importance on public health, the strength of existing global civil society networks and the stage of industrialisation of many Asian countries, however, does suggest that we are likely to see Asian actors pushing successfully for a more flexible global IP regime.

Notes

1 We define 'developing countries' as low- and middle-income countries, as classified by the World Bank.
2 Patents are state-granted monopolies that allow the patent-holder to block others from making, using, selling, or offering to sell a product for a fixed period of time. During the patent term, the monopoly enables patent-holders to charge the highest price the market will bear, which allows the inventor to recoup investments in research and development (R&D), but can also render a product unaffordable to those who cannot pay monopoly prices.
3 The lowest generic price of US$350 for a triple-combination of ARVs in 2001 was offered by Cipla, an Indian generic firm. By 2010, the price of this combination had dropped to as low as US$67. We provide the 2001 price here, as it most accurately represents the potential cost-savings available to governments in the early 2000s when political debates on patents and access to medicines arose on the global public agenda.
4 Indonesia and the controversy over virus-sharing for avian flu vaccine was also a significant development in this context; we do not cover it here since it is the focus of several other chapters in this volume.
5 Nor were Asian countries the only ones active in global IP debates. The government of Brazil has been recognised has having exerted strong influence on IP rules, as well as South Africa, Argentina, Kenya and others.
6 Thai Baht converted to US$ based on average January 1998 exchange rate of 53 THB/US$ (www.oanda.com/currency/historical-rates).
7 Based on the exchange rate of 32.3 THB/US$ on 3 August 2010 (www.oanda.com).
8 Dreifuss was also the former chair of the WHO Commission on Intellectual Property, Innovation and Public Health (CIPIH), which issued its influential report in 2006 (Commission on Intellectual Property Rights, Innovation and Public Health, 2006). The CIPIH launched the two-year Intergovernmental Working Group on Public Health, Innovation and Intellectual Property, which culminated in the adoption of a Global Strategy and Plan of Action for WHO and its Member States. The Global Strategy explicitly calls for exploring the use of alternate incentive mechanisms, outside of traditional IP, to generate innovation targeted towards the needs of developing countries (World Health Organization, 2008b).

9 Global health research governance

An Asian perspective on the need for reform

Sara Bennett, Tikki Pang, Somsak Chunharas and Thaworn Sakhunpanit

Introduction

While certain aspects of global health research governance (GHRG) have received substantial attention, notably in the area of intellectual property as it applies to drug development, there have been few attempts to examine the array of governance functions necessary in the critical areas of research investment and priority-setting, equitable partnerships and capacity-building. Research governance faces many similar (and some different) challenges to that of global health governance. Ultimately, the products of research form the foundations for sustainable health improvement and human development. Thus research, and how it is governed, has ramifications far beyond the research world; research can play a critical role in conceptualizing issues, framing policy debates and setting policy agendas.

Health research is increasingly conducted by cross-border collaborations. This trend towards globalization has led to a growing sentiment that more effective mechanisms for global health research governance are required. The issue of GHRG has been implicit in research discussions for many years, but preparations for the International Conference on Health Research for Development 2000 brought this topic to the forefront and led to an attempt to examine global mechanisms for health research governance. Issues of GHRG were raised and debated again at the Mexico Summit on Health Research in 2004 (World Health Organisation, 2004c), where growing concerns about transparency and 'lack of trust' in health research were highlighted. The 2004 Mexico Summit called for international and national agencies to address this issue through strategies such as the establishment of a global register of clinical trials. Since then, issues of transparency and trust in health research have made headlines, with the now infamous Hwang Affair in which a prominent South Korean scientist falsely claimed in an article published in *Science* that his team had succeeded in creating the world's first cloned human embryonic stem cell line (Kim, 2009).

Transparency and trust have not been the only concerns with respect to GHRG. The refusal of the Indonesian government to share H5N1 viral samples with World Health Organization (WHO) and other international actors over concerns about the future availability of the vaccines to its own population illustrates sensitivities regarding respect for sovereignty as well as fundamental concerns about equity in health research (Xinhuanet, 2007; Sedyaningsih *et al.*, 2008). Additional concerns have been voiced about unethical practices by pharmaceutical companies, the growing significance of and lack of accountability of external non-governmental funders for health research (Peoples Health Movement, 2008), and persistent inequities, both in health research funding and in health research capacity between developing and developed countries.

As the foremost international health agency, the WHO has a natural leadership role to play in GHRG. However, as this chapter will argue, in practice, the norms and standards for GHRG are set and enforced by many different actors, including a range of international agencies, publishers and funders of health research, global public–private partnerships for health research, and professional organizations.

This chapter aims to:

- Document the current need for GHRG and how well the existing structures for GHRG measure up to the need.
- Assess the implications of growing economic, scientific and political power in Asia and emerging health research challenges and their implications for GHRG.
- Propose key next steps to strengthen GHRG, in a fashion that supports a more appropriate role for Asian stakeholders in research governance.

As this chapter is one of a series looking at different aspects of global health governance, it also seeks to apply three lenses common to the S. T. Lee research project, namely:

- Changing Asian concepts and powers
- Institutional diversity
- Sovereignty in the context of health research.

Chapter 8 in this volume, by Moon and Szlezák, focuses exclusively upon the tension between global governance of intellectual property and developing country access to new drugs and technologies, and the innovative mechanisms currently being explored to address this tension. Accordingly, this chapter does not address the question of intellectual property and access to drugs in any depth.

Methods

The chapter used a mixed-methods qualitative approach that included a literature review, semi-structured interviews with key informants in Asia and mini case studies of initiatives or research collaborations that shed light on GHRG and Asian approaches to research governance.

Literature review

While there is a substantial literature about national health research governance, particularly issues concerning the application of ethical research standards, very few articles on global governance exist. GHRG is a new and growing field, hence there is not an extensive body of literature from which to draw. Literature searches across PubMed, Web of Science and JSTOR combined the following sets of terms: (i) research or science; (ii) governance; (iii) health, biomedicine, clinical, stem cell, medical; and (iv) global, Asia, India, China. Those that were found were often quite specific in their scope, addressing, for example, the application of ethical research standards, or methods for research priority-setting, rather than considering the broad needs for GHRG.

Mini case studies

A series of mini case studies were undertaken to identify and examine promising models of research governance in the Asian context. The case studies were selected through discussion between members of the research team, and included examinations of the Asian Partnership on Emerging Infectious Diseases Research (APEIR), Southeast Asian Ministers of Education Organization Regional Tropical Medicine and Public Health Network (SEAMEO-TROPMED) and the Mekong Basin Disease Surveillance (MBDS). The case studies were completed through document review and supplementary interviews, where necessary.

Interviews with Asian stakeholders

Semi-structured interviews were conducted by telephone and in person with senior Asian stakeholders, including policy makers, leaders within the health research community and Asian funders of health and medical research. Questions addressed in the interviews focused on the three objectives of the chapter. The list of interviewees was designed to reflect differences in: geographical location (South Asia, South East Asia and East Asia); role (funders of health research, researchers and policy makers); and type of research conducted (biomedical, clinical, operational). A total of nine interviews were conducted. Half of the interviews were recorded and fully transcribed. For the other interviews detailed notes on the interview were taken.

Ethical approval for the research was received from the national Thai Ethical Review Committee.

The following section of this chapter explores what types of functions need to be performed as part of GHRG. Subsequently it describes how the GHRG landscape has evolved over the past 40 years since the establishment of special global programs on health research, as well as the actors and mechanisms currently active in this field. The chapter then considers Asian perspectives on GHRG, notably Asian perceptions of current governance arrangements and the implications of emerging Asian power, before presenting general conclusions.

What role for the global governance of health research?

There is no agreed definition of what GHRG is or what it encompasses. One definition of health research governance, used at the national level by the Government of the United Kingdom, focuses on public confidence in research, stating that 'the public has a right to expect high scientific, ethical and financial standards, transparent decision-making processes, clear allocation of responsibilities and robust monitoring arrangements' (Department of Health, 2005). Lee and Mills offer a broad definition of GHRG: 'Governance of health research concerns the means and rules by which relevant stakeholders set and achieve their agreed research goals. This includes decisions about what kind of research should be supported, by whom and for what ends' (Lee and Mills, 2000).

While this definition provides a broad framework for understanding GHRG, this chapter takes the view that the systems and processes of GHRG should seek to maximize the benefits of health research for the world as a whole, and, as such, need to promote the relevance, equity and ethical practice of health research. Importantly, GHRG needs to address equity issues, in terms of how different nations contribute to, and benefit from, the fruits of health research.

Health research is governed at multiple levels: national, regional and global. Many research governance functions take place at the national level; ethical review, priority-setting, capacity-building and establishment of norms and standards are all functions that can be and are implemented by national governments. The need for global governance, in addition to national governance, arises from three core reasons.

First, scientific enquiry is increasingly international in nature. Even if teams are not directly collaborating on a research project, there are substantial interdependencies: for example, a research team in one country may procure stem cells from a stem cell bank in another country, which may in turn purchase these from a company in another country (Waldby and Salter, 2008). In this globalized context, the articulation of global standards, both for codes of research conduct and technical norms, is critical to the advance of science.

Secondly, the major inequities remaining between countries in terms of their research capacity and their access to the benefits of research give rise to governance needs. The 1990 report of the Commission on Health Research Development focused global attention on this inequity, labeling the mismatch between global investment in health research and the burden of illness, the 10/90 gap (Commission on Health Research for Development, 1990). Today only 5 percent of global scientists live and work in non-Organization for Economic Cooperation and Development (OECD) countries. Research in developing countries accounts for only 4 percent of the global total (Rweyemamu *et al.*, 2006). Linked to this is the existence of inequitable research partnerships (Jentsch and Pilley, 2003; Sack *et al.*, 2009) and the imposition of knowledge derived by Western researchers on country policies and practices without due recognition of varying contexts. Imbalances in terms of the type of research supported and gaps in research coverage also occur, typically with a dominance of biomedical/clinical research, which can lead to new products and technologies, compared to health systems and policy research, which facilitates local decision making (Leroy *et al.*, 2007).

Further, inequities between countries compound the problems of transparency and ethical issues. For example, while it has been estimated that 30–40 percent of clinical trials involve low income and lower-middle income countries, only about 3 percent of the trials currently included in the Clinical Trials Search Portal involve participants from such countries, suggesting significant under-recording of such trials (Ghersi and Pang, 2008). Such lack of transparency enables those conducting clinical trials to only partially disclose findings if negative evidence emerges or adverse events occur. Issues also arise with respect to human subject research. Clinical trials are increasingly being shifted to low- and middle-income countries, where costs are lower and affected populations may be larger, easier to recruit and less tainted by use of other drugs than Western populations (Petryna, 2005; Benatar and Vaughan, 2008). In this context there has been substantial criticism of the ethics of trials of new regimens aimed at preventing the vertical transmission of HIV for including a placebo arm, rather than 'the best proven treatment' which would be available in developed countries (Benatar and Singer, 2000; Petryna, 2005). Such issues raise complex ethical questions: in contexts where, for financial reasons, there might not be access to 'the best proven treatment', what treatments should be provided as part of clinical trials, and how long should these treatments be financed for? GHRG needs to provide answers to questions like these.

Thirdly, some (though not all) health research can be viewed as a global public good, that is 'a good which it is rational, from the perspective of a group of nations collectively, to produce for universal consumption, and from which it is irrational to exclude an individual nation' (Woodward and Smith quoted in Smith and Mackellar, 2007). Economic theory suggests that left to private markets, without government intervention, such global public goods will be under-produced. While patents can provide financial incentives to promote some types of research investments, there are likely to be insufficient incentives for private actors to invest in research that primarily benefits the poor. This suggests that there may be a role for GHRG mechanisms in ensuring appropriate levels of investment in health research, particularly those targeting the needs of the poor, and health policy and systems research, where the financial returns are limited.

These challenges point to a number of core functions needed for a system governing health research at the global level.

Norms and standards

International norms and standards for health research are required, as well as mechanisms to enforce these standards. Such norms and standards may cover, for example, ethical aspects of health research, transparency and access to results, as well as a code of conduct for North–South research partnerships. They may also be important in standardizing practices and definitions across researchers in different countries.

Priority-setting mechanisms

Priority-setting is likely to occur at multiple levels, from individual research teams, to national governments, to the global level. Global governance mechanisms need to identify where research priorities lie, help channel funding into these areas in a balanced and coordinated manner, promote accountability for the use of such research funds and equitable access to the results/outputs of health research so as to ensure that research contributes to addressing priority health needs.

Funding for research as a global public good

Traditionally research that can provide international benefits has been funded through multinational organizations. However, in recent years, and as discussed further below, multiple innovative funding mechanisms for global health research have developed.

Capacity development for research institutions in developing countries

Given the major imbalance between capacities to conduct research in high-income countries and those in many low- and middle-income countries, there is a need to enhance research capacity in biomedical research, as well as health system and policy research. Capacity must also be developed for translating research into policy. Capacity development is needed in terms of individual skills, institutional capacities and the development of health research systems.

Advocacy and monitoring of health research

While many governments and private actors appreciate the importance of health research, there are others who do not. There is a strong need for advocacy on behalf of investment in health research; monitoring, reporting and evaluating the nature of research conducted and research impacts. Such reports can highlight neglected areas, or inequities between north and south, as well as demonstrate the return on research investment.

The evolving landscape

During the 1970s, the dominant response to the need for GHRG was an intergovernmental one. Special programs for health research were set up by multilateral agencies; these included the Special Program for Research and Training in Tropical Diseases (TDR) and the Special Program on Human and Reproductive Health Research (HRP), both hosted by the WHO. Their mandate was to invest in health research in their respective fields that was relevant to the needs of developing countries. Recent evaluations of these programs have documented how much the funding environment has changed since the programs were established

(Carucci and Gottlieb, 2008; Daar *et al.*, 2008). While some foundations that traditionally fund health research, such as the Wellcome Trust, have increased the resources they direct towards research in low- and middle-income countries (Trust, 2005), by far the bigger increase has come from new players, particularly the Bill and Melinda Gates Foundation (BMGF). It is estimated that the BMGF spends about US$1 billion per annum on health, with a sizeable chunk of this for health research (Daar *et al.*, 2006). During the period 1999–2006, it is estimated that the BMGF spent US$570 million in the field of R&D for malaria, second only to the Government of the United States of America (*The Seattle Times*, 2007). Increased funding brings with it increased influence in terms of determining the research agenda.

Formerly, UN-administered special programs were the primary mechanism to channel funding for neglected research areas. However, some research funders have sought alternative, more nimble funding vehicles due to increasing distrust of UN administrative systems and perceptions of overly bureaucratic processes (Daar *et al.*, 2006). Since 2000, this has led to a proliferation of new public–private partnerships aimed at developing particular drugs or technologies, including the Medicines for Malaria Venture (MMV) and the International AIDS Vaccine Initiative (IAVI), among others (Szlezák and Moon, 2010). While some research on public–private partnerships is extremely positive regarding development of new drugs, others have sounded a more cautious note, highlighting the fact that partnerships with the private sector are often market-driven, and questioning the likely governance implications of these arrangements (Buse and Walt, 2000).

Table 9.1 shows the array of mechanisms and actors engaged in GHRG across the five different functions of global health research described above. It also distinguishes between intergovernmental agreements and actions based on cooperative agreements, or private actions. Very few of the governance arrangements operate through legally binding agreements, the main exceptions being the International Health Regulations (and the mechanism therein for verifying information relating to disease outbreaks and public health emergencies), and WTO agreements, which relate primarily to the protection of intellectual property rights. Instead, governance functions are executed through a plethora of soft international agreements that lack legal force, cooperative action (including the actions of public–private partnerships) and actions by individual private bodies. There has been no concerted effort to review or re-structure GHRG mechanisms, while over time there has been a proliferation of entities that play a role in GHRG. Many of the partnerships and initiatives focus on specific diseases or services, such as malaria or HIV/AIDS, and seek within their field of focus to provide a full range of global governance functions, including priority setting, funding of global public goods and advocacy. In practice there are not impermeable boundaries between the different sub-fields of health research; scientists often engage in research on more than one disease and laboratory capacity can be used to investigate different microbes, thus the remits of different agencies are frequently overlapping.

Table 9.1 Mechanisms and actors involved in global health research governance functions

	Norms and standards	*Priority setting*	*Funding for global public goods*	*Research capacity development*	*Advocacy and monitoring*
Hard international agreements	World Trade Organization–TRIPS (intellectual property) International Health Regulations (e.g. virus-sharing)				
Soft international agreements, declarations, international organization guidelines and resolutions	Multiple international declarations and codes of conduct (Universal Declaration on Bioethics and Human Rights) International Clinical Trials Registration Platform, WHO WHO and UN Special programmes (TDR, HRP) guidelines on specific aspects of research practice	UN Special Programmes – priority setting within sub-fields (TDR, HRP)	UN Special Programmes (TDR, HRP)	UN Special Programmes, (TDR, HRP)	WHO reports, hosting of ministerial summits and meetings. World Health Assembly Resolutions (WHA58.34) UN Special programmes (TDR, HRP)
Cooperative action by government and/or non-government actors, e.g. self-regulation	Professional codes of conduct, (e.g. International Council of Nurses code of ethics, Singapore Statement on Research Integrity) Public–private partnerships (IAVI clinical trial database)	Public–private partnerships Medicines for Malaria Venture (MMV), International AIDS Vaccine Initiative (IAVI), Drugs for Neglected Diseases (DNDi)	Public–private partnerships (MMV, IAVI, DNDi)	Public–private partnerships (MMV, IAVI, DNDi)	Public–private partnerships (MMV, IAVI, DNDi)
Private action	Funders, with respect to open access, ethical review, open datasets. Journals, with respect to clinical trial registration, ethical review UK stem-cell bank standards		Private foundation funders (BMGF, Wellcome Trust)	Private foundations (Wellcome Trust, African Institutions Initiative) NGOs (COHRED)	NGOs (Global Forum for Health Research, Council on Health Research for Development [COHRED])

Further, the rise of alternative funding mechanisms has blurred public–private boundaries. The former dichotomy between publicly funded global health research organizations linked to international (UN) organizations, which epitomized a state-centric, traditional approach on the one hand, and private investment by pharmaceutical companies on the other, has given way to a much more complex reality. Not only have there been a multitude of new organizational forms, and increasing engagement by civil society organizations, but also a proliferation of new initiatives that aim to apply market mechanisms at the global level to achieve social goals. These include, for example, advanced market commitments, patent buy-outs and patent pools (Szlezák and Moon, 2010).

The proliferation and fragmentation of both funding and implementation mechanisms for global health research have led to the emergence of extremely complex accountability structures. For example, public–private partnerships are often accountable to a board. Board composition varies according to the organization, but typically reflects funders and, to some degree, beneficiaries. The strength of such accountability structures is not clear. Further, many research partnerships operate within the WHO, or are very closely linked to the WHO, creating even more confusing lines of accountability, with reporting obligations both through the WHO to the World Health Assembly, and to their own boards. Behind these new structures are funders, who are themselves only weakly accountable. The BMGF is the most frequently questioned of these, largely because of its size and lack of board structure (Peoples Health Movement, 2008), but other foundations also operate under similar arrangements.

The GHRG system as it currently exists exhibits more governance mechanisms and greater diversity in terms of actors involved in governance than ever before. In this fragmented environment, the WHO's role has been continuously challenged. In 2007, WHO member states requested that the WHO develop a research strategy, a version of which was approved by the Executive Board in January 2009, and finally fully approved by the World Health Assembly in May 2010. This research strategy focuses not only on the WHO's role in research, but also on the role of research within the WHO. It is based on three principles (quality, impact, inclusiveness) and has four pillars (strengthening capacity, priority-setting, translation of research and standards setting). However, while the WHO is commonly seen as being a major player in terms of GHRG, it is unlikely that it alone will be able to address the broad array of current GHRG concerns.

Asian perceptions of current governance arrangements

All but one of the Asian stakeholders interviewed questioned whether it was fair to suggest that there were global governance arrangements for health research:

> I'm not sure that there is a global (health research) governance mechanism. There are parts of systems for governing health research but not really an overarching one.
>
> Interviewee 6

> The problem is I'm not really sure that there is a global (health research) governance arrangement! A global (health research) governance arrangement would imply that there is a structure around global (health) research that represents countries or that countries empathize with. Although there is a structure within WHO that influences WHO research it absolutely does not determine research strategy outside of the Organization.
>
> Interviewee 2

Interviewees perceived that there has never been a concerted effort to establish a global governance structure for health research. Instead the existing arrangements had developed in an ad hoc fashion, which in turn had led to extremely fragmented arrangements. Further, some respondents argued that large global funders of health research (such as National Institutes of Health, the BMGF and the Wellcome Trust) have no incentive to help create a stronger governance mechanism. 'Nobody wants to be strategic around this, nor do they want to openly share, although there is some interest to see if we can define some overlapping areas and avoid duplication' Interviewee 2.

Thus part of the problem in terms of the development of global governance arrangements could also be viewed as one of power imbalance between international organizations such as the WHO, which many interviewees saw to be the natural home for global governance, and the more powerful players who today have increasing influence over the shape and nature of global health research. Being primarily a public health, rather than a research funding, agency, WHO was perceived by respondents to lack resources (Interviewee 1); be poorly organized and too bureaucratic (Interviewee 3, Interviewee 8); and to be insufficiently prepared to leverage the resources of other powerful international actors, such as the Global Fund, the World Bank and GAVI (Interviewee 4).

Opinions varied regarding the creation of a unified global architecture for governing health research, or whether the existing fragmentation is inevitable. Typically respondents from higher-income countries were more skeptical about the feasibility of creating a unified architecture.

> The idea of an overarching architecture for governance of global health research is unrealistic – there are too many different organizations with different remits. Any attempt to do this will just lead to other arrangements coming up to further confuse matters.
>
> Interviewee 1

> I don't think there will ever be one architecture for global health research governance – it will always be pluralistic. There is the commercial sector, then WHO and the other global bodies play a role, then academia has its own subsystem, and then a lot of national funders and foundations. There will always be multiple players performing different roles in global governance, though they might work together better.
>
> Interviewee 6

One respondent (Interviewee 9) argued that it is no longer possible to conceive of governance as a top-down process; instead, norms and standards for the responsible conduct of research need to be negotiated and agreed through collaboration and partnership. Other respondents were clearly supportive of efforts to create a stronger and more unified architecture for GHRG, for example calling for an 'apex of responsibility' (Interviewee 4) in this area.

'We need a Boeing 747 jumbo jet with one captain where the passengers are the "players" – and not 40 Cessnas going for a joy ride' (Interviewee 5).

Some respondents gave more moderate opinions, indicating that while it was unrealistic to expect a single unified structure for GHRG, improved coordination was desirable (Interviewee 8).

The very varied perceptions among respondents of the need for, and feasibility of, a unified architecture for GHRG may in part reflect the scope of issues that respondents thought might fall under the remit of a global governance body. The needs for global governance with respect to biotechnology research undoubtedly differ substantially from those within the health systems or health services research field, for example. Those respondents who were more accepting of fragmentation in this field sometimes highlighted the multiple mechanisms through which research is currently governed at the global level. The policies adopted by journals can influence what is acceptable in terms of ethical review and research standards. Research funders such as the NIH and the Wellcome Trust, which have adopted policies that require open access publishing, have been critical players in terms of the drive towards open access publishing (Delamothe and Smith, 2004), as well as open access datasets. There are also several examples where professional groupings have developed some form of self-regulation, at the global level. Box 9.1 illustrates this through the UK Stem Cell Bank.

While some progress has been made in terms of determining standards (the International Clinical Trials Registry Platform, for example), often the global mechanisms for enforcing these standards are weak. With reference to clinical trials, for example, the strongest enforcement mechanism at this point appears to be a resolution from journal editors that clinical trials must be registered at their onset if they are to be published (Godlee, 2006), although some national ethics review committees are also requesting trial registration prior to reviewing ethical aspects of the proposed research. While standards for and approaches to enforcing standards on human subject research are well defined at the national level, more remains to be done in terms of considering the implications for multi-country studies. Finally, while some compilations of best practice have been created to guide research collaborations between developing and developed countries, there are not widely accepted norms and standards regarding the nature of research partnerships (Swiss Commission for Research Partnership with Developing Countries, 1998).

Several interviewee comments demonstrated recognition that health research has gone beyond governments and researchers; a diverse array of actors now exist, including private sector funders (both foundations and commercial companies), NGOs and advocacy groups. In the eyes of some respondents, this proliferation of stakeholders meant that any governance mechanism has to be inclusive, reaching out to multiple parties, and able to act as an '*honest and neutral broker*' (Interviewee 4).

While none of the respondents directly expressed concern that existing governance mechanisms impinged on national sovereignty, there was a strong theme to discussions of the need for inclusive, consensus-oriented governance. Respondents spoke of the need to get 'buy-in' from many actors involved in research (Interviewee 2), and to pursue governance through collaborative, partnership-oriented approaches (Interviewee 9). Such approaches stand in contrast to more autocratic, hierarchical approaches to governance that are more likely to cause concern with respect to national sovereignty. Indeed the closing comments of the

Box 9.1 New actors in global governance: the UK Stem Cell Bank

The UK Stem Cell Bank is a British organization established to act as a clearing house for stem cell lines within the UK and ensure enforcement of UK regulatory standards on stem-cell research. Investment in stem-cell research has grown rapidly, outpacing the development of international standards on stem-cell research. The UK Stem Cell Bank has, through a number of different initiatives, stepped into this vacuum and supported the development of standards concerning both the social and ethical aspects of stem-cell research, as well as basic aspects of stem-cell classification. For example, stem cells are very fragile and volatile, so the Stem Cell Bank has played a role in coordinating standards for handling and transferring stem cell lines. Similarly the Stem Cell Bank's Steering Committee also determines whether stem cell lines deposited with the bank have the proper information, and have appropriately protected donors.

The UK Stem Cell Bank directly controls all stem cells that UK researchers work on, but as the Bank also accepts stem cells from depositors outside the UK and supplies researchers outside the UK, the norms and standards that it applies are increasingly becoming global ones. Furthermore, the Stem Cell Bank has supported the International Stem Cell Initiative, which is a voluntary, collaborative initiative to standardize the classification of stem cells. This initiative has been successful despite intense competition in the field of stem cell research. Its success comes, in large part, from recognition among researchers for this kind of standardization as a prerequisite to global collaborative research.

This example illustrates both how national level entities can influence global norms and standards, as well as the scope for the collaborative negotiation of standards between professionals within the field.

Source: Waldby and Salter (2008).

paper by Sedyaningsih and colleagues, which was co-authored by Dr Supari, the former Indonesian Minister of Health, emphasize that in pursuing the H5N1 virus: 'the work must be conducted side by side with mutual trust, transparency and equity as global citizens and professionals, taking into consideration the elements of human dignity and solidarity' (Sedyaningsih *et al.*, 2008).

This statement implies that procedural issues in global governance, particularly concerning respect between nations, are critically important; perhaps as important as the final outcome (in this instance access to vaccines).

Implications of emerging Asian power

Growing Asian engagement in health research

The rapid economic development in Asia has both contributed to, and in part been driven by, research investments. China and India have sought to position themselves as competitive players in the commercial health research arena, particularly in terms of biotechnology (Salter *et al.*, 2006, 2007). At the same time, pharmaceutical and biotechnology companies have increasingly sought to outsource to lower-cost research and development groups located in Asian countries. Both the Chinese and Indian governments have made major public investments in the biotechnology field. For example, it is estimated that over a five-year period the Ministry of Science and Technology in China planned to spend between US$63 and US $250 million on stem cell research (Salter *et al.*, 2006). China was the only developing country to participate in the Human Genome Project (and recently completed sequencing of the entire genome of a Chinese national).

Much less is known about the level of investment by Asian governments in non-commercial fields of health research. Over the past two decades, the Thai government has established an array of institutions to address different types of health research. In 2006, the Thai government invested approximately US$14 million, with around half going to biomedical research and the other half to health services/system and policy research. The Indian government has committed about US$14 million to the establishment of the Public Health Foundation of India. But these amounts appear relatively small compared to the magnitude of government investment in commercially oriented health research.

Again there is little data to illuminate the extent of collaboration on health research between teams within the Asian region. Certainly there are some long-standing regional initiatives that have sought to stimulate regional collaborations (see Boxes 9.2 and 9.3 on APEIR and SEAMEO-TROPMED, respectively). However, it seems likely that the strongest research partnerships are with high-income-country research groups, particularly those where Asian researchers received their postgraduate training. Even the large and rapidly developing Asian countries, such as China and India, continue to send large numbers of students overseas for postgraduate training. For example in 2001, 28.7 doctorates were awarded to Chinese students studying in the US for every 100 awarded within China (Salter *et al.*, 2006). Many Asian students stay on to conduct postdoctoral studies in the US, although in recent years there have been concerted efforts to lure the diaspora back home. A bibliometric analysis of patterns of collaboration in the field of health systems research, for example, found that only 21 percent of multi-country studies involved South–South collaboration, whereas international collaborations were more typically led by authors based in high-income countries (Gonzalez Block, 2006).

During the past few years there have been efforts to engage Asian countries in the existing GHRG mechanisms. For example, both China and India now have seats on the Joint Coordinating Board of the Special Program on Tropical Disease Research, however Asia remains relatively weakly represented with just four representatives on the Board out of a total of 34. Further, while China, India, Malaysia and Thailand all now contribute to the running expenses of TDR, their contributions constitute a tiny fraction of the total. China's contribution runs at just over 1 percent of TDR's total receipts, whereas the contributions of each of the other three countries are less than one tenth of a percent. For the new public–private partnerships, such as IAVI, the situation appears to be no better. While IAVI receives some funding from the Government of India, none of the other institutional or government funders named on its website are Asian. This picture is corroborated by Tucker and Magkoba, who found that of the nine product development partnerships that they surveyed, the chief executives, board and advisory board members were overwhelmingly from developed countries (Tucker and Makgoba, 2008).

All of the large foundations that are now playing increasingly influential roles in global health research are 'Western' (including the BMGF, the Rockefeller Foundation and the Wellcome Trust) with perhaps the sole exception being the Latin American Carso Health Institute. While there are an increasing number of Asian foundations with the resources to play a role, their activities in this field have been fairly limited. India, perhaps, forms the main exception to this, where private benefactors have played a major role in the establishment of the Tata Institute, the Indian Institute of Health Management Research and the Public Health Foundation of India. There has been no systematic enquiry regarding the extent to which Asian philanthropy has or could have played a more active role in

Box 9.2 Asian Partnership on Emerging Infectious Diseases Research (APEIR)

The vision of the Asian Partnership on Emerging Infectious Diseases Research is to catalyze efficient and timely generation of knowledge, and capacity-building for multidisciplinary collective research on emerging infectious diseases in the most severely affected Asian countries, comprising Thailand, China, Cambodia, Laos PDR and Vietnam. The Partnership seeks to develop a trust-based voluntary network among researchers, donors and policy makers within and among member countries and with other networks.

The collaboration started through discussions between Canada's International Development Research Centre (IDRC) and research institutes in Thailand. The Thai Health Systems Research Institute (HSRI) and IDRC hosted the first international meeting between delegates from the four countries and international partners in December 2005 (Silkavute, 2008).

While many of the key institutions in the Partnership are government entities, such as the Chinese Academy of Sciences, Ministry of Public Health of Thailand and the Ministry of Science and Technology of Vietnam, their role is limited to providing research clearances to allow budget disbursements from IDRC. A steering committee with two representatives from each country and development partners is responsible for setting the strategic direction of the partnership, and for appointing and guiding the activities of the Coordinating Office. IDRC supports at least 50 percent of the operating cost of the coordinating office and country partner institutes, while other development partners contribute the rest (APEIR, 2006).

The APEIR has helped to develop real collaboration among research funding agencies, research institutes, research users and policy makers in the region, bridging animal and human health. Six initial research priorities were identified:

1 migratory bird surveillance;
2 socio-economic impacts;
3 backyard poultry;
4 policy analysis;
5 control measures; and
6 risk behavior.

To date, five regional collaborative researches have been conducted. The voluntary nature of the network, the exchange of information between institutions, the development of trust and the strengthened collaboration within each member country are seen as being key factors for success.

Sources: APEIR (2006) Silkavute (2008).

Box 9.3 The SEAMEO TROPMED network

Vision and mission

The SEAMEO TROPMED network is a regional network under the South East Asian Ministers of Education Organization to conduct education, training and research in tropical medicine and public health. The SEAMEO TROPMED Project was officially approved by the Southeast Asian Ministers of Education Organization Council (SEAMEC) in Manila in November 1966 and formally established in 1967.

While initially the network's focus was on tropical diseases, in 1993, SEAMEO TROPMED decided to expand its role to encompass health and development in South East Asia. At the same time, the network also expanded its collaborations with other institutions in developed countries, and to all developing countries in the Asia-Pacific region (Chongsuphajaisiddhi and Salazar, 1998).

Funding and Organization

During 1967–1970, the primary source of funds for SEAMEO TROPMED operations came from a US government grant and from 1971–1992, the US Government continued to contribute financially. Since 1992, SEAMEO operations have been sustained by country contributions and some specific grants, including those from private organizations. Member countries support both the operational budget of the TROPMED central office and a special fund for research and training.

The SEAMEO TROPMED network agreed to operate through a cooperative network of existing national centers rather than through creating a new entity, as it was thought that this strategy would be more cost-effective and allow SEAMEO TROPMED to address the range of endemic diseases in the region through already established institutions. The network comprises a Central Coordinating Board and eight National Centres of Tropical Medicine and Public Health (Harinasuta, 1972). The centres in each country specialize in different fields.

TROPMED member countries have also committed to develop and upgrade their respective national centres. The network is governed by a board, and representatives are nominated by the Minister of Education of each member country.

Achievements and successes

The national and regional centres have done much to build health manpower capacity through short course training, the exchange of personnel and postgraduate degree courses. The SEAMEO TROPMED Network supports research and also publishes the *Southeast Asian Journal of Tropical Medicine and Public Health*, a quarterly publication.

The guiding principles behind SEAMEO TROPMED have been the Asian values and spirit of working together and of mutual, harmonious reliance.

Sources: Harinasuta (1972); Chongsuphajaisiddhi and Salazar (1998); Waikagul (2006).

global health research, or the extent to which research leaders from Asia can play a role in shaping the direction and practices of global research partnership.

Views of Asian stakeholders

Respondents were fairly cautious in terms of how they approached questions regarding an emerging role for Asian stakeholders in GHRG. Many prefaced their comments by referring to the remarkable recent economic growth in Asia, and indicating that it was obvious and necessary that over time Asian countries would come to play a greater role in GHRG. However, respondents were much more cautious in terms of the specifics of what might be done with regard to GHRG. First, many did not believe that it made sense to talk about 'Asia' as a single region; they pointed out the great heterogeneity within the region and the presence of a number of regional alliances, and suggested that it makes better sense to distinguish between different parts of the region. This lack of a cohesive identity has been exacerbated in the field of health research by the fact that Asia is divided among three different WHO regional offices (SEARO, WPRO and Eastern Mediterranean Regional Office of the World Health Organization [EMRO]).

Secondly, respondents held mixed views concerning the standing of Asian countries in the field of health research. One respondent, for example, asserted that Asians had made significant contributions at multiple levels in terms of health research, but questioned what impact Asians were truly able to have (Interviewee 5). Another suggested that while Asia had come a long way in terms of developing its research capacity, it still had a 'lot of catching up to do' (Interviewee 8). Several respondents suggested more or less explicitly that in the immediate future the focus needed to be on the development of domestic health research capacity rather than engagement at the global level (Interviewee 7, Interviewee 8). Respondents appeared to be more willing to take on regional responsibilities than global ones: 'There are organizations that could play a clearing house or coordination role for Asia. But whether we should play this role for the whole world? . . . I am not sure what that means' (Interviewee 8).

Some respondents argued that the most important aspects of GHRG actually concerned stimulating greater regional collaboration (Interviewee 9). Finally, there was a line of questioning as to whether the lack of Asian involvement in GHRG was attributable to a lack of appetite on the part of Asian stakeholders, or an attempt to retain control of the global agenda by stakeholders in the West. One respondent for example spoke of a 'glass ceiling' for Asian health research leadership and felt that GHRG structures do not reflect Asian views and are still largely 'Euro-centric' (Interviewee 5).

There was clearly no consensus among respondents as to what Asian values or perspectives might bring to the GHRG agenda. Some respondents thought that Asian countries valued more applied social science-driven health research over more commercially oriented health research – others thought the opposite. Regional bodies, such as ASEAN and APEC, were perceived not to have fulfilled their responsibilities in terms of promoting improved coordination within the region, in contrast, for example, to the European Union which has played a significant role in developing regional capacity for health research (Barben, 2001).

Discussion and suggestions for improving GHRG – Asian perspectives

Health research governance is an important function at the national, regional and global levels. Given the impacts of globalization, and increasing tendency towards transnational research, the challenges for GHRG are growing in significance. What can be learnt from this analysis in terms of the three cross-cutting themes of research, and future directions for GHRG?

Changing Asian concepts and power

From the interviews conducted so far, Asian stakeholders seem reluctant to engage at the global level, and are perhaps more concerned with strengthening national capabilities for health research. This might well make sense as a near-term strategy. Other analysts have suggested that the national level is likely to play the dominant role in research governance, but the regional level is of increasing importance (Barben, 2001). For example, the European Union has played an active role in research governance, mainly as a way to promote research competitiveness, innovation and capacity development within the region. Further, Barben suggests that research governance at the global level may be most important in terms of mediating the relationship between the global north and the south. This formulation of the role of global governance is one that appears inherently to reflect power imbalances between the north and the south. High-income countries are unlikely to invest in the efficient functioning of GHRG structures if they believe that the main role of such structures is to control their behavior in relation to the conduct of research in low- and middle-income countries.

In light of this, an Asian strategy to focus on developing national capacity and regional linkages for health research, so as to be able ultimately to engage in more equitable negotiations regarding research governance at the global level, may make sense. There have been several successful regional initiatives, such as those documented in this chapter which, although dependent upon external funding for support, have been successful in creating truly regional initiatives to address local priorities and strengthen research capacities. However, concerns remain regarding a lack of involvement in this field by key regional entities (notably ASEAN). Activating more formal regional mechanisms for health research coordination may help to build regional capacity and competitiveness as well as potentially reducing reliance on collaborations with high-income countries.

Institutional diversity

While there is clearly frustration with the decentralized global marketplace for health research, there is also a pragmatic recognition that creating a single streamlined GHRG structure is not feasible. Instead, initial steps for improvement should focus on improving transparency and developing 'light touch' coordination mechanisms that reach out to the wide array of different actors now active in health research. More modest attempts to coordinate or streamline specific subsets of governance structures, such as those linked to the WHO (Rottingen *et al.*, 2009), may make sense. What is critical, however, is to focus on improving the accuracy of information on sources, levels and nature of global health research spending, the status of national health research systems, measures of inequity in research between countries and between types of global health research. Such information can help highlight gaps and channel funding towards critical research areas and support capacity-building. Platforms or fora that bring together diverse actors and facilitate exchange and dialogue about research standards and norms, perhaps relying primarily on voluntary codes of conduct, appear more feasible than regulation.

Sovereignty

Concerns about the implications of GHRG structures for sovereignty were not clearly voiced by Asian respondents. However, interviewees expressed some concerns about the responsiveness of research governance structures to Asian stakeholders, and frequently asserted the need for inclusive governance structures that facilitated coordination across countries rather than autocratic approaches. While it appears that Asian stakeholders were not well represented, for example, on the boards that govern many global partnerships concerned with health research, the resources at the disposal of such entities is often relatively insignificant compared to the levels of investment that Asian governments are now making in public–private partnerships in the global health research field. Thus Asian stakeholders may be making a rather rational decision to focus on developing appropriate national and regional health research environments and governance approaches, rather than engaging at the global level.

Finally, at the global level, further progress on developing GHRG structures would be supported by clearer and more far-reaching analyses of the multiple mechanisms through which GHRG is currently exercised. To date, our understanding of the nature of interactions between the multiple organizations and institutions that together make up the global health research system is somewhat limited (Matlin and Samuels, 2009). A clearer understanding is needed of the relative importance of, and interactions between, different types of governance mechanisms, journal requirements, funder requirements, international agreements and professional codes of conduct in each respective research field. A stronger empirical assessment of the various components of the GHRG could lead to more effective governance strategies in the future.

Part 4

Cross-cutting perspectives on Asia and global health governance

10 Complexity and institutional diversity in global health governance

Implications for Asia

Mathias Koenig-Archibugi

Introduction

Asian policy-makers are in the process of redefining their relationship to a system of global health governance (GHG) shaped principally by actors outside of the region, most notably Western governments. The way in which Asian policy-makers define this relationship – by choosing lukewarm or wholehearted support, passive or active resistance, pressure for change from within or the creation of alternative institutions – will be a key determinant of how GHG will evolve over the next decades. Whatever their choices, they will have a major impact on human health and well-being in Asia and beyond.

Asian policy-makers will no doubt focus on the *content* of global health policies. This includes key questions such as: which rules should be supported, accepted, enforced and complied with? Which kinds of resources should be transferred and for what purposes? Which ideas should be promoted, contested, accepted or rejected? These questions are crucial to three key dimensions of global governance: regulative (development, negotiation and enforcement of rules), allocative (extraction, transfer and distribution of material resources) and discursive (generation and diffusion of ideas).

But Asian policy-makers also have to consider what can be called the *form* of GHG. This is more about who the actors are than what they do, and especially about the patterns of interaction among those actors. Clearly, content and form are intimately related; actors enter into specific relationships because they want to pursue specific goals and in turn the relationships they have influences their goals and what they can expect to achieve. However, the distinction between content and form can be useful to gauge the role of certain aspects of the problem while keeping others in the background.

This chapter is concerned with a specific *formal* characteristic of governance: its *complexity*. Complexity is an ambiguous term and yet is it frequently used by practitioners as well as observers of global governance. For instance, after noting that 40 bilateral donors, 90 global health initiatives, 26 UN agencies and 20 global and regional funds work in global health, the UK Department of International Development deplored that the system was 'over-complex' (cited by McCoy *et al.*, 2009: 414). Policy pronouncements on governance complexity seem to suggest that it can be an obstacle to effective policy-making and at the same time that it can be reduced or managed through appropriate institutional design. Calls for institutional reforms are often framed in terms of giving GHG an overarching 'architecture' that it currently lacks (see Fidler, 2007 for a discussion of the metaphor, and Charnoz and Severino, 2008 for a more general discussion of these themes). Asian governments thus face the following questions: assuming that governance complexity is not an inescapable 'fact of nature', how should they relate to it? Considering their needs, is the current system of GHG too complex, not complex enough, or 'just right'? Would a different kind of complexity be more appropriate to the interests and values of Asian countries? How much leeway do they have in promoting changes in the extent and form of governance complexity?

Thinking about these issues raises a range of difficult questions. Analysts of GHG can help placing policy-making on more solid grounds by tackling at least three important research challenges.

First, how can we subject to systematic scrutiny the widespread perception that GHG is becoming more complex? How can complexity be defined and operationalized in such a way as to provide a precision tool for qualitative, quantitative, comparative and historical research?

Secondly, what are the consequences of complexity? To what extent does more complexity – more precisely, specific forms of complexity – have a positive or negative impact on outcomes, such as infant mortality, overall mortality rates, immunizations, disability-adjusted life expectancy, government spending on health, measures of health inequality, etc.? Are certain forms of complexity more beneficial or harmful than others, and is their impact linear or nonlinear? To be sure, policy-makers are not interested only in improving health outcomes when they assess current and possible GHG structures, since a whole range of political, economic and cultural factors play a role as well. But researchers should investigate impacts on health outcomes under the assumption that they are, and will be, important for Asian policy-makers.

Thirdly, to what extent can the level and form of complexity be modified by deliberate policy choices? Answering this question requires a broader analysis of the *causes* of complexity and an assessment of the relative importance of structural and policy-controlled causes in explaining existing levels and forms of governance complexity. The analysis should also assess to what extent both state and non-state actors are likely to resist attempts to 'rationalize, centralize, and harmonize' their involvement in global health and limit their freedom of action (Fidler, 2007), or even to promote further governance complexity in order to better assert their values and interests (Drezner, 2009; Benvenisti and Downs, 2007).

The next section addresses the first task, while the third section of this chapter considers the consequences of complexity. The empirical material presented here reflects, to a large extent, what Western countries are doing in the global health domain, since they bear the primary responsibility for the current levels and forms of governance complexity, and the response of Asian governments facing this status quo. The chapter will also refer to examples from Asian countries, to the extent that they provide some indication on how their policies are affecting governance complexity in global health.

Defining and operationalizing complexity in GHG

According to a general definition, complex systems are 'made up of a large number of parts that interact in a nonsimple way', in the sense that, 'given the properties of the parts and the laws of their interaction, it is not a trivial matter to infer the properties of the whole' (Simon, 1962: 468). In global governance, complexity can be seen a function of various elements, including (a) the number of actors who 'produce' governance; (b) the degree of diversity in their properties; and (c) the degree of diversity in their regulative, discursive and allocative relationships. Complexity is thus related to what has been called the 'unstructured plurality' of global health (Fidler, 2007).

For analytical purposes, it seems useful to operationalize complexity in GHG in relation to the three dimensions mentioned in the introduction – allocative, regulative and ideational – even though in actual fact most governance relationships combine the three dimensions in more or less complex ways. For each of these dimensions, I will first present some concepts and then some empirical illustrations.

With regard to the allocative dimension, in the analysis of development aid for health it is usual to refer to 'donors' and 'recipients', and those terms are adopted here as a shorthand. McCoy *et al.* (2009) provide a more rigorous conceptualization by distinguishing between the actors 'providing' funds for global health, actors 'managing' those funds and actors 'spending' them. They also note that several actors perform all three functions simultaneously. Governance complexity can thus be seen as having a number of components:

1 The number of donors that provide aid for health;
2 The number of collaborative initiatives among donors for the management of those funds, whatever institutional form they make take;
3 The number of organizations that spend funds for health. Another cluster of components refers to the institutional diversity of providers, managers and spenders;
4 The institutional diversity between donors. Obviously the distinction between governments and non-governmental actors is important, but there are also important differences among governments, and among non-governmental actors. With regard to the former, differences that have a direct impact on governance complexity are the number of veto points in the political system (democratic countries tend to have more) and more specifically the degree of internal fragmentation and competition among the government departments that are involved more directly in the regulative, discursive and allocative aspects of GHG. Among non-governmental actors, member-based non-governmental organizations (NGOs) with extensive representative structures are likely to behave differently than more hierarchical foundations, or companies.
5 The institutional diversity among collaborative initiatives among donors. These can range from traditional multilateral organizations to more informal 'private–public partnerships'. Relevant diversity can occur across many

institutional dimensions, which is why researchers proposed a number of different typologies (e.g. Koenig-Archibugi 2002).

Further components of governance complexity concern the relationship between donors and recipients. Development aid specialists have introduced the concept of aid proliferation to indicate the degree to which a donor distributes aid widely among many recipients, and the concept of aid fragmentation to indicate the degree to which a recipient obtains aid from a wide range of sources.

An attempt to define and operationalize complexity in the allocative dimension of GHG would be incomplete if it did not include mechanisms through which policy-makers attempt to reduce or manage this complexity. Complexity could be reduced through specialization, which entails donors voluntarily concentrating their aid on a limited number of recipients, or a limited number of policy sectors. Collaborative health initiatives can specialize as well, for instance, on specific diseases. But this form of specialization does not necessarily reduce complexity since this typically entails a larger number of separate health initiatives.

Complexity can be managed through coordination, either among donors or collaborative health initiatives. An increase of the proportion of aid that is channelled through multilateral organizations (as opposed to provided bilaterally) is likely to reduce complexity, although this is not necessarily the case if the multilateralization of aid is accompanied by a proliferation of multilateral initiatives.

If these components are used as indicators to assess to current arrangements for development aid for health, what can be said about the current situation and historical trends? It should be noted that systematic knowledge about global health funding is hampered by serious data collection problems, but a number of studies have attempted to present an overall picture (Ravishankar *et al.*, 2009; McCoy *et al.*, 2009; Lu *et al.*, 2010)

There is much discussion at present on the significance of so-called 'emerging donors', i.e. countries that did not provide significant amounts of development aid until recently and, in some cases, were or still are recipients of development aid, such as Brazil, China, India and Thailand (Woods, 2008). The debate on emerging donors tends to focus on the alleged specificities of their policies (for instance with regard to targeted sectors, the mix of grants and loans, conditionality, tied aid, etc.), although some worry about their (lack of) 'coordination' with other donors. In contrast to the established donors that are members of the Organisation for Economic Co-operation and Development (OECD) Development Assistance Committee (DAC), there are significant gaps in the publicly available information on the magnitude and sectoral distribution of aid provided by emerging donors. Kharas (2009) estimates that in recent years new bilateral donors provided about US$10 billion annually, while DAC members provided about US$73 billion bilaterally (see Figure 10.1).

Information about the amount of *health* aid provided by non-DAC donors is still scarce, although other chapters in this volume provide valuable data on this issue. Further work is needed to ascertain the extent to which the new donors have made a noticeable difference in the health sector. The available evidence suggests

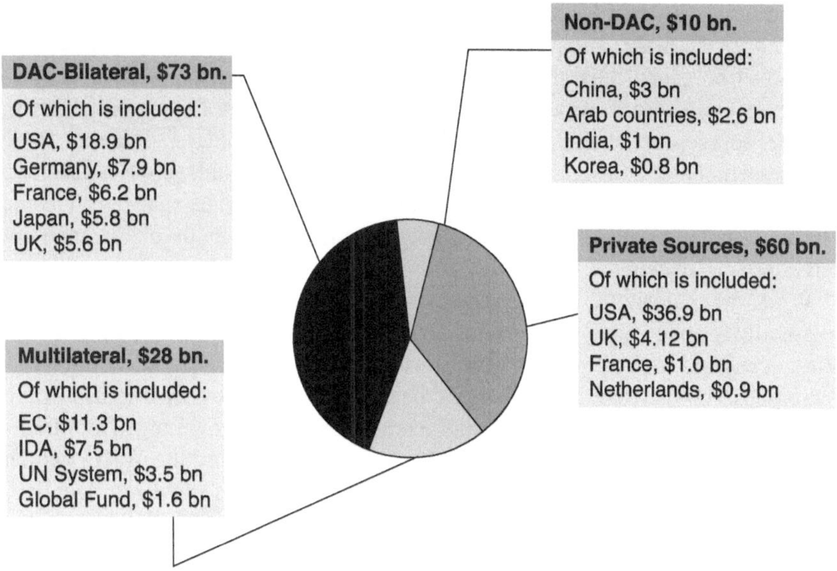

Figure 10.1 Sources of development aid.

Source: Kharas (2009). Reprinted with permission.

that emerging donors have concentrated their resources on non-social sectors, and specifically on infrastructure projects. For instance, a study of the involvement of four emerging Asian donors (China, India, South Korea and Thailand) in Cambodia shows that they mainly financed infrastructure using concessional tied loans (Sato *et al*., 2010). Wang and colleagues (Chapter 3 this volume) report that China has undertaken only 33 health aid projects providing health equipment and medicine in the 2000s, 3 in the 1990s and 2 in the 1980s, although the number of Chinese Medical Teams deployed in poor countries is significant, and China also provided training to foreign health workers and contributed to the construction of health facilities abroad.

Another component of complexity mentioned above refers to the fact that state donors (and recipients) are not 'unitary actors' but governments composed of departments with different, sometimes competing, agendas. It has been reported that in the United States, 12 departments, 25 different agencies and nearly 60 government offices are involved in foreign assistance programmes, and that the main agency, USAID, oversees only 45 per cent of US foreign aid (Frot and Santiso 2010). Pilcavage (Chapter 2 this volume) notes that Japan's Official Development Assistance (ODA) is administered among the Cabinet Office and 12 ministries and agencies, with no independent international development agency in charge. While the US and Japanese governments may display an unusually high level of fragmentation, this issue is likely to affect emerging donors as well. Wang and colleagues (Chapter 3 this volume) note that, in addition to the Ministry of

Commerce and its Department of Aid to Foreign Countries and Department of International Trade and Economic Affairs, a further 22 ministries and commissions under the State Council participate in Chinese foreign aid programmes.

Studies on global health financing stress the increasing importance of non-governmental sources. As estimated by Kharas (2009) (see Figure 10.1 above), private sources account for almost as much foreign aid as bilateral DAC governmental aid, and significantly more than multilateral aid, across all sectors. For the health sector, McCoy and colleagues (2009) estimate that by 2006 the Gates Foundation had become a bigger international health donor than all governments, except the US and the UK.

While the majority of official development assistance for health is channelled bilaterally – about three-quarters for DAC countries, more for non-DAC countries, according to McCoy *et al.* (2009) – the number of multilateral channels has increased. The increase in number has been accompanied by an increase in the institutional diversity of aid-managing institutions, which now range from traditional multilateral organizations, such as the World Bank and the WHO (which are themselves organized very differently), to hybrid but formalized agencies, such as the Global Fund, to less formal private–public partnerships that are often disease-specific. McCoy *et al.* (2009) note that some public–private partnerships are primarily funding agencies, while the majority of them are implementing agencies, although the complexity of allocative arrangements is further increased by the fact that some of the latter also transfer resources to other actors.

These trends have produced a significant increase in the fragmentation of development aid. Over the past 40 years, projects have increased dramatically in number and become smaller in size. Since countries no longer target their aid to a small number of countries of post-colonial strategic or economic interest, recipients tend to obtain aid from a large number of donors, some of which only provide a small percentage of total aid. In 1960, the average OECD donor disbursed aid each year to an average of 20 countries, while in 2006 it did so to more than 100. Aid budgets did not rise at the same rate as the number of recipients, resulting in increasing levels of fragmentation (Frot and Santiso, 2010). In 2002, 25 official bilateral donors, 19 multilateral donors and about 350 international NGOs were operating in Vietnam, and they collectively accounted for over 8,000 projects (Acharya *et al.*, 2006). Globally, over the past 40 years projects have increased dramatically in number and become smaller in size.

Fragmentation is associated with the proliferation of monitoring and accountability structures. For instance, Cambodia reportedly has 121 parallel project implementation units, and 358 donor missions, reviews and studies are said to have taken place in a single year (Sato *et al.*, 2010). The DAC suggests that fragmentation constitutes a serious problem when 15 or more donors combined provide just 10 per cent of country programmable aid, and it published the information shown in Figure 10.2 to highlight the 32 countries falling into this category.

In general, donors from Asia do not appear to contribute to fragmentation more than donors from other regions, but there are significant differences among them. In 2001–2008, DAC-member Japan gave aid to 143 countries, and 50.6 per cent

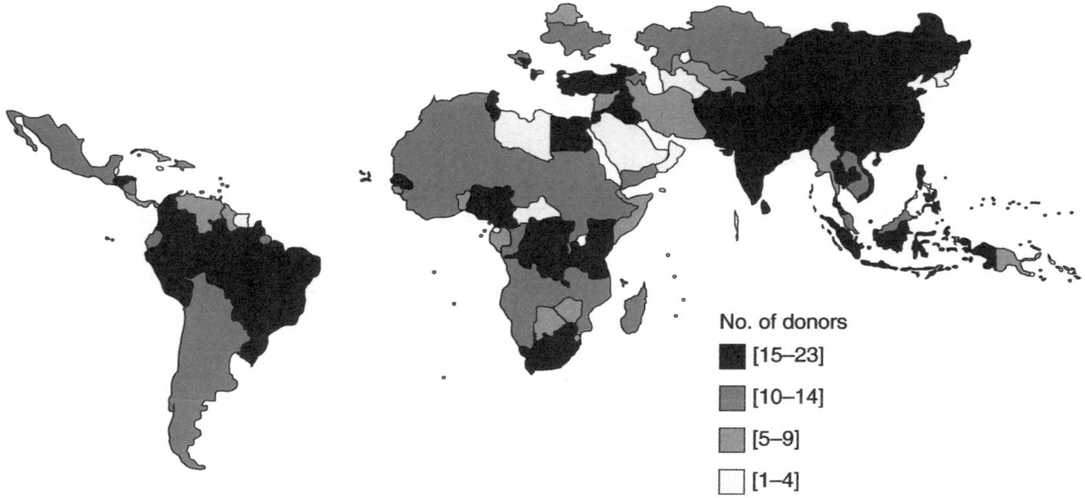

Figure 10.2 Opportunities to concentrate: number of donors together accounting for less than 10 per cent of aid (Gross disbursements of CPA, 2005–06).

Source: OECD DAC (2008) *Scaling up: Aid fragmentation, aid allocation and aid predictability*. Report of the 2008 Survey of Aid Allocation Policies and Indicative Forward Spending Plans. www.oecd.org/dataoecd/37/20/40636926.pdf Reprinted with permission.

of its aid went to its top 5 recipients.[1] Korea, not a DAC member until 2009, gave aid to 160 countries, and 45.7 per cent of its aid went to its top 5 recipients. These levels of proliferation are broadly similar to those of Western donors, such as the United States (143 recipients, 44 per cent to top 5) or Germany (143 recipients, 34.3 per cent to top 5). By contrast, non-DAC-member Thailand gave aid only to 14 countries and almost all of it (95.2 per cent) was concentrated on the top 5 recipients (Dreher *et al.*, 2010). Comparable measures are not available for China and India, but Guntupalli and Nachiappan (Chapter 4 this volume) show that India's foreign aid is more highly concentrated. In 2007–2008 the bulk of India's foreign aid went to four countries: Bhutan, Afghanistan, Bangladesh and Nepal.

Fragmentation across all aid sectors should be distinguished from fragmentation in a specific aid sector, such as health. For illustrative purposes, Table 10.1 shows the fragmentation of health aid in Vietnam in comparison to total aid and aid for economic infrastructure projects. Health aid is less fragmented than total aid but more fragmented than infrastructure aid. This pattern is a typical one, because projects in health and other social sectors tend to be smaller on average than non-social projects. Frot and Santiso (2010) calculated that globally in 2007 recipient countries had, on average, ten donors in the health sector, of which five provided collectively less than 10 per cent of total health aid. This is less fragmentation than in the education sector, but significantly higher than in economic and productive sectors (in transport and communications, for instance, the average number of donors is only five, of which three provide collectively less than 10 per cent of aid for that sector). This also indicates that emerging donors, who appear to prefer infrastructure projects, contribute less to fragmentation than established donors.

Table 10.1 illustrates the potential role of sectoral specialization in reducing fragmentation. Austria is Vietnam's smallest donor overall (0.04 per cent of all aid) but it is the third-largest donor in the health sector (9.3 per cent). Specialization can be 'unilateral' or the outcome of explicit coordination. Over the past decade, donors and recipients have repeatedly committed themselves to reduce fragmentation and increase coordination, most notably in the Paris Declaration of 2005 and in the Accra Agenda for Action in 2008. But proliferation and fragmentation continue to be high despite such public commitments (Aldasoro et *al.*, 2010). Woods (2008: 1218) remarks that

> The paradox about coordination is that established donors have created so many institutions to enable better coordination among themselves, and yet have simultaneously sidelined them . . . Multilateralism in the international development assistance regime is weakening; and there are very few incentives in the existing governance structure of multilateralism to give emerging donors an incentive to engage.
>
> (Woods, 2008: 1221)

At a minimum, emerging donors would need to be reassured that they would not be put under pressure to comply with principles, such as specialization, when such principles are not actually implemented by established donors themselves.

Table 10.1 Country programmable aid in Vietnam

Country level			*Health*			*Economic Infrastructure*		
Donor	*CPA share %*	*Cumulative %*	*Donor*	*CPA share %*	*Cumulative %*	*Donor*	*CPA share %*	*Cumulative %*
Japan	34.5	34	Japan	22.9	23	France	22.8	23
IDA	18.3	53	United States	18.6	41	Japan	21.8	45
AsDF	10.0	63	Austria	9.3	51	Germany	15.3	60
France	5.8	69	France	6.7	57	Denmark	6.4	66
United Kingdom	4.2	73	EC	6.1	64	Belgium	6.1	72
Denmark	3.5	76	Germany	5.8	69	Netherlands	5.4	78
Germany	3.0	79	The Global Fund	5.4	75	EC	4.2	82
Netherlands	2.9	82	Luxembourg	4.1	79	Sweden	3.9	86
Canada	2.6	85	United Kingdom	3.0	82	Switzerland	3.8	90
Australia	2.4	87	Finland	2.5	84	Norway	2.5	92
Sweden	2.1	89	Belgium	2.5	87	Australia	1.9	94
EC	2.1	91	UNICEF	2.4	89	Canada	1.6	96
United States	1.6	93	IDA	2.2	91	United Kingdom	1.4	97
Finland	0.9	94	Sweden	2.1	94	Finland	1.0	98
Belgium	0.9	95	Netherlands	2.0	95	United States	0.9	99
Switzerland	0.9	96	Spain	1.1	97	Ireland	0.5	99
Norway	0.7	96	Canada	0.9	97	Luxembourg	0.4	100
Spain	0.7	97	New Zealand	0.7	98	New Zealand	0.1	100
Luxembourg	0.5	98	Ireland	0.7	99	Spain	0.0	100
The Global Fund	0.4	98	Norway	0.4	99			
IFAD	0.4	98	Australia	0.4	100			
UNFPA	0.3	99	Denmark	0.2	100			
UNDP	0.3	99	UNAIDS	0.2	100			
Ireland	0.3	99	Switzerland	0.0	100			

(Continued)

Table 10.1 (Continued)

Country level			*Health*			*Economic Infrastructure*		
Donor	*CPA share %*	*Cumulative %*	*Donor*	*CPA share %*	*Cumulative %*	*Donor*	*CPA share %*	*Cumulative %*
UNICEF	0.2	100						
New Zealand	0.2	100						
Italy	0.1	100						
GEF	0.1	100						
Austria	0.0	100						
Total CPA (US$ millions)	1,996		Total health (US$ millions)	111		Total economic infrastructure (US$ millions)	61	

Countries in italics together provide less than 10% of aid in that sector/in total.

Source: OECD DAC 2008. Reprinted with permission.

Beyond this, they are likely to expect some 'special and differential treatment' that takes into account their own development needs. Not surprisingly, Sato *et al.* (2010) show that emerging donors display significant diversity with regard to coordination goals: Thailand and Korea, for instance, declare acceptance of DAC principles, whereas China and India do not actively seek international coordination.[2]

The cumulative effect of the proliferation of bilateral, multilateral and hybrid donors produces what many consider a very high level of complexity at all levels of governance. Figure 10.3 takes a global perspective and summarizes the flows of health funding in 2006 according to the estimates by McCoy *et al.* (2009). Figure 10.4 takes a country-level and disease-specific perspective and illustrates the relationships between international and national actors involved in addressing HIV/AIDS in Tanzania.

The second dimension of global governance, the regulative aspect, can also be broken down into a number of components. A first component is the number of actors who take an *active* part in the negotiation of international rules, notably international treaties. A second component is the diversity of those actors, and specifically the role of non-governmental actors in setting the agenda, formulating and approving rules and monitoring compliance. A third component is the number of treaties and other legal agreements that have been negotiated, ratified and need to be monitored. A fourth component is the number of rules negotiated between non-state actors that create legal or quasi-legal obligations. A fifth component is the extent to which the provisions of one international treaty or agreement overlap and possibly clash with the provisions of other agreements. This issue has been examined by the legal literature on norm collision in international law (e.g. Fischer-Lescano and Teubner, 2006; Benvenisti and Downs, 2007). Political scientists are increasingly interested in the issue of international regime complexity and fragmentation (e.g. Benvenisti and Downs, 2007; Alter and Meunier, 2009; Biermann *et al.*, 2009; Drezner 2009). An important aspect of this issue is whether the overlapping/collision of rules crosses policy domains as they are traditionally conceived, such as health and trade (Lee *et al.*, 2009). Cross-sectoral overlapping or collision increases complexity because it promotes the interaction of policy-makers with different backgrounds, goals, cognitive orientations and acquaintance with different policy networks. A sixth component is closely related to the fifth: the presence or absence of a legal framework that can claim some sort of priority over the others and that can 'reduce complexity' by providing authoritative solutions to possible conflicts between rule systems, or at least a 'focal point' that helps negotiate a solution.

What is the situation in relation to health governance? In comparison to other policy sectors, there are few international agreements that create legally binding obligations for states. In the environmental domain, for instance, there are over 1000 legally binding multilateral agreements, 1500 bilateral agreements, and 250 agreements between governments and international organizations or non-state actors (as opposed to other governments) (Mitchell, 2002–2010). Such a dense system of 'hard law' is lacking in the global health domain.

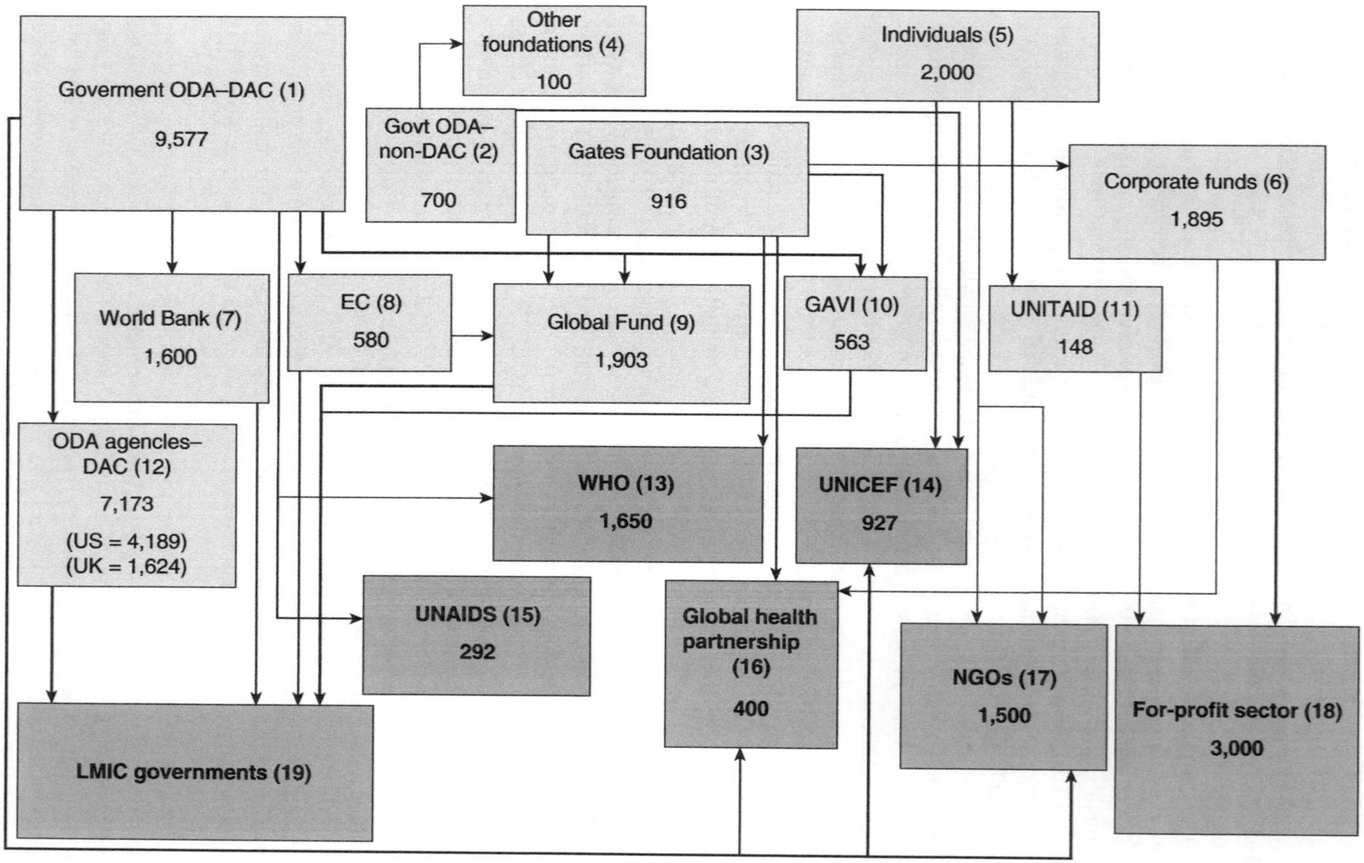

Figure 10.3 Overview of the main blocks of global funding for health in 2006. Figures are in US$ millions.

Source: McCoy *et al.* (2009). Reprinted with permission.

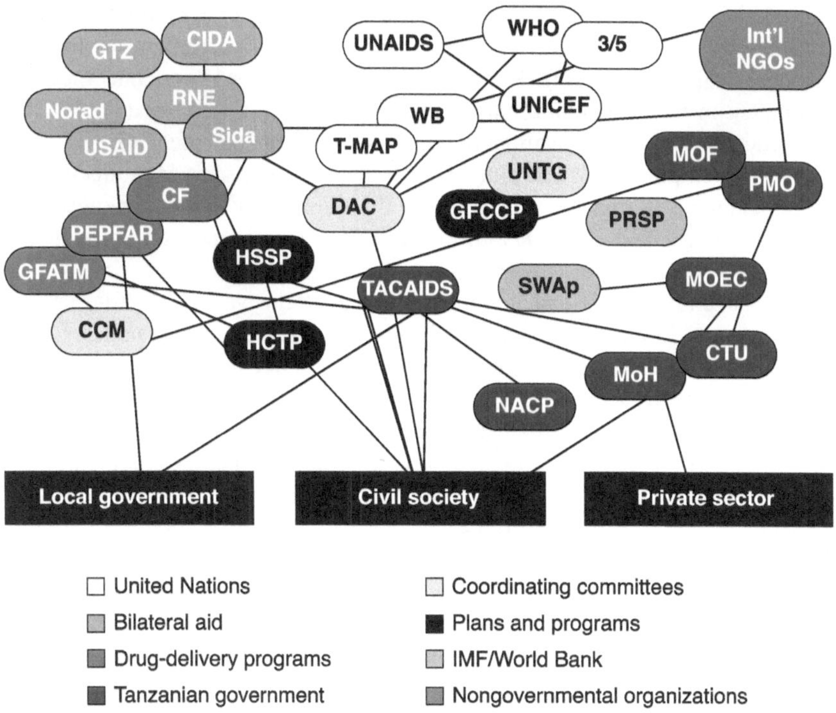

Figure 10.4 The relationship between various stakeholders in Tanzania.
Source: UNAIDS 2005. Reprinted with permission.

Other chapters in this volume indicate that treaty creation processes in the health domain vary considerably in the degree of diversity of their participants. Lee and Kao (Chapter 7 this volume) show that the WHO's Tobacco Free Initiative facilitated the access by civil society organizations to the negotiation process, and non-state actors played a key role in all stages of the process leading to the Framework Convention on Tobacco Control. Among Asian countries, Thailand was a particularly vocal supporter both of stringent tobacco control policies and of the involvement of NGOs without links to the tobacco industry. Kamradt-Scott *et al.* (Chapter 5 this volume) show not only that non-state actors played a much lesser role in the negotiation of the International Health Regulations of 2005, but also that governments exercised a tight control over their participation, by voting to exclude all NGOs from the November 2004 meeting of the Intergovernmental Working Group (IGWG) and then accepting a limited role for those organizations in the IGWG's February 2005 meetings.

Finally, the third dimension of GHG – discursive – is more difficult to operationalize, because patterns of ideational influence are more diffuse, ambiguous and volatile than flows of material resources or formal rules. The field is characterized by broad discursive formations, for instance the biomedical model, social medicine, economism and the 'health security' paradigm in the field of global health (Lee, 2009). As noted above, this chapter is not concerned with the content of the ideas that are transmitted globally, but with the complexity of interaction patterns that constitute the discursive dimensions of GHG.

The key components of this dimension relate to the key sites of production and the key channels of transmission of global discourses, which include knowledge, ideas and norms. The global health research governance analysed by Bennett *et al.* (Chapter 9 this volume) is an important part of this discursive dimension. A very broad understanding of governance includes the validation, filtering and transmission of knowledge, as well as its production. If this broad understanding is accepted, then the number of institutions that produce health research, and the number of links between them in global research networks, are key components of governance complexity. Another component is the number of formal collaborative initiatives among research institutions, which sometimes coincide with the 'partnerships' providing funding discussed earlier. Channels of transmission are probably more difficult to pin down with any degree of precision, as they include diffuse phenomena such the media, networks of researchers and the transnational migration of professionals, such as doctors and nurses. But other channels are more amenable to systematic analysis, notably the number of intergovernmental organizations and the number of NGOs that are active in global health – or, more precisely, the total number of memberships in intergovernmental organizations (IGOs) and international non-governmental organizations (INGOs) across all countries and the number of links between countries that are created by shared IGO and INGO memberships. IGOs and INGOs are not just channels for the transmission of information, but often also the context of deeper socialization processes that modify identities and interests. Finally, a determinant of complexity is the degree to which one or a few organizations play a central role in the validation, selection, diffusion and promotion of health information, ideas and norms.

Bennett *et al.* (Chapter 9 this volume) note that currently only 5 per cent of global scientists work in non-OECD countries. But they also note that China and India are seeking to develop globally competitive health research capabilities, particularly in the area of biotechnology. Moon and Szlezák (Chapter 8 this volume) note that the Chinese government aims to attract 2 per cent of global pharmaceutical research and development spending, and has promoted partnership between multinational companies and Chinese research centres. Pharmaceutical companies such as AstraZeneca, Novartis, GlaxoSmithKline and Sanofi-Aventis have established research and development structures in India, China and Singapore. While the dispersion of research activities beyond the OECD is still in an early stage, the dynamics of pharmaceutical research have changed as a result of the involvement of actors besides companies and governments. Civil society organizations have placed the question of global access to medicines on the policy agenda and large foundations (specifically the Gates Foundation) have channelled new resources into research relevant to the concerns of low and medium income countries. For instance, Bennett *et al.* (Chapter 9 this volume) report that the Gates Foundation was the world's second-biggest funder of research and development for malaria from 1999–2006. As Szlezák and Moon (2010) note, many new initiatives for the development of drugs or technologies take the form of public–private partnerships, such as the Medicines for Malaria Venture (MMV), the Drugs for Neglected Diseases Initiative (DNDI), the Global Alliance for TB drug development, and the International Aids Vaccine Initiative (IAVI). They conclude that 'the era is long past in which states or intergovernmental organizations are the sole, or even leading, actors in addressing the problem of how to produce accessible innovations that address global health needs'.

The complexity created by the proliferation of collaborative research initiatives is not being reduced or managed through a more or less centralized governance structure. According to the policy-makers interviewed by Bennett *et al.* (Chapter 9 this volume), 'there had never been a concerted effort to establish a global governance structure for health research. Instead the existing arrangements had developed in an ad hoc fashion, which in turn had led to extremely fragmented arrangements.'

Kamradt-Scott and Yoon (Chapter 6 this volume) assessed the degree of networking among Asian governments on public health issues in general and pandemic influenza preparedness in particular, and found that most Asian governments seem more interested in building national capabilities than investing in regional initiatives. They also note that the approach chosen in the Asian region may not be distinctive in global comparison.

Institutionalized communication among governments is obviously not the only channel for the diffusion of ideas and strategies to address public health issues. INGOs may be important mechanisms of discursive interdependence across borders. According to the *Yearbook of International Organizations*, over 2600 INGOs were concerned with health, out of about 55,000 INGOs in existence in 1999. While their role is likely to be very substantial in a number of health domains, this is not necessarily the case in others. For instance, Kamradt-Scott and Yoon (Chapter 6 this volume) find little evidence that they played a significant role in pandemic influenza preparation, preparedness and response matters in Asia, apart from isolated exceptions such as the faith-based Muhammadiyah organization in Indonesia.

Effects of governance complexity on health policies and health outcomes

What are the consequences of complexity for the ability of GHG to improve health outcomes and promote substantive health policies that are perceived to be conducive to better outcomes? More precisely, which components of complexity have what effect on health outcomes and health policy? These questions raise a number of difficult methodological issues, not least the choice of terms of comparison. Governance complexity might be reduced by excluding certain actors from policy-making, by increasing coordination among existing actors and by concentrating power in one or few dominant actors; for instance, Sridhar, Khagram and Pang (2008–2009) discuss a number of proposals for increasing the coherence of GHG. There is no reason to expect that all these potential changes would have the same kind of effect on health outcomes.

It is not obvious that complexity per se should have either desirable or undesirable consequences. Many analysts point at harmful consequences. For instance, McCoy *et al.* (2009: 7) argue that

> While the increase in number of global health actors may positively reflect the greater amount of resources and attention for global health, it may lead to an uncoordinated and competitive environment that is problematic for governments and CSOs in [low and middle-income countries]. Many transaction costs come attached to the proliferation of global health actors and initiatives and to the convoluted channels of financing.

See Sridhar (2010) for an elaboration. Several policy-makers, such as the UK's Department for International Development (DfID), tend to agree. Initiatives such as the Sector-Wide Approach (SWAp), the Paris Declaration on Aid Effectiveness, the Accra Agenda for Action, and the International Health Partnership (IHP+) are reactions to the perceived costs of uncoordinated action. Also within the UN there is concern about the proliferation of health initiatives originating from different UN agencies and programmes, such as UNAIDS, UNICEF, WHO, UNFPA, and the UNDP (United Nations, 2006). But the balance of costs and benefits of complexity, and the discrimination of fruitful and harmful forms of complexity, remains a matter of contention.

At the most abstract level, the benefits and costs of complexity can be related to the distinction between 'exploration' and 'exploitation'. 'Exploration includes things captured by terms such as search, variation, risk taking, experimentation, play, flexibility, discovery, innovation. Exploitation includes such things as refinement, choice, production, efficiency, selection, implementation, execution' (March, 1991: 71). While every functioning system must exploit existing certainties as well as exploring new possibilities, often there is a trade-off between the two orientations. High complexity, in the sense elaborated in the previous section, provides many opportunities for exploration, but possibly at the cost of making established policies less efficient. For instance, there is no simple relationship between the degree of competition among institutions and actors promoted by international regime complexity on the one hand, and negative or positive effect on efficiency on the other hand (Alter and Meunier, 2009: 19; Biermann *et al.*, 2009).

Various strands of research offer insights on the effects of global governance complexity on outcomes of interest, and the following provides a very selective overview of findings.

Starting with the allocative dimension of GHG, there is some debate on whether development aid for health has any significant impact on health outcomes. Several studies have examined statistically the effects of health-sector specific ODA and reached diverging conclusions. Wolf (2007) finds that the share of ODA that is provided for health has a positive impact on health outcomes. Similarly, Mishra and Newhouse (2009) find that official health aid decreases infant mortality and increases domestic health spending per capita. By contrast, Williamson (2008) examines five health indicators – infant mortality, life expectancy, death rate and immunizations (diphtheria/pertussis/tetanus and measles) – and finds that health foreign aid has no effect on them. It should be noted that these studies do not provide direct insights on the consequences of health funding complexity – for instance, they focus on ODA and do not consider other channels of health funding. A partial exception is the recent study by Lu *et al.* (2010), which found that development assistance for health to governments has a significant negative effect on domestic government spending on health, whereas development assistance for health to the non-governmental sector had a significant positive effect on domestic government health spending (see also the comments by Ooms *et al.*, 2010 and Sridhar and Woods, 2010).

A strand of research that is more directly relevant to the issue of complexity focuses on aid proliferation and fragmentation. Acharya *et al.* (2006) hypothesize that the proliferation of aid channels increases direct transactions costs (absorption of the scarce energies and attentions of relatively senior government staff) and indirect transactions costs (dysfunctional bureaucratic and political behaviour). This decreases aid efficiency. On the other hand, Frot and Santiso (2010) argue that too little fragmentation may also be problematic, noting that 'Ideally one would like to have some competition, to not have developing countries depending on a single country for aid, but not so much competition that the costs of administering all the partnerships become unmanageable.' Similarly, on the basis of experiences in Cambodia, Sato *et al.* (2010) note that 'a greater number of donors with diverse institutional characteristics (in their values, strategies and modalities) encourages healthy donor competition and thus may contribute to the development plan of the Cambodian government'.

Some cross-national statistical studies found that fragmentation has a negative impact on economic growth (Kimura *et al.*, 2007; Djankov *et al.*, 2009; Annen and Kosempel, 2009) and bureaucratic quality (Knack and Rahman, 2007), but these studies do not specifically focus on health aid or health impacts.

An important study of the impact of NGO aid on development outcomes is by Masud and Yontcheva (2005), which is noteworthy also because it specifically includes impacts on health outcomes. Masud and Yontcheva only examine projects proposed by European NGOs and co-financed by the European Union between 1990 and 2001, and find that NGO aid reduces infant mortality in recipient countries. On the other hand, the same authors find no significant impact of total bilateral ODA on infant mortality, nor any evidence that either total bilateral aid or NGO aid has an impact on the share of spending on health care in total expenditure.

Research into the regulative dimension of global governance has equally yielded mixed findings with regard to the effects of complexity. Alter and Meunier (2009: 14) usefully summarize the current state of knowledge as follows:

> Sometimes complexity empowers powerful state actors, while at other times NGOs and weaker actors gain from the overlap of institutions and rules. Sometimes overlap introduces positive feedback effects that enhance cooperation and the effectiveness of any one cooperative regime. Sometimes, however, complexity introduces unhelpful competition across actors, inefficiencies, and transaction costs that end up compromising the objectives of international cooperation and international governance.

An assessment of which of these effects tends to prevail in GHG is hindered by the scarcity of legally binding international treaties on health matters. The IHR 2005 and the FCTC entered into force only in recent years and evaluations of their effectiveness are still tentative. Lee and Kao (Chapter 7 this volume) cite a Chinese official according to whom the FCTC process galvanized a nascent tobacco control movement in China and helped it gain political impetus. They also note how support for a strong FCTC by the Indian government interacted with the promotion of strong domestic legislation in a mutually reinforcing way. On the other hand, the experience with pre-2005 versions of the IHR indicates that the status of binding international law does not guarantee an actual effect. Kamradt-Scott *et al.* (Chapter 5 this volume) found substantial differences among Asian countries in the level of attention and commitment devoted to the implementation of the IHR 2005.

As stressed in the previous section, the discursive dimension is a very important aspect of GHG (Lee, 2009). While a number of scholars have pointed at the deleterious effect of certain *contents*, notably neoliberal discourses on global health (e.g. Kay and Williams, 2009), we know much less on whether the multiplication of actors propagating global health discourses is good or bad for health. Research has shown that territorial contiguity helps policy innovations to spread from country to country (Shearer *et al.*, 2010), but less is known about the relative importance of different vectors – bilateral government contacts, interaction within IGOs, transnational networking among NGOs, the mobility of health professionals, etc. It can be hypothesized that national and local policy-makers and officials who interact with a larger number of transnational actors (representatives of NGOs, IGOs and foreign donors) are more likely to select and implement more effective health policies, in line with the alleged benefits of a vibrant 'marketplace of ideas'. But we do not have yet the evidence necessary for a rigorous assessment of this hypothesis, or the opposite hypothesis.

This gap in knowledge can be addressed by a research agenda that exploits the potential of innovative statistical approaches, notably social network analysis and spatial econometrics. These techniques are particularly suited to capture the complex processes of interdependent policy-making that characterizes a diffuse governance complex such as global health. From the perspective on individual governance units, researchers can try to establish whether the degree of network centrality and embeddedness of territorial units affects health outcomes within those units.[3] Two networks deserve special attention: first, the network of intergovernmental organizations concerned with health or with related social issues;

secondly, the network of transnationally active NGOs concerned with health issues. Moreover, researchers could establish whether the health policies of governments (specifically health spending) are influenced by what other governments do, and which governments are particularly influential: hegemonic centres, or 'peer groups' identified on the basis of frequent interactions within the same IGOs, or linked by the same INGOs. The outcome of such investigations would provide important new information on whether and how involvement of actors in global discursive networks affects their ability to address health challenges.[4]

Concluding remarks

This chapter has discussed a number of concepts that can help policy-makers in Asia and elsewhere to think systematically about the nature of governance complexity in global health, and ultimately to design more effective global health policies – e.g. aid proliferation and fragmentation, and network centrality and embeddedness. Social researchers have also produced knowledge on the consequences of those complexity indicators, for instance, by highlighting the negative impact of aid fragmentation on economic growth, or the positive impact of non-state actors on outcomes such as government health budgets, funding for specific diseases and the creation of international law. However, there are still major gaps in our knowledge of the consequences of governance complexity on health outcomes and related goals. What is missing is not only the analysis of specific aspects of the problem – for instance, cross-national statistical studies of the relationship between fragmentation of *health* aid and *health* outcomes, or of the role of NGOs in the diffusion of immunization policies – but also a comprehensive examination of how all these relationships *interact* to shape the dynamics of GHG as we know it today and as it may evolve in the future. A research agenda that, within a broader polycentric approach to global policy (Koenig-Archibugi 2010), uses complexity as a central analytical category can provide policy-makers with tools that are especially valuable in times of transition such as the current one.

Notes

1 Pilcavage (Chapter 2 this volume) notes that the long-term trend in Japanese foreign aid consisted in shifting from a focus on Asia towards a greater diversification of recipients: the Asian region received 98.2 per cent of Japanese ODA in 1970 and 49.6 per cent in 1996.

2 Some limited initiatives to reduce fragmentation are initiated by recipient countries. An example is India under the National Democratic Alliance government, which announced in 2003 that it would accept bilateral aid only from UK, Japan, Germany, Russia, the EU and the US. The list was later extended to Canada, France, Italy and the Scandinavian countries (Guntupalli and Nachiappan, Chapter 4 this volume).

3 An important application of social network analysis to environmental policy outcomes is Ward (2006).

4 For a study that has begun to implement this research agenda, see Han *et al.* (2012).

11 Asia and global health governance

Power, principles and practice

David P. Fidler

Introduction

Global health governance (GHG) is an increasingly significant area of focus within the fields of global health and international relations. Though the literature and discourse on GHG has expanded, to date there has been little work examining the perspectives and roles of Asian countries and GHG (see, e.g., Stevenson and Cooper, 2009). Analyzing Asian perspectives and participation in GHG represents a difficult task because of Asia's political, economic and cultural complexity as well as the quantity and diversity of problems addressed through GHG mechanisms. This chapter analyzes Asian countries' conceptions of and contributions to GHG. My analysis attempts to provide a framework for thinking about the Asian approach to and impact on GHG, which hopefully will contribute to more sophisticated conceptual and empirical work on Asia and GHG.

This chapter contains four analytical sections. First, it examines the simultaneous 'rise of Asia' and 'rise of health' in global affairs. While the rise of Asia has little to do with the rise of health as a foreign policy and diplomatic issue, the increased economic, political and strategic importance of Asia is significant for exploring how Asian governments conceptualize global health challenges and what contributions Asian states have made or can make to GHG.

Secondly, the chapter analyzes more specifically how the shift of power and influence towards Asia affects GHG and potential Asian contributions to GHG in the future. This power shift has positive and negative implications for Asia's role in GHG. How Asian countries view their new power and influence will significantly shape how they conceptualize global health as an issue, and how they approach GHG.

Thirdly, the chapter looks at normative ideas that characterize Asian approaches to foreign policy and international cooperation. The key norms are the Five Principles of Peaceful Coexistence (Five Principles), first articulated in 1954 by China, India and Burma, but which have become bedrock tenets of Chinese and Indian foreign policies and Asian regional efforts, especially within the Association of Southeast Asian Nations (ASEAN) (see Box 11.1). The Five Principles apply to health issues as to other policy topics, and thus have potentially significant impact on how Asian countries think about collective action toward health issues, including GHG.

Box 11.1 Five Principles of Peaceful Coexistence

1 Mutual respect for territorial integrity and sovereignty
2 Mutual non-aggression
3 Mutual non-interference in internal affairs
4 Equality and mutual benefit
5 Peaceful co-existence

Fourthly, the chapter considers existing Asian practices on international health cooperation, which include bilateral relations, regional efforts and participation in multilateral organizations. Asian diplomatic activity includes health issues in all these contexts, but the activity tends to be state-centric and utilizes traditional, sovereignty-sensitive mechanisms of international cooperation. Asian countries have not been prominent in more innovative GHG mechanisms developed in the past 10–15 years. The analysis of Asian practices also considers some Asian-specific controversies involving GHG and GHG's potential future in an Asian-centric international system.

The chapter ends with preliminary conclusions about Asian conceptualizations of and contributions to GHG. A key conclusion is that, to date, there is nothing distinctive about Asian conceptualizations of or contributions to GHG. Asian power, shared principles and diplomatic practices have not been a driving force in the recent transformations of health as a foreign policy issue or in the way GHG has emerged and evolved. The chapter raises some possibilities for a more pronounced or distinctive Asian role in GHG. It also highlights potential obstacles to Asian countries, especially China and India, in blazing an Asian-oriented path for GHG.

Rise of Asia and the rise of health in world affairs

The past 10–15 years have witnessed the 'rise of Asia' and an increased profile of health issues in foreign policy, diplomacy and global governance. For the most part, the relevant literatures on Asia's new importance and on global health's novel political prominence do not overlap, meaning that experts do not explain these phenomena as being interconnected. This reality has important features for Asian conceptualizations of and contributions to GHG.

The lack of connection between the rise of Asian countries in global politics and the unprecedented importance global health has achieved suggest that Western countries, particularly the United States and European nations, triggered the transformation of global health into a foreign policy and diplomatic issue. This observation is consistent with the S. T. Lee Project Study Group on Global Health Governance's sense that the majority of contributions to GHG have come from Western developed countries (S. T. Lee Project on Global Governance Study Group on Global Health Governance, 2009).

Asian countries' increasing influence has produced debates about 'Asian values', an 'Asian way' of policy-making and diplomacy, the 'ASEAN way' of regionalism and contributions to international law by Asian civilizations and cultures (see Box 11.2). None of these conversations have involved much, if any, attention to Asian attitudes towards health domestically or globally. Asian countries have addressed global health challenges during Asia's rise to greater political and economic prominence, but these efforts at health diplomacy have not led or characterized the larger phenomenon of the shift of power and influence towards Asia.

Box 11.2. The 'Asian Way'

> So is there an 'Asian way' of approaching global governance? The positive aspects of this approach to diplomacy and governance include respect for diversity, consensus-building over conflict, pragmatic approaches rather than lofty principles, and gradualism rather than abrupt change. The negative aspects can be that the desire to avoid confrontation prevents meaningful agreements being concluded in a reasonable timeframe, or that the appearance of consensus merely masks the true politics at work.
>
> Mahbubani and Chesterman (2009: 6)

The lack of focus on health in Asia's political emergence raises the question of what Asia's trajectory of increasing importance means for health diplomacy and GHG. In geopolitical terms, the rise of Asia will change the structure and dynamics of the international system, moving the world away from the quasi-hegemonic, American-centric, post-Cold War system into an Asian-influenced multipolar arrangement in which China and India continue to emerge as great powers. This still-unfolding change in the structure of the international system reminds us that the transformations in health diplomacy and GHG in the post-Cold War period may simply reflect the system that prevailed during those years. In other words, the changes seen in health as a diplomatic and global governance issue over the past 10–15 years are not permanent.

In the new, emerging system, the dynamics of international relations will reflect both multipolarity and continued globalization. Put another way, nations will continue to face many collective action problems exacerbated by globalization, including health challenges, but reaching cooperative solutions will be harder in a multipolar context. The US National Intelligence Council (2008: 81) referred to this more difficult diplomatic and governance context as potentially exhibiting 'multipolarity without multilateralism'. This situation means that what China, India and other Asian countries want will matter more in terms of power and ideas, but Asian preferences may not prevail if opposed by other geopolitical heavyweights.

Cooperation may only be effective on problems, such as virulent and mobile infectious diseases (e.g., pandemic influenza), where countries share strong common, reciprocal interests. More complicated GHG problems, such as improving the social determinants of health (e.g., poverty, education, gender equality) within countries as called for by the World Health Organization (WHO) Commission on the Social Determinants of Health (2008), could face greater difficulties. In short, the emerging multipolarity may limit the ability of Asian countries to influence GHG significantly should they attempt to do so.

Asian power and global health governance

The 'rise of Asia' refers to the realization in international affairs that material power and political influence are shifting towards Asia. The engine of this shift has been the sustained, significant economic growth achieved by China, India and Southeast Asia. One prominent indicator of this shift in power and influence is the decision to have the Group of 20 (G20) replace the Group of 8 (G8) as the premier international forum for cooperation among the world's most important economic powers. The G8 had only one member from Asia (Japan), but the G20 has five (China, India, Indonesia, Japan and the Republic of Korea). This power shift has positive and negative features for GHG.

Positive features of Asian power for global health governance

In terms of positive features, Asia's economic growth has contributed toward achieving the Millennium Development Goals (MDGs), which include health-specific objectives (e.g., reducing the burden of HIV/AIDS, TB and malaria) and goals on improving key social determinants of health, such as poverty reduction, education and empowerment of women and girls. For example, the United Nations (2009a: 7) reported that '[t]here was a dramatic fall in the poverty rate in Eastern Asia – thanks in large part to rapid economic growth in China, which helped lift 475 million people from extreme poverty'.

These positive health implications of Asian economic growth do not, however, owe anything to instruments or initiatives specific to global health. Asian economic growth has occurred because of, among other things, domestic economic reforms in Asian countries, negotiation of bilateral and regional trade and investment agreements, foreign investment in Asian economies and Asian participation in the multilateral World Trade Organization (WTO).

A second positive feature of the power shift towards Asia has been that it has, so far, been peaceful. Previous shifts in geopolitical tectonic plates have produced serious tensions, hostile rivalries and armed conflict. Both China's and India's increased material power and political influence have caused nervousness, suspicions and some balancing behavior regionally and globally, but, to date, this historic shift has not triggered armed conflict or threats of war, which is good for global health given how devastating war is for individual and population health. Asia has not been free of armed conflict in the past 10–15 years, but the conflicts that have occurred (e.g., the Indo–Pakistan conflict in 1999; the Tamil Tiger insurgency in Sri Lanka; the Taliban/Al Qaeda insurgency in Pakistan; the Naxalite insurgency in India) relate to problems that have little, if anything, to do with Asia's emerging geopolitical heft. However, the lack of armed conflict related to Asia's rise has nothing to do with health diplomacy or GHG.

A third positive feature is more speculative, but it is still worth mentioning. As China and India emerge as great powers, they may wish to compete more effectively with the United States, Japan and other powers in the 'soft power' arena of global health. Already, the United States and China view health activities as part of their soft-power efforts in Africa (Cooke, 2009; Hackbarth, 2009; Huang, 2010). Multipolarity could trigger more competition for global health leadership, with different initiatives and increased money being applied to address various global health problems. Such soft-power competition could bring additional attention, political capital and economic resources to global health. The potential downsides for GHG would be that (1) such a 'health race' would continue to fragment GHG instead of contributing to a more consolidated strategy; and (2) global health would become increasingly a policy space to pursue narrow, national interests rather than collective action that improves health globally.

Negative aspects of Asian power for global health governance

There are three negative implications of the power shift to Asia for global health governance. First, the health benefits of economic growth depend on such growth continuing, which, as the great global recession of 2008–10 has proved, is not guaranteed. Although China and India seem to have weathered the global economic and financial crisis better than others, the crisis took a terrible economic toll that set back achievement of the MDGs around over the world (United Nations, 2009a).

Secondly, the power shift means that multipolarity will become the new structure for the international system, which, as noted above, may make effective cooperation on global health problems more difficult. A soft-power 'health race' among the great powers would not necessarily produce effective collective action, and could simply multiply global health initiatives without an overall GHG strategy. In addition, the multipolarity that emerges may not be stable; rivalries may develop (e.g., China vs. United States) that result in political and economic resources being expended in ways that do not benefit global health.

Thirdly, the growth of Asian material power and influence has not eliminated massive domestic problems Asian countries face, especially China and India (Lo, 2010; Fidler and Ganguly, 2010). To maintain their great power status, China and India may focus more on their own serious domestic political and social problems, including health, and not scale up their support for or take leadership roles in global health initiatives or GHG. Improvements in domestic health conditions in China and India would, given the sheer size of their respective populations, benefit global health outcomes, but these improvements would not rely on GHG mechanisms. Similarly, the United States may be forced to focus on domestic problems, including reform of its dysfunctional healthcare system and ballooning budget deficits.

Asian principles and global health governance

Despite Asia's political, economic and cultural diversity, Asian countries have exhibited solidarity on basic normative ideas for the conduct of international relations as described in the Five Principles of Peaceful Coexistence. The importance of the Five Principles in Asian nations' foreign policy, regional efforts and participation in multilateral forums is well-documented, and the Five Principles constitute the normative framework Asian countries, at present, want to utilize as material power and political influence move their way (see Box 11.3), and have provided no indication that global health falls outside the scope of the Five Principles. Thus, the Five Principles are important for how Asian countries conceptualize GHG now and in the foreseeable future.

Box 11.3 Asia and the Five Principles of Peaceful Coexistence

> Pan-Asian support for the [Five Principles] has deep roots in the emergence of Asian societies from imperialism, and the Five Principles have resonated strongly in Asia to the present day. The Five Principles laid the basis for the Association of Southeast Asian Nations (ASEAN) in 1967 and were reinforced in the 1994 creation of the ASEAN Regional Forum on security issues. More recently, the first India-ASEAN summit in 2002 explicitly referred to the Five Principles, and China and India jointly celebrated the fiftieth anniversary of the Five Principles in 2004. Outside Asia, both China and India have used the Five Principles to shape their relations with countries across the Middle East and Africa.
>
> Kim, Fidler and Ganguly (2009: 58)

The principles of sovereignty and non-intervention

If applied to global health, the ideals of the Five Principles run counter to trends in GHG over the past 10–15 years. For example, support for a strong sovereignty principle clashes with many arguments made in global health that traditional notions of sovereignty are a serious obstacle to progress, and that effective GHG requires less emphasis on sovereignty and more internationalized or globalized governance approaches. In this vein, Stevenson and Cooper (2009: 1380) argued that the actions of Asian countries in global health episodes (e.g., China and SARS, Indonesia and avian influenza A [H5N1] and Burma and HIV/AIDS) illuminate 'sovereignty as an impediment to progressive global health governance'.

GHG discourse also contains frequent assertions that states must be held increasingly accountable domestically and internationally for their performance in public health and health care. Such accountability requires, logically, the ability for the international community to scrutinize and, if necessary, interfere in the domestic affairs of states unable or unwilling to protect and promote health effectively. This increasing demand for accountability is connected with renewed efforts to emphasize the human right to health (Committee on Economic, Social and Cultural Rights, 2000), but it is perhaps most dramatically seen in the development of a purported new principle of international law called 'the responsibility to protect' or R2P (International Commission on Intervention and State Sovereignty, 2001). The Asian preference for a strong principle of non-interference in the domestic affairs of sovereign states stands athwart this movement for global accountability of governments for health in their territories, and opposes the responsibility to protect principle and similar interventionist notions connected with concepts of human rights and humanitarian imperatives.

GHG literature also contains arguments that the capabilities and authority of international organizations, especially the WHO, should be strengthened and expanded. Moving in this direction requires greater institutionalization of global health policy and, potentially, greater legalization through adoption of more binding rules, for example, in the mould of the WHO's Framework Convention on Tobacco Control (FCTC) and International Health Regulations (2005) (IHR, 2005) (World Health Organisation, 2003c, 2005).

However, Asian application of the Five Principles has, especially in the regional context, demonstrated preferences for weak institutions and utilization of non-binding solutions. As Mahbubani and Chesterman (2009: 3) observed, the Asian 'preference is still for consultative, non-binding forums that avoid issues of national sovereignty'. ASEAN provides the best example of this Asian predilection because this regional organization 'is associated not with sovereignty-reducing integration but with the "ASEAN Way": a process of consultation and consensus that is identified with many of the cultures in the region' (Ginsburg, 2010: 36).

Another characteristic of GHG in the past 10–15 years has been the increased involvement of non-state actors, especially non-governmental organizations (NGOs) and philanthropies (e.g., the Bill and Melinda Gates Foundation). Although the Five Principles are not overtly hostile to non-state actors, they are state-centric principles, indicating a belief that states remain the primary interlocutors of world affairs. The activities of NGOs, especially those engaged in human rights advocacy and philanthropic foundations endowed with substantial resources, can be conduits for outside interference in a state's domestic affairs. The stress on non-interference in the Five Principles creates a somewhat more skeptical view of non-state actor involvement in global health politics than has appeared in GHG discussions elsewhere.

The importance of non-interference creates other potential problems for Asian perspectives on GHG. A number of global health problems stem from practices, traditions and systems deeply embedded within countries, forcing solutions to involve significant changes in domestic affairs. For example, inadequately regulated economic activities, such as lax biosecurity and biosafety standards in industrial-scale poultry production, contribute to global health problems, including the spread of zoonoses and antimicrobial resistance (Institute of Medicine, 2009). Health-systems reform, a leading concern in global health (World Health Organisation, 2007b), requires transformation of domestic medical, healthcare and regulatory arrangements in many countries. Bringing about the progressive realization of the human right to health often involves the need for significant domestic policy reform across a range of sectors.

Similarly, addressing the increasing prevalence of non-communicable diseases (NCDs) within countries, such as those associated with tobacco consumption, requires interventions within domestic societies. Reducing corruption to achieve 'good governance' – both important goals for improving health systems' performance (Lewis, 2006) – involves alterations to political and legal systems. Improving social determinants of health in many nations cannot be achieved without transformations in aspects of government and society, including the conditions that produce poverty, poor education, discrimination against females and environmental degradation (Commission on the Social Determinants of Health, 2009). Preventing and mitigating the health-related impact of climate change will necessitate serious changes within greenhouse gas-producing countries (Costello *et al.*, 2009).

The tenet of non-interference in the Five Principles creates potential problems for GHG actions to stimulate needed reforms for health-related challenges that are embedded in the domestic politics, economics, regulatory capabilities and governing cultures of sovereign states. As explored further below, this observation does not mean that Asian countries avoid cooperation on these challenges; rather, it means that the Asian commitment to non-interference limits GHG on health problems tightly intertwined with the domestic affairs of states.

The principle of equality and mutual benefit

The principle of equality and mutual benefit also creates potential complications for GHG. This principle harkens back to the unequal treatment and exploitation many Asian countries experienced at the hands of Western imperial powers. This heritage makes Asian governments particularly sensitive to developments that threaten to treat them unequally or inequitably, or that produce benefits mainly for other countries.

This sensitivity has been prominent in the controversy sparked by Indonesia's stance on avian influenza A (H5N1) virus-sharing and access to benefits, such as vaccines, developed through research on such strains (Fidler, 2007). Concern about the unequal impact and benefits of patent protection on pharmaceuticals within the WTO and bilateral trade agreements also reveal this sensitivity. The principle of equality and mutual benefit informs China's and India's stance on climate change – namely that the Western industrialized countries caused the problem and should take greater responsibility, rather than demanding that developing countries limit their economic development. This perspective can be found in the Copenhagen Accord negotiated in December 2009, which provides that developed and developing countries should

> cooperate in achieving the peaking of global and national emissions as soon as possible, recognizing that the time frame for peaking will be longer in developing countries and bearing in mind that social and economic development and poverty eradication are the first and overriding priorities of developing countries.
>
> (Copenhagen Accord, 2009)

The gap between Asian principles and the trajectory of global health governance

The examples discussed above reflect a gap between the post-sovereignty mindset present in GHG discourse and the post-colonial insistence on sovereignty and non-interference as principles in international relations. The emergence of China and India as great powers in a multipolar system has two additional effects with respect to the potential impact of this gap.

First, as great powers, China and India will increasingly be able to deflect criticisms of their domestic behavior and proposals for health-related outside intervention in their domestic affairs. An example of this ability to shrug off criticism can be found in China's aggressive measures against influenza A (H1N1), such as quarantines of travelers, which created controversy but which China sustained and increased as other countries scaled back their responses in light of new information (Huang, 2010).

Secondly, Chinese and Indian commitment to the Five Principles will shape their relations with other countries, which may prefer the Five Principles approach to more demanding, interventionist ideas prevalent in Western thinking (see Box 11.4). The efforts of governmental and non-governmental actors advocating for serious domestic changes could be undermined if China or India increased their soft power and opened channels of potential political influence in other countries.

Box 11.4 The appeal of Five Principles-based assistance

> China's respect-for-sovereignty rhetoric still resonates for many Africans. China's often expressed respect for sovereignty and territorial integrity and its policy of noninterference resonate for obvious reasons with many African leaders. But they resonate too with many Africans who view Western lecturing on human rights, economic liberalization, and democracy as condescending and hypocritical. The lack of conditionality or broad consultation attached to Chinese assistance and loans allows projects to be implemented quickly, with visible and often immediate results.
>
> Cooke (2009: 27)

Asian practices and global health governance

Understanding Asian conceptualizations of and contributions to GHG also requires comprehending how Asian countries go about health cooperation in their foreign affairs. Actual diplomatic practices can reveal wrinkles in governmental attitudes towards collective action that may indicate important differences and possibilities not reflected in rhetoric about power, sovereignty and non-interference. The level of Asian countries' participation in collective action on health matters is significant. However, this participation tends to be very state-centric through the predominant use of traditional diplomatic approaches. This approach to health cooperation is consistent with the general pattern associated with the diplomacy of Asian countries.

Asian participation in global health cooperation

Asian countries have included health concerns in their diplomatic activities in bilateral, regional, identity- or status-based and multilateral cooperative endeavors. Health cooperation has featured in both Chinese and Indian relations with Africa (Forum on China–Africa Cooperation, 2009; India–Africa Forum Summit, 2008). Sino-American and Indo-American bilateral relations include joint activities on health (White House, 2009a, b). Japan has made efforts to be a global health leader by increasing its support for health initiatives in its diplomatic activities (Kondo, 2009).

Regionally, health cooperation features on the agendas of numerous regional organizations in Asia, including ASEAN, Asia Pacific Economic Cooperation (APEC) forum, South Asia Association for Regional Cooperation and Shanghai Cooperation Organization. Asian participation in identity- or status-based intergovernmental organizations, processes, and initiatives – such as the G8, Organization of the Islamic Conference, and South–South collaborations – also includes health issues. Table 11.1 provides some examples of health activities under these regional and identity- or status-based intergovernmental organizations.

Asian countries also participate in multilateral organizations important in GHG, such as the United Nations, WHO (including its relevant regional offices), UNAIDS, International Vaccine Institute (located in South Korea), the World Bank and the WTO. Asians have served as the Director-General of WHO: Hiroshi Nakajima (Japan), Jong-wook Lee (South Korea) and Margaret Chan (China). In terms of WHO legal instruments important in GHG, many Asian countries have become States Parties to the FCTC, and all Asian members of WHO are States Parties to the International Heath Regulations (IHR) 2005. Indonesia and Thailand were founding members of the Foreign Policy and Global Health initiative launched in 2007 (Oslo Ministerial Declaration, 2007).

In terms of more innovative GHG efforts made in recent years (e.g., public–private partnerships), representatives from Asian countries participate or have participated as board members on the Global Fund to Fight AIDS, Tuberculosis and Malaria and the GAVI Alliance. Asian countries have not, to date, become

Table 11.1 Regional organizations and health cooperation

Organization	*Example(s) of health cooperation issues*
Regional organizations	
APEC	• Health Ministers' Meetings • Health Working Group (influenza preparedness, HIV/AIDS, improving health through health information technologies) • Infectious disease surveillance
ASEAN	• HIV/AIDS • SARS • Avian influenza A (H5N1) • Influenza A (H1N1)
Shanghai Cooperation Organization	• Pandemic influenza • HIV/AIDS • Tuberculosis • Malaria
South Asia Association for Regional Cooperation	• Information-sharing on infectious disease outbreaks • Sharing of health knowledge and expertise • Sharing of drug manufacturing capacities • Adopting regional standards on drugs and pharmaceuticals
Identity- or status-based organizations and initiatives	
G8	• Access to antiretrovirals for HIV/AIDS • Malaria • Tuberculosis • Avian influenza A (H5N1) • Polio • Bioterrorism • Improving health systems
Organization of the Islamic Conference	• Polio • Malaria • Tobacco control • Pandemic and avian influenza • Health equity in the Islamic *Ummah*
South–South collaborations	• Health care delivery • Food security • Child labor • Hunger • Poverty

donors in the International Finance Facility for Immunization (2010) or the Advance Market Commitment for Pneumococcal Vaccines (2010).

Although Asian participation in global health cooperation is impressive, this level of participation is not distinctively Asian. The increased importance of global health in foreign policy, diplomacy and global governance in the past 10–15 years reveals that many countries and regions have scaled up their participation in global health affairs in the same way Asian countries have (UN Secretary-General, 2009; World Health Organisation, 2009a). As argued above, the rise of Asia has not been linked with global health's increased political importance, indicating that Asian participation in health cooperation has not been considered seminal to the changes that have reshaped health as a foreign policy, diplomatic and global governance issue. Nor does the level of Asian participation provide insight into whether the participation has produced effective, sustainable results.

Perceptions of Asia as a source of global health problems

Instead, Asia has been more associated with problems that challenge or threaten progress on global health and GHG. These episodes include Asian countries being (1) the origin and epicenter of dangerous disease outbreaks, especially SARS and avian influenza A (H5N1); (2) threatened by the continued spread of HIV/AIDS, AIDS-associated sequela (e.g., TB), malaria and dengue fever; and (3) at risk from adverse health consequences predicted to accompany climate change.

Several serious global health controversies indicate that the rise of Asia and application of the Five Principles may hamper the evolution of GHG. For example, Asian opposition to the application of the R2P principle blocked efforts to advance the health and other humanitarian concerns of Western nations and NGOs in the aftermath of Cyclone Nargis in Myanmar (*The Economist*, 2008) and the Sri Lankan government's defeat of the Tamil Tiger insurgency (Asia-Pacific Centre for the Responsibility to Protect, 2008). Similarly, Indian, Chinese and ASEAN refusal to interfere in Myanmar's domestic affairs has allowed that failing state to multiply domestic and cross-border health harms (e.g., HIV/AIDS, malaria, illicit drug use and trafficking) that degrade national, regional and global health (Stevenson and Cooper, 2009).

Asian support for Indonesia's 'viral sovereignty' over avian influenza A (H5N1) virus strains collected in Indonesian territory challenged the legitimacy of WHO's Global Influenza Surveillance Network, undermined global efforts at H5N1 surveillance and produced a new intergovernmental negotiating process on virus and benefit-sharing that has yet, as of this writing, to reach any mutually satisfactory solution (Leboeuf, 2009; Scoones and Forster, 2009). As noted above, the Indonesian stance and Asian backing for it reflected long-standing Asian concerns about unequal, potentially exploitative regimes and practices in international relations.

Negotiations of the IHR 2005 were almost damaged severely by differing perspectives on sovereignty by China and Taiwan (Fidler, 2005; Huang, 2010). Taiwan wanted to use the principle of universal application in the IHR 2005 to heighten its legitimacy as a sovereign state, while China maintained its position that it holds sovereignty over Taiwan. Of course, the China–Taiwan problem is not unique to global health, but it revealed that a matter as critical as global health does not outweigh claims of sovereignty.

Concerns about Asian perspectives on human rights also have arisen in global health. One source of these concerns was the acrimonious 'Asian values' debate in the 1990s that pitted assertions about Asian cultural understandings of rights against the more universalist perspective of human rights advocates and international bodies. Ginsburg (2010: 33) has argued that '[t]he greatest conceptual innovation of Asian states in international law in the past several decades has been a regressive one, namely the idea that "Asian values" offered an alternative to liberal universalism'. Although the Asian values debate did not focus on health issues, it raised concerns among those who believe that universal human rights form part of fabric of GHG.

Another source of discomfort in the human rights area flows from the weakness of human rights institutions and processes in Asia. Unlike other regions, Asia has no regional human rights machinery. The closest thing to such machinery is the ASEAN Intergovernmental Commission on Human Rights, which ASEAN formally established in October 2009. This new development has generated controversy; many question whether the ASEAN members really intend to create a robust human rights mechanism. The Commission has been called the 'world's most toothless human-rights body' (*Wall Street Journal*, 2009) and 'remarkable and . . . an essential first step toward ASEAN's stated goal of respecting and protecting human rights' (Kelsall, 2009).

Although it is too early to judge the ASEAN's new human rights mechanism, the strong ASEAN and Asian adherence to the principles of sovereignty and non-interference make the potential development of an effective regional human rights regime questionable. The fulfillment of human rights relevant to health is, under the Five Principles, largely a matter of a country's domestic affairs in which other states or international organizations cannot interfere.

China and India have also generated controversy in global health for, so far, refusing to negotiate binding reductions in greenhouse gas emissions as part of a needed global agreement on climate change. China and India were key players in the negotiation of the Copenhagen Accord in December 2009, a non-binding political agreement under which they and other countries agreed to make voluntary commitments to reduce greenhouse gas emissions (United Nations, 2009b). Assessments of the Copenhagen Accord and its future impact on climate change vary significantly (Levi, 2009; Stavins, 2009; Greenpeace, 2010). Failure to make progress on preventing climate change and preparing to mitigate the anticipated damage climate change may cause could be a tragedy of enormous magnitude for global health and GHG (World Health Organisation, 2009c).

In sum, Asian practices reveal high levels of Asian engagement with health issues bilaterally, regionally and globally, as well as Asian involvement in controversies that threaten global health and the development of GHG. Both themes are consistent with application of the Five Principles in the global health context. The Five Principles do not prevent Asian countries from engaging in significant levels of collective action and, thus, contributing to GHG through bilateral, regional, and multilateral efforts. As one analysis put it, '[t]he vast majority of Asian governments now understand that collective action does not erode, but instead protects sovereignty' (Mahbubani and Chesterman, 2009: 2).

In this respect, Asian practices are similar to those of countries in other regions that have increased their foreign policy and diplomatic activities on global health.

Asian countries appear, thus, to be reacting to global health challenges and contributing to GHG in ways similar to many non-Asian nations. Thus, locating distinctive Asian attributes in Asian participation in GHG proves a difficult and potentially misleading exercise. To date, most Asian involvement in GHG mechanisms reflects the Asian preference for traditional collective action strategies that do not create significant sovereignty problems.

However, the interpretation and application of the Five Principles by Asian countries are not fixed and static, and Asian use of the Principles in the future might not resemble their use during decolonization and the Cold War. In those earlier periods, Asian countries deployed the Five Principles predominantly in defensive ways that reflected the countries' political and economic weaknesses, and their vulnerability to outside pressure and interference from more powerful states. Although prickliness over perceived outside intervention still occurs, as seen in Chinese and Indian bristling over human rights criticisms, many Asian countries, such as the Asian members of the G20, no longer equate, for example, economic interdependence with threats of foreign intervention.

Asian countries and societies have become more globalized through their sovereign choices to integrate into global markets for goods, services, technologies and investment capital. The most dramatic examples of change in this regard are China and India, both of which avoided interconnections with Western market economies for decades after World War II in favor of autarkic political and economic development. Today, China's and India's emerging power and influence come from rejecting autarky in favor of deeper levels of political cooperation and economic interdependence.

These dramatic changes have also helped Asian countries realize their vulnerability to many global problems, such as the spread of infectious diseases, financial crises and the dangers of climate change, which require international cooperation to address. The globalization of Asian policy-making now makes Asian countries less wary about collective action from the perspective of the Five Principles than they once were.

Put another way, as Asia increasingly becomes politically and economically important to international relations, and achievement of Asian national interests plays out in global terms (and requires significant efforts at collective action), the Five Principles may operate differently. The stronger Asian countries may be experiencing what other rising powers have experienced: a decrease in anxiety about sovereignty and non-intervention proportional to an increase the country's power and influence in the international system. The United States underwent such a shift, evolving from wary young state concerned about interference from the European great powers (e.g., the Monroe Doctrine) to a confident superpower sure of its global influence.

Historically, great powers' attitudes shift from an unwavering commitment to the principles of sovereignty and non-intervention, and bend increasingly to reflect their foreign policy objectives. Controversies involving Asian countries may reflect diverging national interests rather than the application of the Five Principles. Although the Five Principles are a distinctive feature of Asian approaches to international relations, diverging national interests in global health and other areas are driven by complex motivations. The United States, for example, does not embrace the Five Principles but, nevertheless, has been involved in its share of global health controversies when US interests diverge from the interests of other countries.

Caution is also warranted because invocation of the Five Principles might represent rhetorical cover for material interests Asian states have for their actions, such as gaining or maintaining access to markets or supplies of essential natural resources. Thus, Asian conceptualizations of global health might not reflect the Five Principles as much as it reflects subordination of some global health problems to other strategic, political, and economic interests that Asian countries have. Such an outcome, however, is hardly limited to Asian practices in global health.

Conclusion

While more research is necessary to provide an accurate picture of the impact of Asian power, principles and practices on GHG, this chapter's analysis offers some preliminary conclusions about Asian conceptualizations of and contributions to the field.

First, Asian conceptualizations of and contributions to GHG show few distinctive features. The shift of material power and influence towards Asia is moving the world closer to multipolarity – a systemic, structural phenomenon that is not 'Asian' in nature. More importantly, this power shift has little, if anything, to do with Asian participation or leadership in global health generally or GHG specifically. Neither China nor India – the two emerging great powers in Asia – has been identified as a global health leader in their respective developments into geopolitical heavyweights.

Secondly, Asian commitment to the Five Principles affects Asian countries' conceptualization of and contributions to GHG. These principles, and Asian application of them, are conservative compared to themes in GHG literature that discount sovereignty and seek more government accountability for their domestic health performance. The Five Principles embody post-colonial attitudes and do not reflect the post-sovereignty currents running through GHG debates. In short, the conceptualization of global health through the Five Principles is not innovative and does not account for the increased interest in GHG, its differences from past forms of international health governance, or its future evolution.

Thirdly, Asian practices in the realm of health diplomacy and GHG reveal significant participation by Asian countries on a range of issues in many diplomatic venues. However, as noted earlier, the same type of participation can be found in non-Asian countries and regions, which reflects the general increase in global health's importance in foreign policy, diplomacy and governance. Asian practices that have caused, or been involved in, global health controversies may reflect application of the Five Principles, but they also may indicate that the national interests of states simply diverge – hardly a phenomenon that should be associated with things distinctly Asian.

These preliminary conclusions do not mean that Asian countries have little opportunity to develop more distinctive conceptualizations of and contributions to GHG. Three possibilities come to mind. First, China or India could decide it wants to become a leader in global health, both through how it handles its own domestic health problems and how it supports collective action among nations. This possibility would involve harnessing Asian power productively to advance the cause of global health. In fact, experts have identified global health as an area in which Asian countries generally, and China specifically, could show more leadership (Mahbubani and Chesterman, 2009; Lo, 2010).

Secondly, Asian countries could show more flexibility on sovereignty or even carve out a global health exception to the Five Principles. China has demonstrated some increasing flexibility on its sovereignty claims to Taiwan in the global health context, allowing, for example, Taiwan to have observer status at the World Health Assembly in 2009 (Huang, 2010). Another possible precedent is Asian acceptance of the provisions in the IHR 2005 that subordinate sovereignty to global health interests, particularly the provisions allowing the WHO to use non-governmental sources of surveillance information to declare a public health emergency of international concern – even over the objections of the countries involved in the disease event – and issue temporary recommendations that may have adverse political and economic costs for affected states. However, any Asian global health flexibility within or exception to the Five Principles would have to be narrow given the potential for GHG concerns to produce frequent interference in domestic affairs.

Thirdly, Asian countries could focus more attention on making their involvement in health cooperation more effective. Asian countries could make sure their policies and practices in global health include follow-up and follow-through so that commitments made have positive impacts on health. One frequent complaint about many recently made health commitments, such as those made by the G8, is that the commitments are rarely fulfilled. Asian countries could aim to reduce the gap between rhetoric and reality in terms of health cooperative endeavors in which they are involved. In this respect, an excellent starting point for Asian countries would be to make sure global health becomes an effective part of the emerging agenda of the G20.

A number of obstacles stand in the way of Asian countries making a distinctive contribution to GHG. The shift toward multipolarity only means that the dynamics of international politics will change; it does not mean that China, India, or other Asian countries will be able to do what they please. Thus, multipolarity could blunt Asian power and act as a significant structural constraint on any Asian country or group of countries attempting to seize global health leadership. In a multipolar world, it may become harder to achieve sustainable collective action on matters related to individual countries national interests, especially those of non-Asian great powers.

In addition, China and India may not have the ability to test multipolarity's constraints on better GHG because they have to address massive and growing internal problems involving health. The requirement for a significant domestic focus might limit the interest of China and India in making global health a signature feature of their emergence and interests as great powers. Improvements in domestic health in China, India and the Asian region would contribute much to global health because of the sheer size of the populations concerned, but such domestic health advances would not necessarily have to rely on or need GHG mechanisms.

More conceptually, the Five Principles, consistently applied, may create sovereignty and non-interference barriers for strengthened collective action on global health problems deeply embedded in domestic affairs, including NCDs, health system reforms, human rights, good health governance and improving the social determinants of health. In addition, Asian countries might use the Five Principles to avoid controversy on global health issues in their relations with non-Asian nations, such as those in Africa, in order to maintain good political relations, economic opportunities, access to natural resources and strategic influence vis-à-vis potential rivals.

Thus, the power, principles and practices of Asian countries may truncate the space for 'global governance' and move global health politics back to a more state-centric, conservative mode of addressing international health problems. As Mahbubani and Chesterman (2009: 3, 6) argued:

> [T]he Asian style of consensus and consultation may fail when confronted with the need for bold, collective action. Appealing to the lowest common dominator produces *wide*, but not *deep* commitments to change. The result is that many Asian want change at the same time as wanting things to remain the same . . . The danger in such an approach is that decisions may not be made, or that those made will fail to resolve fundamental political challenges by putting rhetoric ahead of substance.

How Asian countries and regional bodies respond to the existing and future challenges of GHG remains to be seen, but one thing is certain: how Asian countries respond will carry more political weight and normative significance than at any other time in the history of the modern international system. Responding effectively to these GHG challenges has now become Asia's burden and opportunity.

12 Global governance for health

Ten proposals for Asian leadership and influence

Lawrence O. Gostin

Most Asian[1] countries have been relatively passive players in global governance for health – more often the recipients than the funders of global health assistance, and more often the subjects than the shapers of global health policy. Powerful countries such as the People's Republic of China and India, of course, exercise considerable diplomatic (Huang, 2010) and political power (Chan *et al.*, 2008). China, for example, has bolstered its economic presence through financing and concessional loans for infrastructure projects and large economic investments in Africa, Latin America and Southeast Asia (Lum *et al.*, 2009). Still, Asian impact on global institutions such as the World Health Organization (WHO), World Trade Organization (WTO), and Global Fund has not risen to the level that it could.

This relative passivity is at once understandable and remarkable. It is understandable because of the crushing burdens of disease within the region. Countries such as Afghanistan, China, India, Russia and Sri Lanka suffer deep and multiple health challenges ranging from AIDS (Acquired Immune Deficiency Syndrome), malaria and tuberculosis, to maternal and infant morbidity and mortality, through to non-communicable diseases (NCDs) compounded by smoking, high-fat diets, and sedentary lifestyles – often fueled by the inexorable processes of globalization. Even in rapidly developing Southeast Asia, along with increasing development and longevity, there are widening socioeconomic and health inequalities (Engelgau *et al.*, 2011).

However, the passivity is also surprising given the rise in economic and political clout of emerging Asia. The region has more than 60 percent of the world's inhabitants; one of the highest combined GNPs (gross national product); and at least four massive armed forces with nuclear capabilities (Eberstadt, 2006). The geostrategic importance of the region is clear, and it could become a major force in pushing the world's health and trade agendas toward equitable burden- and benefit-sharing among the world's rich and poor.

Leadership in global governance for health would afford Asia a major voice in, and influence over, global health strategies and resources. If the region set as its goal a dramatic reduction in unconscionable health inequalities, it would reap enormous benefits – not only in health but also in economic productivity and political stability. But what are the most effective pathways to achieving this objective? Here, I offer critical proposals on how Asia could powerfully alter the world's health and trade agendas to benefit low- and middle-income countries.

Certainly, emerging political and economic powers, such as the BRIC group of countries (Brazil, Russia, India, China), are already adopting many of the strategies proffered in this chapter (Fidler, Chapter 11 this volume). China and India, for example, have embarked on ambitious health system reforms (Ho and Gostin, 2009), while Russia is championing the NCD high-level summit at the United Nations.[2] But my intent is to push the region harder and to sharpen its focus. First, it will be helpful to explain what I mean by global governance for health. Next, I will offer ten recommendations for Asian leadership and engagement in global governance for health. Finally, I will provide an illustrative case study of the kind of innovative campaign that the region could lead – the Joint Action and Learning Initiative on National and Global Responsibilities for Health (JALI) – with the aim of a United Nations Framework Convention on Global Health (Gostin, 2008).

Global governance for health: a definition and differentiation

What does global governance for health (GGH) mean, and how can it be differentiated from similar concepts such as international health law generally and global health governance in particular? I define GGH as the collection of norms, institutions and processes that collectively shape the health of the world's population (Gostin, forthcoming). It encompasses structures at the international level, such as the norms created by major treaties in the health (e.g. the International Health Regulations and Framework Convention on Tobacco Control) and related sectors (e.g. TRIPS and the Kyoto Protocol); the international organizations that affect global health (e.g. WHO, World Bank and World Trade Organization); and global decision-making bodies and processes (e.g. the World Health Assembly and Global Fund grant-making process).

Global governance for health encompasses the dynamic relationship between global structures and forces and those at regional, national, and sub-national levels: how they interrelate and influence norms, institutions and processes at all levels, including at the community level. GGH also includes how, in turn, more local structures affect global structures and processes. For example, virtually all states have infectious disease laws that must comply with the International Health Regulations (IHR). The IHR, in turn, also feeds into national and local structures, for example, by mandating capacity-building with international cooperation and assistance.

Scholars sometimes use global governance for health interchangeably with global health governance, but the former term is broader and therefore more desirable. Global governance for health refers to the broader governance system's influence on health outcomes, including multiple sectors such as health, trade, food, labour, human rights and the environment. Global health governance, on the other hand, refers to the narrower form of governance that is encapsulated by the boundaries of the health sector.

Rules play a critical role in global governance for health. Such rules can range from legally binding agreements (e.g. public international law relating to human rights or trade) to non-legally binding instruments, such as declarations, codes of conduct and memoranda of understanding (e.g. WHO codes of practice), through to institutional bylaws (e.g. the organizational structure of the Global Fund or GAVI Alliance). Understanding, applying and shaping the law is therefore central to the task of formulating more effective GGH. These international legal instruments, in turn, are implemented through and otherwise influence laws and legal structures within countries, effects that are also central to understanding the idea of GGH.

Governance does not operate in a vacuum, but is shaped by multiple forces, including politics (globally and nationally); power dynamics (between and among countries of the global North and South); the influence of vested interests (e.g. corporations) and economic power (e.g. the Gates Foundation); security interests (human security and more traditional national security); changing circumstances (evolving disease burdens and the changes driven by globalization and market liberalization); knowledge and learning (lessons from how present structures are affecting global health); and values (e.g. human rights and global ethics). Civil society-led social movements, which are of particular importance in the quest of social justice, also powerfully shape governance.

A comprehensive understanding of GGH and how to wield this potentially powerful tool as a source for better health for all and for health equity should inform the political agendas of emerging Asian powers.

Ten proposals for Asian global governance for health leadership

1 Frame strategic objectives on the human right to health

What makes the human right to health – and related entitlements such as the right to food, clean water and adequate sanitation – a compelling framework to guide Asian GGH leadership is that it has wide international acceptance. Although other powerful paradigms inhabit the space of GGH discourse, such as global goods for health (Smith *et al.*, 2003) and the human security framework (Takemi *et al.*, 2008), the right to health alone is grounded in binding international law. Every country has ratified at least one treaty recognizing the human right to the highest attainable standard of physical and mental health (United Nations, 2010). Under the human rights framework, individuals can claim their rights from government, changing power dynamics and instilling a sense of dignity and self-worth.

Although the right to health offers a critical framework for GGH leadership, it also suffers from obvious limitations, such as insufficient specificity, monitoring and enforcement. Unlike civil and political rights, the right to health is 'progressively realizable', rather than immediately actionable. Yet these structural limitations can be overcome. The main treaty body, the UN Committee on Economic,

Social and Cultural Rights (CESCR), and the Special Rapporteur can develop clear and enforceable standards and press states harder toward implementation, as the CESCR has done with General Comment 14 on the Right to Health. The text of the main treaty, the International Covenant of Economic, Social and Cultural Rights, itself requires states immediately 'to take steps' to achieve 'the full realization' of the right to health. The CESCR affirms that states must 'move as expeditiously and effectively as possible towards full realization'.[3]

The all-important capacity problem can be overcome through the treaty's insistence on states using 'the maximum of [their own] available resources', and the international community providing 'assistance and co-operation, especially economic and technical'. As General Comment 14 explains

> If resource constraints render it impossible for a State to comply fully with its Covenant obligations, it has the burden of justifying that every effort has nevertheless been made to use all available resources at its disposal in order to satisfy, as a matter of priority, its obligations.[4]

Taken together, international law requires collective cooperation for development as an obligation of all states, with particular duties on richer countries to provide global health assistance.[5]

2 Lead the WHO reform agenda

In May 2011, The World Health Assembly supported reforms that could bring the most significant changes in the agency's 63-year history (Butler, 2011). Yet member state leadership is virtually impossible to ascertain, with Asian states largely sitting on the sidelines. Although perhaps over simplistic, powerful states in Australia, Western Europe and North America exercise inordinate control over WHO's agenda through the power of the purse. The global South plays a vital role in the Executive Board and Assembly but has done little either to alter the power dynamics or ensure sustainable funding. In short, member states – South and North – have not acted as genuine stakeholders in the agency.

The WHO suffers from a crisis of leadership amidst a dramatically altered global health landscape that includes multiple politically and economically powerful global health actors ranging from the Global Fund, the Gavi Alliance and Gates Foundation to the US President's Emergency Plan for AIDS Relief (PEPFAR). It is not simply that the agency experienced a US$300 million deficit in 2010 or that the World Health Assembly (WHA) set its two-year budget nearly US$1 billion less than the US$4.8 billion requested by the Secretariat. More fundamentally, member states increasingly insist on eschewing mandatory contributions in favor of discretionary 'extra-budgetary' funding, which now constitutes some 80 percent of the agency's budget. Extra-budgetary funding has transformed the WHO into a donor-driven organization, restricting its ability to direct and coordinate the global health agenda. The rationale for the shift towards extra-budgetary funding is clear: by tying funding to specific programs, donors ensure that their resources influence the activities and direction of the organization (Sridhar and Gostin, 2011).

Extra-budgetary funding, moreover, skews global health priorities. Assessed contributions are more aligned with the actual global burden of disease than extra-budgetary funding. For example, WHO's extra-budgetary funding is primarily for infectious diseases (60 percent), with negligible allocations for NCDs (3.9 percent) and injuries (3.4 percent). Yet NCDs account for 62 percent of all deaths worldwide, and injuries account for 17 percent of the global burden of disease.

Asia should get behind a fundamental reform of the WHO, pushing member states to become genuine shareholders in the WHO's future, acting collectively and refraining from exerting narrow political interests. Certainly, Asian countries that can afford it, such as China, India, Indonesia, Russia and Turkey, as Margaret Chan urges, should contribute more generously a fair share to WHO's budget. Politically, they ought to push the WHA to set significantly higher mandatory contributions.

There is no substitute for a strong WHO with sustainable funding and normative leadership. The agency could become a powerful force for global health equity, rebounding to the benefit of Asia and its partners in the global South.

3 Use the power of WHO treaties

Symptomatic of the WHO's lack of leadership has been its reticence to exercise its formable treaty-making powers vested in the WHO Constitution. In its 63-year history, the WHO has negotiated only two major treaties – the Framework Convention on Tobacco Control (FCTC) and the International Health Regulations (IHR). While pushing the agency to be bolder and more innovative in exercising its normative powers, Asia could use existing international health law to benefit its population.

Multinational tobacco corporations – supported by high-income countries and empowered by international trade and investment treaties – have shifted the global tobacco market from industrialized countries (where smoking rates have substantially declined) to the less-regulated markets of Asia and Latin America, where the tobacco market is spurred by rising incomes, trade liberalization and intensive marketing. By 2030, developing countries will account for about 80 percent of the projected eight million-plus annual deaths from tobacco. China alone accounts for one-quarter of the world's smokers. And when Indonesian children as young as nine years old smoke Philip Morris International (PMI) cigarettes, something is badly wrong.

The tobacco industry, moreover, is aggressively using international law to defend its economic interests in Asia and beyond. In the Thailand-Cigarette Case (1990), for example, the United States challenged Thailand's decision to ban the importation of cigarettes. Thailand argued that US cigarettes contain chemicals and other additives that make them more harmful than Thai cigarettes, a claim affirmed by the WHO. The GATT dispute panel, however, found that Thailand's import ban violated international trade rules.

More recently, on 19 February 2010, PMI used the Swiss-Uruguay Bilateral Investment Treaty (BIT) to challenge Uruguay's tobacco control regulations requiring 80 percent of the surface of cigarette packs to be devoted to pictures and warnings about the dangers of smoking. PMI claims the regulations limit the space on packages available for branding, preventing the company from effective use of its intellectual property in the form of trademarks. Although the case is ongoing, it represents a pivotal moment in tobacco control under international law.

International law, however, can cut both ways, and developing countries should exercise their prerogatives under the Framework Convention on Tobacco Control. More than 170 countries have ratified the FCTC, covering 87 percent of the world's population. The FCTC affords states parties the power, and the responsibility, to implement demand- and supply-side rules to dramatically decrease tobacco consumption, including rules that cover taxation, marketing restrictions, smoking bans and smoker education and treatment. Developing countries, however, have not effectively used this WHO treaty to systematically adopt known, effective tobacco control measures that would vastly improve the health of their populations (Lee and Kao, Chapter 7 this volume). Some Asian countries are merely the target of unconscionable marketing by the tobacco industry, including targeting women and children as consumers. But in others, such as China, there is a domestic tobacco industry that undermines public health campaigns and policies to reduce supply and demand.

The same strategies could also apply to the other main WHO treaty, the International Health Regulations (Kamradt-Scott and Simon, 2012). The IHR requires all states to engage in effective surveillance and response to public health emergencies of international concern, such as the 2009/10 Influenza (A) H1N1 pandemic. Most importantly, the IHR requires states to build capacity in resource-poor countries – a rule that has largely not been implemented effectively. Asian countries could use the IHR to demand a fair sharing of resources for surveillance, public health response and therapeutic countermeasures such as vaccines and antiviral medications.

4 Fight for predictable, sustainable and scalable funding

Resource-poor states lack capacity to ensure all of their people even core health goods and services, much less a fuller realization of the right to health. Countries in a position to assist are obliged to do so under principles of international law and global social justice. All countries have mutual responsibilities towards ensuring the health of the world's most disadvantaged. Yet richer countries have not come close to fulfilling their pledge to devote 0.7 percent of gross national product on official development assistance. Even when countries make specific commitments, they often fail to follow through. For example, only one month after countries at the 2010 United Nations (UN) Millennium Development Goals (MDG) Summit committed to provide 'adequate funding' for the Global Fund to Fight AIDS, Tuberculosis and Malaria, pledges at the replenishment conference fell billions of dollars short. The Summit called for accelerated development assistance for health, though the rate of increase in assistance dropped during the global recession. Budget shortfalls in the aftermath of the financial downturn further threaten assistance levels.

At the same time, Asian governments themselves frequently do not devote sufficient resources to building strong health systems domestically. Overall, the percentage of GDP devoted to health is much lower in low- and middle-income countries in Asia than it is in Europe or North America. Worse still, there is an observed 'substitution effect' whereby resource-poor countries reduce domestic spending for each dollar they receive in international development assistance for health.

Predictable and sustainable funding, scalable to health needs, is badly needed. Not only is funding necessary for the development and maintenance of health goods and services, it is also important that budgets are predictable and stable so health ministers can plan for the long term.

Asia should seek to transform the paradigm for global health funding – moving from 'health aid' to global social justice. Framing the global health endeavor as health aid provided by the affluent to the poor is fundamentally flawed. This suggests that the world is divided between donors and countries in need. This is too simplistic. Collaboration among countries, both as neighbors and across continents, is also about responding to health risks together and building capacity collaboratively – whether it is through South–South partnerships, gaining access to essential vaccines and medicines, or demanding fair distribution of scarce life-saving technologies. New social, economic and political alignments are evident, for example, with the emergence of health leadership from Asian countries such as China, India, Indonesia and Thailand.

5 Become global donors as well as recipients

If it is true that global social justice is a better paradigm for global health funding, then what does this mean for emerging powers in Asia that have resources as well as needs? It should mean that countries that are rapidly developing should give as well as receive international assistance. This role-shift is already beginning to occur in countries such as China, India, Brazil, Mexico, South Africa and Thailand, but the change in mindset is slow and incomplete.

Human health is a globally shared responsibility reflecting common risks and vulnerabilities – an obligation of health justice that demands a fair contribution from everyone, North and South, rich and poor. Global governance for health must be seen as a partnership, with financial and technical assistance understood as an integral component of the common goal of improving global health and reducing health inequalities.

6 Demand fair trade policies

Earlier, I explained that there are many international regimes that impact health beyond the health sector. Among the most important are trade and intellectual property. Although free trade advocates believe that trade liberalization will lift the prospects of the poor as well as the rich, there remain deep concerns that the trade system favors the North, while impeding development and health in the South – leaving the poor in no better, and perhaps worse, shape economically.

The global rich, of course, benefit from trade liberalization and particularly international protection of intellectual property. However, poorer countries, which lack scientists, entrepreneurs, investment and industrial capacity, are often left behind. For rapidly developing countries with a highly educated, technologically savvy elite, such as China and India, the effects of trade liberalization are decidedly mixed. India, for example, has been supplying the developing world with generic medications of high quality, although that role may be severely restricted due to implementation of intellectual property rules. Nevertheless, for those concerned with equity and social distribution, there is a fear that trade liberalization places rich countries and multinational corporations' interests ahead of the health and lives of the world's poor.

The WTO process, more importantly, marginalizes developing countries. Developing countries find it difficult to veto a proposed decision that is widely accepted by the more influential member states. The process can stifle opposition, as developing countries fear retaliation by more powerful member states. Developing countries face additional barriers to participating fully and on equal terms in WTO decision-making processes. They also may not possess the necessary expertise to negotiate effectively at the WTO, given the complexity of the legal issues underlying its agreements.

Coalitions have been used by developing countries to enable more effective representation (see Recommendation 9 below). For example, the Group of 77, established at the United Nations Conference on Trade and Development in June 1964, serves as the largest coalition of developing states in the UN. More recently, developing countries have also turned to issue-based coalitions.

Asia could be a global leader in fighting unfair trade rules that disadvantage the region and other resource-poor regions of the world. By leading developing country coalitions, Asia could use its considerable political clout to alter trade rules to improve health, development and prosperity for all.

7 Demand fair intellectual property rules to ensure affordable access to essential vaccines and medicines

The TRIPS Agreement (Trade-Related Aspects of Intellectual Property Rights) affords protection to a variety of IP rights including trademarks, copyrights and designs. This enables biotechnology firms to charge monopoly prices for a period of time, rendering essential vaccine, medicines and other technologies unaffordable for the poor.

The TRIPS Agreement allows countries to issue a compulsory license in a public health emergency; a legal vehicle whereby a government grants to itself or a third party the right to produce or import a patented product without authorization of the patent holder. In the aftermath of TRIPS, many developing countries began resisting the restrictive concessions required by the agreement. As a result, the international community gradually became more sensitive to the public health concerns of developing nations, lessening international support for the harsh intellectual property demands of the United States and other industrialized nations.

Although compulsory licensing was designed to provide the flexibility necessary protect the public's health, the HIV/AIDS pandemic brought its shortcomings into stark contrast with its goals. To ensure greater access to life-saving medications for resource-poor countries, the WTO Ministerial Conference promulgated the Declaration on the TRIPS Agreement and Public Health in November 2001 (the Doha Declaration).[6] The Declaration called for the TRIPS Agreement's 'flexibilities' to be used to protect the public's health by promoting access to essential medicines: countries have the right to determine what constitutes a national emergency and the grounds on which compulsory licenses are granted.

Countries with the manufacturing capacity, such as Brazil, India and Thailand, can make generic antiretroviral medications for their populations. But the Doha Declaration left an important problem unresolved. Most countries could not produce the generic drugs that they need for the public's health. To date, this problem has never been resolved, leaving developing countries in the lurch. This is an area of potentially major impact for Asian leadership. Asia could also support alternatives to the TRIPS agreement, such as the Impact Fund, an arrangement that gives incentives to the industry to produce affordable drugs that have a major beneficial effect on common diseases.

8 Find innovative ways for equitable burden- and benefit-sharing for essential biotechnologies

The discussion on trade and intellectual property regimes demonstrated the unfairness of the current WTO system. Yet even beyond WTO, there are major concerns about global equity in the fair distribution of health burdens and benefits throughout the world. The North–South divide on global justice could not have been starker than in the global outbreaks of novel strains of influenza – first, H5N1 in 2006 and then, H1N1 in 2009.

During the avian influenza A (H5N1) outbreaks, Indonesia refused to share virus specimens with the WHO, claiming it was unfair to give pharmaceutical companies access. Indonesia argued that the pharmaceutical industry would use its viruses to patent vaccines and antiviral medications that Indonesia could not afford. Indonesia asserted sovereignty over viruses isolated within its territory, grounded on the Convention on Biological Diversity (CBD). Indonesia also argued that the IHR did not require states to share H5N1 viruses. The international community feared that Indonesia's refusal to share would impede surveillance and response, particularly because Asia was the epicenter of the global H5N1 outbreak. Serious health and political repercussions would result if states failed to cooperate when confronting a common threat. The H1N1 pandemic deepened developing-country mistrust because vaccines were not equitably shared. After nearly four years of arduous negotiations, the WHO's Director-General announced the Framework for benefit- and burden-sharing on 16 April, and the World Health Assembly (WHA) approved it in May (Fidler and Gostin, 2011).

The Indonesia virus-sharing dispute was indicative of the deep problems of equitably sharing technological benefits, including life-saving vaccines and antiviral medications. The final WHO agreement required pharmaceutical companies to make specific contributions toward developing country capacity in exchange for sharing virus specimens. But notably absent from the agreement, and characteristic of WHO member states, governments were not required to contribute anything, such as donating a specified percentage of vaccine purchases to developing countries. Asian leadership is vital in this regard. It is clear that in the event of a mass catastrophe in which the rich live and the poor die, there could be dire diplomatic, political and security implications; thereby creating deep tensions between the global North and South. Asian leadership is, therefore, badly needed.

9 Form south–south partnerships and alliances

Highly developed countries have effectively used economic and political alliances, such as the G8, to pursue their interests in areas such as trade, IP and security. Military alliances, such as NATO, have been equally effective in advancing the West's interests. Although later to the game, developing countries are beginning to wake up to the power of South–South alliances. Asian countries are represented in the BRIC countries (Russia, India and China), as well as the Oslo-7 Health and Foreign Policy Group (Indonesia and Thailand).[7] Notably, China and India help lead developing country trade coalitions, such as the Group of Twenty (G20) Developing Nations, to push the WTO toward more affordable access to essential vaccines and medicines.

South–South alliances on issues of major import to Asia, such as agriculture, trade and IP – all focused around a right to health and development agenda – would give the region much greater influence and focus than it presently has. Given Asia's growing economic and political power, joining with other like-minded regions, such as Latin America (e.g., Argentina, Brazil and Chile) and Africa (e.g., Nigeria and South Africa), could make these emerging economies a powerful force for the common good.

10 Embrace civil society movements

Civil society movements are central to securing and ensuring global health equity. Such movements have spurred momentous transformations in health. Advocates changed the world's response to AIDS from one marked by discrimination to one focused on empowering marginalized people and scaling up HIV services. The Campaign to Ban Landmines drove a process that culminated in a treaty banning this indiscriminate weapon. Civil society campaigns for the right to health, such as those through the People's Health Movement, are already underway.

Many governments distance themselves from social activists, and some Asian countries, such as Burma and China, even persecute them. At the international level, innovative governance arrangements have begun to meaningfully engage with civil society, such as the Global Fund and UNAIDS. The WHO, as an intergovernmental organization, has not had a tradition of civil society participation, and the WHA even has failed to adopt a proposal for a Committee C comprised of non-state actors. But this is beginning to change. The recent WHO reform agenda includes a global forum that will bring non-state actors together to closely advise the Executive Board.

The neglect of civil society by governments and international organizations is a mistake. Civil society can enhance and add precision to the effectiveness of international human rights law, which could in turn reinforce civil society efforts to hold their own governments to account. Governments should adopt universal human rights-based principles of transparency, honesty and accountability. By drawing on the voices of civil society and disadvantaged communities, Asian governments could gain the legitimacy and the political support to transform global governance for health.

A case study on civil society and the right to health: the Joint Action and Learning Initiative (JALI)

Recently, a coalition of civil society and academics launched the Joint Action and Learning Initiative on National and Global Responsibilities for Health (JALI). JALI seeks to develop a post–MDG framework for global health, one rooted in the right to health and aimed at securing universal health coverage for all people. JALI's goal is a global agreement, such as a Framework Convention on Global Health that sets priorities, clarifies national and international responsibilities, ensures accountability and develops corresponding institutions, such as a Global Health Fund. JALI is southern-led and accumulating critical civil society support. For the four defining questions posed by JALI, see the Box (Gostin *et al.*, 2010).

JALI's four defining questions for global health

JALI posed four defining questions for global health that will be the subject of action and research:

1. *What are the services and goods guaranteed to every person under the human right to health?* The World Health Organization (WHO) has placed universal health coverage high on the global health agenda (WHO, 2010g).[8] The human right to health provides critical insight into how states should work towards universal coverage. Core obligations offer benchmarks to assess progress towards universal coverage (such as non-discrimination, equitable distribution of health facilities and essential services for all), including those addressing underlying determinants of health.

The core principle of equality requires states to prioritize covering 100 percent of their populations. The right to health framework militates against a narrow definition of 'key' services. Rather, these should encompass the WHO's health system building blocks (e.g., services, workforce, information, financing and governance); essential vaccines, medicines, and technologies; and fundamental human needs (e.g., sanitation, nutritious food, potable water, safe housing, vector abatement, tobacco control and healthy environments). These core entitlements – health systems, essential vaccines and medicines, and fundamental human needs – would represent a significant step towards achieving the highest attainable standard of health.

2. *What responsibilities do all states have for the health of their own populations?* The right to health places the primary responsibility on governments to ensure the health needs of all their inhabitants. National responsibility includes health sector funding, addressing the socioeconomic determinants of health and good governance.

   National health responsibilities should comply with well-defined, measurable international standards, balanced against the flexibility necessary to respect national priorities, health profiles, and needs.

   States also have a responsibility to govern well, derived from central human rights tenets such as participatory processes, transparent and accountable government, and non-discrimination and equality. Well-designed legal rules and institutional arrangements can facilitate honest administrations, openness and accountability, along with meaningful civil society and community participation in decision-making. The law, moreover, should guarantee equality and non-discrimination on the basis of race, sex, religion, disability and other statuses. Measures to enhance accountability to communities in India's National Rural Health Mission, for example, offers instructive lessons.

3. *What duties do states owe to people beyond their borders in securing the right to health?* Resource-poor states lack the capacity to ensure all of their people access to even core health goods and services, much less a fuller realization of the right to health. Countries in a position to assist are obliged to do so under principles of international law and global social justice. All countries have mutual responsibilities towards ensuring the health of the world's most disadvantaged.

   Beyond development assistance, coordination and coherence is required across sectors, as global health can be improved or harmed through state and international policies and rules that govern areas such as trade, intellectual property, health worker migration, international financing and debt relief. These responsibilities extend to the exercise of state power and influence over multilateral institutions such as the World Bank, International Monetary Fund and World Trade Organization.

4. *What kind of global governance for health is needed to ensure that all states live up to their mutual responsibilities?* Translating a shared understanding of national and global responsibilities into new realities requires effective and democratic global governance for health. Notwithstanding the Paris Declaration on Aid Effectiveness, global health faces challenges of weak leadership, poor coordination, under-funded priorities and a lack of transparency, accountability and enforcement.

   Innovative global governance and enhanced funding would empower the WHO to exercise effective leadership in the health sector and persuasive advocacy on agriculture, finance and trade. Moreover, state policies (e.g., agricultural subsidies, intellectual property and foreign affairs) can powerfully affect health in resource-poor countries. States, therefore, should adopt a 'health-in-all-policies' approach where all ministries address the health impacts of their policies and programs. Effective governance must include active citizen participation to ensure transparency, collaboration and accountability while maximizing creativity and resource mobilization by states, international organizations, businesses and civil society.

   Most importantly, the global health architecture must hold stakeholders accountable, with clear standards for success, monitoring progress and enforcement – all of which have been lacking. Lack of sufficiently precise obligations and compliance mechanisms under the right to health hinders accountability.

   An empowered human rights sector could learn from international regimes with more vigorous adjudication and enforcement mechanisms, such as trade. Actions to ensure that social movements and voters are well-informed about their countries' commitments could strengthen political accountability. The Global South, where most of the world's least healthy people reside, should lead in shaping global governance for health policies, where community priorities drive global action. New governance requires the full participation of, and support for, marginalized populations.

   The framework of mutual responsibilities that emerges from JALI should prove attractive to both Southern and Northern governments, creating incentives to develop a far-reaching global health agreement. Mutual responsibilities come with mutual benefits. Southern countries would benefit from increased respect for their strategies, greater and more predictable funding from more coordinated and accountable development partners, reform of policies that harm health, such as those in trade and agriculture, and most importantly, better health for their populations. Countries in the North would benefit from increased confidence that development assistance is spent effectively and the prospect of reduced financing needs over time as host countries increase their own health spending and build sustainable health systems.

All would benefit from lessons on shared health challenges, from the economic and educational gains that come with improved global health and from increased protection for their populations from global public health threats – and from mutual goodwill derived from participating in an historic venture to make unprecedented progress towards global health equity.

We invite readers to join JALI (www.section27.org.za/2010/11/23/jali) to develop widely shared understandings of national and global responsibilities for health to inform post-MDG commitments and create an innovative global agreement. It is time to define – and to meet – these responsibilities.

Source: Gostin, Friedman, Ooms *et al.* (2011)

In April, the UN Secretary-General Ban Ki Moon urged adoption of the Framework Convention on Global Health (FCGH):

> Countries must commit to global solidarity, built on the tenets of shared responsibility, true national ownership and mutual accountability. Let the AIDS response be a beacon of global solidarity for health as a human right and set the stage for a future United Nations Framework Convention on Global Health.[9]

Yet JALI and the FCGH do not have a state champion. The governments of Brazil, Germany, Norway and India have engaged with JALI. But no government has taken the mantle of leading this broad coalition and supporting the adoption of a binding global health convention. This is a defining moment in global health given the NCD summit, together with the need for momentum in the next phase of the MDGs in 2015. The Global Fund is seeking a broader mission, as the WHO is reforming itself. After a decade of unprecedented engagement and funding of global health, the world has entered a state of financial restraint and retrenchment.

Now is the time for bold global governance for health. Whether it is a binding treaty such as a Framework Convention or softer norms, Asia should emerge as the leader of this movement. It would vastly expand the region's international prestige and, much more important, push the global community toward greater solidarity and equity. Europe and North America defined themselves with trade liberalization. Asia, Africa and Latin America could do the same with global social justice and the international right to health.

Notes

1 I use the term Asia also to include Eurasian countries located within Europe and Asia (e.g., Russia and Turkey) as well as the Indian subcontinent.
2 See United Nations (2011).
3 See United Nations Economic and Social Council (1990).
4 See United Nations Economic and Social Council (2001).
5 See United Nations Economic and Social Council (1990).
6 See Correa (2002) *Implications of the Doha declaration on the TRIPS Agreement and Public Health.*
7 See Ministers of Foreign Affairs of Brazil, France, Indonesia, Norway, Senegal, South Africa, and Thailand (2007).
8 World Health Report (2010).
9 See United Nations General Assembly (2011).

Appendix 1
Deployment of CMT as CHAFC by country and responsible Chinese province (1963–2008)

Region	*Country*	*Responsible province/city*	*Starting year*	*Changes*
Africa	Algeria	Hubei	1963	Withdrawn due to civil war in 1995, returned in 1997
Asia	Laos	Yunnan	1964	Stopped in 1974
Africa	Zanzibar	Jiangsu	1964	
Africa	Somalia	Jilin	1965	Withdrawn in 1991 due to civil war
Asia	Republic of Yemen	Liaoning	1966	
Africa	Congo (Brazzaville)	Tianjin	1967	Withdrawn in 1997 due to civil war, returned in 2000
Africa	Guinea	Beijing	1968	
Africa	Mali	Zhejiang	1968	
Africa	Mauritania	Heilongjiang	1968	
Africa	Tanganyika	Shandong	1968	
Asia	Vietnam	Yunnan	1968	Stopped in 1971
Asia	Republic of Yemen	Anhui	1970	
Africa	Equatorial Guinea	Guangdong	1971	
Africa	Sultan	Shaanxi	1971	
Europe	Albania	Liaoning	1973	Stopped in 1974
Africa	Congo (DRC)	Hebei	1973	Withdrawn for civil war in 1997, returned in 2006; peacekeeping medical team sent by Shenyang military area command
Africa	Sierra Leone	Hunan	1973	Withdrawn for war in 1993, returned in 2003
Africa	Tunisia	Jiangxi	1973	Helped create the first acupuncture centre in Africa in 1994
Africa	Ethiopia	Henan	1974	Stopped in 1979, returned in 1984
Africa	Togo	Shanghai	1974	
Asia	Cambodia	Shanxi	1975	Stopped in 1981
Africa	Cameroon	Shanghai	1975	Stopped in 1979; Shanxi took over the deployment in 1985

Region	*Country*	*Responsible province/city*	*Starting year*	*Changes*
Africa	Madagascar	Gansu	1975	
Africa	Morocco	Shanghai	1975	Jiangxi attended the deployment in 2000
Africa	Senegal	Fujian	1975	Withdrawn in 1996, returned in 2007/9
Africa	Burkina Faso		1976	Withdrawn in 1994 due to a break in diplomatic relations
Africa	Guinea-Bissau	Guizhou	1976	Withdrawn in 1990 due to a break in diplomatic relations; Sichuan took over the deployment in 2002
Asia	Kuwait	Liaoning	1976	
Africa	Mozambique	Sichuan	1976	Returned in 1991
Africa	Sao Tome	Heilongjiang andSichuan	1976	Withdrawn in 1997 due to a break in diplomatic relations
Africa	The Niger	Guangxi	1976	Withdrawn in 1992 due to a break in diplomatic relations; returned in 1996
Africa	Gabon	Tianjin	1977	
Africa	Gambia	Tianjin	1977	Deployed by Guangdong in 1991; Withdrawn in 1995 due to a break in diplomatic relations
Africa	Benin	Ningxia	1978	
Africa	Central Africa	Zhejiang	1978	Withdrawn in 1991 due to a break in diplomatic relations; returned in 1998
Africa	Chad	Jiangxi	1978	Withdrawn in 1979 due to a break in diplomatic relations; returned in 1989; withdrawn in 1997 due to a break in diplomatic relations; returned in 2006; withdrawn for civil war in 2008, returned in May.
Asia	Iran	Jiangsu	1978	Stopped in 1979
Asia	Syria	Academy of Traditional Chinese Medicine (MOH)	1978	Stopped in 1981
Africa	Zambia	Henan	1978	
Africa	Botswana	Fujian	1981	
Africa	Djibouti	Shanxi	1981	
Asia	The United Arab Emirates	Sichuan	1981	
Africa	Rwanda	Inner Mongolia	1982	
Africa	Libya	Jiangsu	1983	Contract not extended in 1994
Europe	Malta	Jiangsu	1983	Began in 1973; formally sent in 1993

(Continued)

Region	*Country*	*Responsible province/city*	*Starting year*	*Changes*
Africa	Uganda	Yunnan	1983	
Africa	Cape Verde	Heilongjiang	1984	Deployed by Sichuan in 1988; later by deployment implemented in Hunan
Africa	Liberia	Heilongjiang	1984	Deployed by Tianjin PLA 254 Hospital in 1986; withdrawn in 1989 due to a break in diplomatic relations; returned in 2005
Oceania	Vanuatu	Shaanxi	1985	
Africa	Zimbabwe	Hunan	1985	
Africa	Burundi	Guangxi	1986	Deployed by Qinghai in 2000
Oceania	Samoa	Anhui	1987	
Africa	Seychelles	Guangxi	1987	
South America	Guyana	Jiangsu	1993	
Africa	Namibia	Zhejiang	1996	
Africa	Eritrea	Henan	1997	
Africa	Lesotho	Hubei	1997	
Africa	Comorin	Guangxi	1998	
Asia	Nepal	Hebei	1999	
Asia	East Timor	Sichuan	2000	
Oceania	Papua-New Guinea	Chongqing	2002	
Asia	Thailand*	Shanghai	2004	Aid during the Indian Ocean tsunami
Asia	Indonesia*	Armed police	2005	Aid during the Indian Ocean tsunami
Asia	Pakistan*	Armed police	2005	
Asia	Sri Lanka*	Beijing	2005	Aid during the Indian Ocean tsunami
Asia	Lebanon*	Chengdu military area command	2007	Chengdu military area command sent peacekeeping medical team
Asia	Mongolia†	Inner Mongolia	2007	
Africa	Angola	Sichuan	2008	Suspended due to housing problems
Africa	Ghana	Guangdong	2008	
Africa	Malawi	Shaanxi	2008	
Asia	Myanmar*		2008	Disaster relief

* Emergency or special aid, not part of regular MOH programs.
† Local government-led aid.

Source: Li (2009: 30–31).

Appendix 2
Facility construction as CHAFC (1978–2008)

Region	*Country*	*Year*	*Facility constructed*
Africa	Madagascar	1978	A pharmaceutical factory
Africa	Mauritania	1979	Selibaby Health Center
Africa	Rwanda	1979	A hospital (20 beds, 486 square meters)
Africa	Rwanda	1989	Kibungo Health School (250 beds, expanding 5,720 square meters for outpatient department, medical technique department and some parts of surgical and gynecological wards, operation rooms and delivery department)
Africa	Togo	1990	Djamde Hospital in Kara City (130 beds, total area of 6774 square meters, 300 person-times per day)
Europe	Malta	1994	The Mediterranean Regional Centre for Traditional Chinese Medicine
Africa	Mauritania	1994	Moflag Hospital (expansion)
Africa	Benin	1995	Lokossa Hospital
Africa	Rwanda	1998	Kibungo Health School (rebuilt 1200 square meters, newly building 2000 square meters, and some basic furniture, teaching and laboratory facilities)
Africa	Angola	1999	A hospital with 100 beds
Africa	Botswana	1999	A project of prevention and control center for sexually transmitted diseases
Africa	Togo	1999	A pharmaceutical factory
Africa	Ghana	2000	Dangme East District Hospital
Africa	Cape Verde	2001	Inpatient Department and Chinese Doctors' Residential Building of Praia Central Hospital
Africa	Eritrea	2002	Olot Hospital
Africa	Rwanda	2002	Six complementary projects (including the gate and walls) of Kibungo Health School
Asia	Afghanistan	2003	Hospital of Republic of Afghanistan (Maintenance)
Africa	Congo (DRC)	2004	Pointe-Noire Hospital
Asia	Afghanistan	2005	New main building (350 beds, total area of 17,000 square meters), Hospital of Republic of Afghanistan

(Continued)

Region	*Country*	*Year*	*Facility constructed*
Africa	Cape Verde	2005	Outpatients Building and Gynecology Inpatient Department of Praia Central Hospital
Africa	Togo	2005	Lome Central Hospital
Africa	Angola	2006	Saint John Hill Health Center
Africa	Central Africa	2006	Friendship Hospital (maintenance)
Africa	Burundi	2007	Anti-malaria center
Africa	Chad	2007	Malaria prevention and treatment center
Africa	Ghana	2007	Ghana General Hospital
Asia	Indonesia	2007	Gunung Sitoli Hospital in Nias Island
Asia	Laos	2007	Luang Prabang Provincial Hospital (Lao-China Friendship Hospital)
Africa	Liberia	2007	Anti-malaria center
Oceania	Tonga	2007	A health center in Tapu Island, Prince Wellington Ngu Hospital in Vava'u Island (expansion)
Africa	Benin	2008	A malaria prevention and control center
Africa	Benin	2008	A hospital with 100 beds
Africa	Cameroon	2008	Anti-malaria center
Africa	Cote d'Ivoire	2008	Gagnoa Hospital
South America	Peru	2008	Loiza Hospital (expanding)
Africa	Rwanda	2008	Rwanda General Hospital

Source: Information provided by the Office of the Preparatory Work for the 30-year History Project: Exhibition on China's Opening Up (2008). Information contained in this volume was originally prepared by the Economic and Commercial Counselor Office of the Chinese Embassy in each recipient country.

Appendix 3
Aid of health equipment and medicine as CHAFC (1978–2008)

Region	*Country*	*Year*	*Donated medical facilities and medicine*
South America	Peru	1986	Medical
Africa	Burundi	1987	21 batches of medicine and apparatus by 2008
Europe	Belarus	1992	Medical instruments and medicine
Africa	Seychelles	1995	A batch of medicine and medical apparatus
South America	Peru	1996	Medical equipment
Africa	Botswana	2000	Furniture and computers for treatment center for sexual transmitted diseases
Africa	Eritrea	2000	Anti-malaria medicine
Oceania	Papua New Guinea	2002	Medical materials and apparatus
Africa	Angola	2003	Manual wheel chairs for the handicapped
Africa	Burundi	2003	Medical instruments for Kamenge Medical School
Africa	Niger	2003	Medicine
Africa	Seychelles	2003	Materials for prevention of SARS
Africa	Niger	2004	Measles vaccinations
Africa	Togo	2004	Medicine for two hospitals
Africa	Burundi	2005	Medicine
Africa	Dijibouti	2005	Anti-malaria medicine
Africa	Niger	2005	Commonly used medicine
Oceania	Papua New Guinea	2005	Medicine and reagents for prevention and treatment of AIDS
Oceania	Tonga	2005	Five small ambulances
Africa	Cameroon	2006	Anti-malaria medicine
Africa	Niger	2006	Anti-malaria medicine
Oceania	Papua New Guinea	2006	Anti-malaria medicine
Africa	Togo	2006	Anti-malaria medicine
Africa	Burundi	2007	Anti-malaria medicine
Africa	Chad	2007	Anti-malaria medicine
Africa	Cote d'Ivoire	2007	Anti-malaria medicine
Africa	Gabon	2007	Anti-malaria medicine, instruments and equipment
Africa	Ghana	2007	Anti-malaria medicine

(Continued)

Region	*Country*	*Year*	*Donated medical facilities and medicine*
Africa	Madagascar	2007	Anti-malaria medicine
Africa	Senegal	2007	Anti-malaria medicine
Africa	Sierra Leone	2007	Anti-malaria medicine
Africa	Somalia	2007	Anti-malaria medicine
Africa	Togo	2007	Anti-malaria medicine
Africa	Burundi	2008	Instruments and apparatus for a laboratory, and anti-malaria medicine
Africa	Central Africa	2008	Anti-malaria medicine
Asia	East Timor	2008	Anti-malaria medicine
Europe	Malta	2008	Medical apparatus
Africa	Niger	2008	Medical equipment and apparatus

Source: Information provided by the Office of the Preparatory Work for the 30-year History Project: Exhibition on China's Opening Up (2008). Information contained in this volume was originally prepared by the Economic and Commercial Counselor Office of the Chinese Embassy in each recipient country.

Appendix 4
Health cooperation agreements signed as CHAFC (1992–2007)

Region	*Country*	*Year*	*Agreement*
Asia	Armenia	1992	Agreement between the Government of the Republic of Armenia and the Government of the People's Republic of China on Cooperation in the Field of Culture, Education, Health Service, Sport and Tourism
Asia	Turkmenistan	1992	Cooperation Agreement on Health between Turkmenistan and China
Asia	Georgia	1993	Cooperation Agreement on Health between Georgia and China
Asia	Brunei	1996	Memorandum of Understanding on Health Cooperation between the Government of the People's Republic of China and the Government of His Majesty the Sultan and Yang Di-Pertuan of Brunei Darussalam
Europe	Russia	1996	The Agreement on Cooperation Against Illicit Trafficking and Abuse of Narcotic Drugs and Psychotropic Substances between Russia and China
Europe	Slovenia	1996	The Agreement of Cooperation in the fields of Health and Medicine between the Government of China and the Government of Slovenia
Europe	Slovenia	1996	The Programme of Cooperation in the Fields of Health and Medicine from 1996-1998 between the Government of China and the Government of Slovenia
Europe	Romania	1997	Convention between the Government of the People's Republic of China and the Government of Romania on Cooperation in the Sanitary Veterinary Field and Animal Quarantine and Health
Asia	Brunei	1999	Plan of Action on Annual Health Cooperation between Brunei and China
Asia	North Korea	2002	Health Quarantine Agreement between the Health Ministry of DPRK and the General Administration on Quality Supervision, Inspection and Quarantine of the People's Republic of China

(Continued)

Region	*Country*	*Year*	*Agreement*
Europe	Macedonia	2002	The Agreement on Cooperation in Public Health and Medicine between the Government of the People's Republic of China and the Government of the Republic of Macedonia
Asia	Malaysia	2004	Memorandum of Understanding on Health and Plant Health Cooperation between the Government of Malaysia and the Government of the People's Republic of China
South America	Argentina	2004	Framework Agreement on Health Issues and Medical Sciences between the Government of Republic of Argentina and the Government of People's Republic of China
Asia	Brunei	2005	Plan of Action on Health Cooperation between the Ministry of Health of the People's Republic of China and the Ministry of Health of the Government of His Majesty the Sultan and Yang Di-Pertuan of Brunei Darussalam
Asia	Brunei	2007	Plan of Action on Health Cooperation between Brunei and China 2007–2008
Central America	Costa Rica	2007	Memorandum of Understanding on Implementation of Health and Plant Health Measures between the Ministry of Agriculture and Ministry of Health of Costa Rica and the General Administration on Quality Supervision, Inspection and Quarantine of the People's Republic of China

Source: Information provided by the Office of the Preparatory Work for the 30-year History Project: Exhibition on China's Opening Up (2008). Information contained in this volume was originally prepared by the Economic and Commercial Counselor Office of the Chinese Embassy in each recipient country.

Appendix 5 WHO collaborating centers in China

Institution name	*City*	*Title*
Shanghai Institute of Cardiovascular Diseases	Shanghai	WHO Collaborating Centre for Research and Training in Cardiovascular Diseases
Guangdong Provincial Cardiovascular Institute	Guangzhou	WHO Collaborating Centre for Research and Training in Cardiovascular Diseases
Shandong Institute of Parasitic Diseases	Jining	WHO Collaborating Centre for Lymphatic Filariasis and Taeniasis/Cysticercosis
National Institute for the Control of Pharmaceutical and Biological Products	Beijing 100050	WHO Collaborating Centre for Drug Quality Assurance
Jiading Primary Health Care Centre	Shanghai	WHO Collaborating Centre for Primary Health Care
Peking Union Medical College Hospital (PUMCH) Chinese Academy of Medical Sciences (CAMS)	Beijing	WHO Collaborating Centre for the Family of International Classification (WHO-FIC)
National Institute of Nutrition and Food Safety	Beijing	WHO Collaborating Centre for Food Contamination Monitoring
Fudan University	Shanghai	WHO Collaborating Centre for Research and Training in Neurosciences
Peking University	Beijing	WHO Collaborating Centre for the Research and Training in Preventive Dentistry
National Institute of Occupational Health and Poison Control, Chinese Center for Disease Control and Prevention (China CDC)	Beijing	WHO Collaborating Centre for Occupational Health
Beijing Neurosurgical Institute	Beijing	WHO Collaborating Centre for Research and Training in Neurosciences
Shanghai Institute of Planned Parenthood Research	Shanghai	WHO Collaborating Centre for Research in Human Reproduction

(Continued)

Institution name	*City*	*Title*
Fudan University	Shanghai	WHO Collaborating Centre for Traditional Medicine
Institute of Acupuncture and Moxibustion, China Academy of Chinese Medical Sciences	Beijing	WHO Collaborating Centre for Traditional Medicine
Shanghai University of Traditional Chinese Medicine	Shanghai	WHO Collaborating Centre for Traditional Medicine
Institute of Chinese Materia Medica, China Academy of Chinese Medical Sciences	Beijing	WHO Collaborating Centre for Traditional Medicine
Institute of Clinical Research and Information, China Academy of Chinese Medical Sciences	Beijing	WHO Collaborating Centre for Traditional Medicine
Nanjing University of Chinese Medicine	Nanjing	WHO Collaborating Centre for Traditional Medicine
Shanghai Centre for Clinical Laboratory	Shanghai	WHO Collaborating Centre for Reagent Production
Fudan University	Shanghai	WHO Collaborating Centre for Occupational Health
Shanghai Health Education Institute	Shanghai	WHO Collaborating Centre for Health Education and Health Promotion
Chinese Academy of Medical Sciences (CAMS)	Beijing	WHO Collaborating Centre for Traditional Medicine
Shanghai Institue of Mental Health	Shanghai	WHO Collaborating Centre for Research and Training in Mental Health
Nanjing Child Mental Health Research Centre	Nanjing	WHO Collaborating Centre for Research and Training in Child Mental Health
Beijing Chaoyang Hospital	Beijing	WHO Collaborating Centre for Tobacco or Health
Suihua Municipal Health Bureau	Suihua	WHO Collaborating Centre for Information Support to Primary Health Care
Sun Yat-Sen University of Medical Sciences	Guangzhou	WHO Collaborating Centre for Rehabilitation
Capital Institute of Paediatrics	Beijing	WHO Collaborating Centre for Child Health
Yuncheng Stomatological Health School	Yuncheng	WHO Collaborating Centre for Oral Health
Shanghai Blood Centre	Shanghai	WHO Collaborating Centre for Blood Transfusion Services
Sichuan Family Planning Research Institute	Chengdu	WHO Collaborating Centre for Research in Human Reproduction
National Center for TB Control and Clinical Medicine, Center for Disease Control of China (CDC China)	Beijing	WHO Collaborating Centre for Research and Training on Tuberculosis

Institution name	*City*	*Title*
Hunan Institute of Parasitic Diseases	Yueyang	WHO Collaborating Centre on Schistosomiasis Control in Lake Regions
Hongkou District Health Bureau	Shanghai	WHO Collaborating Centre for Development of Urban Primary Health Care
Chinese Center for Diseases Control and Prevention (China CDC)	Shanghai	WHO Collaborating Centre for Malaria, Schistosomiasis and Filariasis
Tongji Medical College	Wuhan	WHO Collaborating Centre for Training and Research in Rehabilitation
People's Medical Publishing House (PMPH)	Beijing	WHO Collaborating Centre for the Promotion and Translation of WHO Publications
Institute of Medical Information, Chinese Academy of Medical Sciences	Beijing	WHO Collaborating Centre for Health and Biomedical Information
National Research Institute for Family Planning	Beijing	WHO Collaborating Centre for Research in Human Reproduction
Institute of Basic Medical Sciences, Chinese Academy of Medical Sciences	Beijing	WHO Collaborating Centre for the Community Control of Hereditary Diseases
Peking University	Beijing	WHO Collaborating Centre for Research in Reproductive Health and Population Science
Tianjin Municipal Research Institute for Family Planning	Tianjin	WHO Collaborating Centre for Research in Human Reproduction
Dongcheng District Health Bureau	Beijing	WHO Collaborating Centre for Urban Health Development
Central South University	Changsha	WHO Collaborating Centre for Psychosocial Substance Abuse and Health
Shanghai Medical Emergency Centre (SMEC)	Shanghai	WHO Collaborating Centre for Research and Training for Prehospital Emergency Services
Peking University	Beijing	WHO Collaborating Centre for Research and Training in Women's and Children's Health
Institute of Dermatology, Chinese Academy of Medical Sciences and Pekling Union Medical College	Nanjing	WHO Collaborating Centre for the Prevention and Control of Sexually Transmitted Infections
Second Military Medical University	Shanghai	WHO Collaborating Centre for Gene Synthesis and Expression
Centre for Disease Control and Prevention of Guangdong Province	Guangzhou	WHO Collaborating Centre for Surveillance, Research and Training of Emerging Infectious Diseases

(Continued)

Institution name	*City*	*Title*
Chinese Center for Disease Control and Prevention (China CDC)	Beijing	WHO Collaborating Centre on Community-based Integrated Noncommunicable Disease Control and Prevention
Beijing Hui Long Guan Hospital	Beijing	WHO Collaborating Centre for Research and Training in Suicide Prevention
Health Human Resources Development Center (HHRDC)	Beijing	WHO Collaborating Centre for Human Resources for Health
The Hong Kong Society for Rehabilitation	Hong Kong	WHO Collaborating Centre for Rehabilitation
Fudan University	Shanghai	WHO Collaborating Centre for Health Technology Assessment and Management
Nanjing Medical University	Nanjing	WHO Collaborating Centre for the Prevention of Deafness and Hearing Impairment
China Rehabilitation Research Center for Deaf Children	Beijing	WHO Collaborating Center for Prevention and Rehabilitation of Hearing Impairment
The Hong Kong Polytechnic University (HKPU)	Kowloon	WHO Collaborating Centre for Community Health Services
Beijing Ditan Hospital	Beijing	WHO Collaborating Centre for Comprehensive Management of HIV treatment and care
Beijing Institute of Otorhinolaryngology	Beijing	WHO Collaborating Centre for Prevention of Deafness
Queen Mary Hospital Infection Control Centre of Hong Kong	Hong Kong	WHO Collaborating Centre for Research, Training and Outbreak Response in Infection Control

Source: WHO website.

Appendix 6
Interviewees list on global health governance in China

Interview A: Dr Haichao Liu, Director, Department of Health Policy and Regulation of MOH, Division 2 for Policy Research (November 2009).

Interview B: Ms Guoping Luo, Director, Department of International Cooperation of MOH, Division of Asian and African Affairs (Division of Medical Aid to Developing Countries (November 2009).

Interview C: Dr Lucy Chen, Institute for Global Health (IGH), Beijing University (November 2009).

Interview D: Mr Peilong Liu, Former Director, Department of International Cooperation of MOH (November 2009).

Interview E: Dr Yin Zhou: Population and Development Studies, Shanghai Academy of Social Sciences (February 2010)

Interview F: Dr Bei Tang: School of International and Diplomatic Affairs, Shanghai International Studies University (February 2010)

Interview G: Dr Guoyou Song: Center for American Studies, Fudan University (April 2010)

Interview H: Dr Hai Zhao: Chicago University (April 2010)

Interview I: Dr Wei Da: Associate Professor, Institute of American Studies, China Institutes of Contemporary International Relations (April 2010)

Appendix 7
List of interviewees on the International Health Regulations

Japan

- Dr Kiyosu Taniguchi, Chief, Division 1, Infectious Disease Surveillance Centre, National Institute of Infectious Diseases
- Dr Nobuyoshi Tani, Director – Division of International Cooperation, National Institute of Infectious Diseases
- Dr Teppei Kiuchi, International Health Risk Management Coordinator, Office of Health Emergency Preparedness and Response, Ministry of Health, Labour and Welfare
- Dr Takuya Sugie, Deputy Director for WHO and International Health Affaris, International Affairs Division, Ministry of Labour, Health and Welfare
- Mr Kansuke Nagaoka, Director – Specialized Agencies Division, International Cooperation Bureau, Ministry of Foreign Affairs
- Mr Masaaki Okuma, Specialized Agencies Division, International Cooperation Bureau, Ministry of Foreign Affairs
- Mr Hajime Inoue, Executive Adviser, Chiba Prefectural Government, Health and Welfare Department

China

- Mr Ma Weixing, Section Chief, Health Supervision Section, Entry–Exit Inspection and Quarantine Bureau
- Mr Yan Dehua, Section Chief, The Section of Coordination and Monitor on Food Safety, Department of Health
- Anonymous, Entry-Exit Inspection and Quarantine Bureau
- Anonymous, Department of Supervision on Health Quarantine

Korea

- Dr Lee Han-Sung, Division of Public Health Crisis Response, Korea Centers for Disease Control and Prevention
- Professor Sohn Myongsei, Director – Asian Institute of Bioethics and Health Law, Yonsei University

- Mr Ki-Hyun Hahm, Adviser, Asian Institute of Bioethics and Health Law, Yonsei University

Taiwan

- Dr Chin-Shui Shih, Deputy Director, Bureau of International Cooperation, Department of Health
- Dr Jih-Haw Chou, Deputy Director-General, Centers for Disease Control, Department of Health
- Mr Yu-Chen Hsu, International Cooperation Affairs Planning Division, Centers for Disease Control, Department of Health
- Professor Chang-Fa Lo, Director – Asian Centre for WTO and International Health Law and Policy, NTU College of Law
- Anonymous, Ministry of Foreign Affairs

Thailand

- Dr Supamit Chunsuttiwat, Senior Expert in Disease Control, Department of Disease Control, Ministry of Public Health
- Dr Pasakorn Akarasewi, Country Coordinator, Director, Bureau of Epidemiology Department of Disease Control, Ministry of Public Health

Additional

- Dr Gunael Rodier, Director – International Health Regulations Coordination Programme, World Health Organization
- Dr David L. Heymann, former Assistant Director-General for Health Security and Environment, World Health Organization
- Dr Takasi Kasai, Regional Adviser, Communicable Disease Surveillance and Response, WHO Western Pacific Regional Office, Philippines
- Dr Li Ailan, Medical Officer (IHR), Communicable Disease Surveillance and Response, WHO Western Pacific Regional Office, Philippines
- Mr Vincent Liu, Director (Program), APEC Secretariat
- Anonymous, former delegate, Intergovernmental Working Group on the Revised International Health Regulations

Appendix 8
List of interviewees on the global health governance of pandemic influenza

Thailand

- Dr Kumnuan Ungchusak, Senior Expert in Preventive Medicine, Bureau of Epidemiology, Department of Diseases Control, Ministry of Public Health
- Dr Supamit Chunsuttiwat, Senior Expert in Disease Control, Department of Disease Control, Ministry of Public Health
- Dr Weerasak Putthasri, Senior Researcher, International Health Policy Program, Ministry of Public Health
- Dr Viroj Tangcharoensathien, Director IHPP, International Health Policy Program, Ministry of Public Health

Vietnam

- Dr Dang Quang Tan, Head of Border Health Quarantine Department, Ministry of Health
- Dr Nguyen Hong Ha, Deputy Director, National Institute of Infections and Tropical Diseases
- Mr David Payne, Partnership and Coordination Specialist, Partnership for Avian and Human Influenza, Vietnam
- Captain Michael Iademarco, US Health Attaché, Vietnam
- Dr Tim Meinke, Senior Avian Influenza Technical Advisor, USAID
- Dr Nicole Smith, Epidemiologist, World Health Organization, Vietnam

Indonesia

- Dr Marie Pangestu, Indonesian Minister for Trade
- Professor Agus Purwadianto, Director General, National Institute of Health Research and Development
- Ambassador Dr Makarim Wibisono, Advisor to the Minister of Health of the Republic of Indonesia on International Cooperation
- Dr Martahan Sitorus, Director of Respiratory Infections, Directorate General of Disease Control and Environmental Health
- Dr Sidibyo Markus, Chairman, Muhammadiyah (Indonesia)

China

- Dr Lee Chin-Kei, Medical Officer, Communicable Disease Surveillance and Response, WHO China Office, Beijing
- Dr Dong Jie, Medical Officer, Communicable Disease Surveillance and Response, WHO China Office, Beijing
- Dr Lu Guoping, Deputy Director, Division of Asian and African Affairs, Department of International Cooperation, Ministry of Health, Beijing
- Dr He Xiong, Deputy Director, Centre for Disease Control and Prevention, Beijing
- Professor Wang Wei, School of Public Health and Family Medicine, Capital Medical University

Additional

- Dr Takasi Kasai, Regional Adviser, Communicable Disease Surveillance and Response, WHO Western Pacific Regional Office, Philippines
- Dr Li Ailan, Medical Officer (IHR), Communicable Disease Surveillance and Response, WHO Western Pacific Regional Office, Philippines
- Dr Henk Bekedam, Director Health Sector Development, WHO Western Pacific Regional Office, Philippines
- Mr Wu Guogao, External Relations Officer, WHO Western Pacific Regional Office, Philippines
- Dr Ingo Neu, Senior Planning Officer, Regional Office for Asia and the Pacific, United Nations Office for the Coordination of Humanitarian Affairs
- Dr Jacques Jeugmans, Practice Leader (Health), Office of the Director General, Regional and Sustainable Development Department, Asian Development Bank
- Ms Eliette Dupre Husser, Asia-Europe Foundation
- Ms Sunkyong Lee, Asia-Europe Foundation
- Mr Royce Escolar, Regional Program Manager, Emerging Infectious Diseases Unit, Australian Agency for International Development
- Mr Gerard Oakes, Executive Officer, People Smuggling, Refugee and Immigration Section, Australian Department of Foreign Affairs and Trade
- Anonymous, Australian Agency for International Development

References

ABT Associates (2006) *ABT Associates launches USAID-funded H5N1 Avian influenza surveillance and control project.* www.abtassociates.com/Page.cfm?PageID=40375 (accessed 1 April 2010).

Achadi, A., Soerojo, W. and Barber, S. (2005) The relevance and prospects of advancing tobacco control in Indonesia. *Health Policy*, 72: 333–349.

Acharya, A., Fuzzo de Lima, A. T. and Moore, M. (2006) Proliferation and fragmentation: transactions costs and the value of aid. *Journal of Development Studies*, 42(1): 1–21.

Advance Market Commitment for Pneumococcal Vaccines. (2010) *The pneumococcal AMC: Ready to save lives.* www.vaccineamc.org/pneu_amc.html (accessed 12 March 2010).

Aguinaga Bialous, S., Mochizuki-Kobayashi, Y. and Stillman, F. (2006) Courtesy and the challenges of implementing smoke-free policies in Japan. *Nicotine and Tobacco Research*, 8(2): 1–14.

AEC Health Working Group (2009) *Annual program of work 2009 (working document).* Internal document dated 14 August 2009.

Aldasoro, I., Nunnenkamp, P. and Thiele, R. (2010) Less aid proliferation and more donor coordination? The wide gap between words and deeds. *Journal of International Development*, 22(7): 920–940.

Alter, K. J. and Meunier, S. (2009) The politics of international regime complexity. *Perspectives on Politics*, 7: 13–24.

Annen, K. and Kosempel, S. (2009) Foreign aid, donor fragmentation, and economic growth. *The B. E. Journal of Macroeconomics* 9(1): ISSN (Online) 1935–1690, DOI: 10.2202/1935–1690.1863, August.

APEC Health Working Group. (2009) Annual Program of Work 2009 (working document). Internal document dated 14 August 2009.

APEIR (2006) *Roles and responsibilities: Asia partnership on avian influenza research.* Nonthaburi: APEIR.

Arase, D. (ed.) (2005) *Japan's foreign aid: Old continuities and new directions.* London and New York: Routledge.

Asahi News Service (2000) Switzerland: WHO ends convention hearings; negotiations this week. 18 October, LTDL, Bates 524860005–0006. http://legacy.library.ucsf.edu/tid/uzo03c00/pdf

ASEAN. (2007) *Third Executive Report Progress of Implementation of the ASEAN–Japan Plan of Action.* www.aseansec.org/20462.htm (accessed 4 November 2010).

——. (2010a) *About ASEAN.* www.aseansec.org/about_ASEAN.html (accessed 21 October 2010).

——. (2010b) *The ASEAN Declaration (Bangkok Declaration)*. www.aseansec.org/1212.htm (accessed 20 March).

——. (2010c) *ASEAN Health Ministers Meeting (AHMM)*. www.aseansec.org/19602.htm, (accessed 19 March 2010).

Asia-Pacific Centre for the Responsibility to Protect. (2008) *Cyclone Nargis and the responsibility to protect (Myanmar/Burma Briefing No. 2)*. Brisbane: Asia-Pacific Centre for the Responsibility to Protect.

Asia-Pacific Economic Cooperation (2008) *Health Working Group (Health Task Force)*. www.apec.org/apec/apec_groups/som_committee_on_economic/working_groups/health.html (accessed 16 June 2008).

Asia Pulse Data (2009) *Ratification of FCTC may raise Indonesia's bargaining power*. Asia Pulse Data, 12 July, http://snus-news.blogspot.com/2009/12/indonesia-ratification-of-fctc-may.html

Asian News International (2008) Government bows down to tobacco industry pressures. *Asian News International*, 3 December.

Assunta, M. and Chapman, S. (2006) Health treaty dilution: a case study of Japan's influence on the language of the WHO Framework Convention on Tobacco Control. *Journal of Epidemiology and Community Health*, 60: 751–756.

Asukai, Y., Toril, Y. and Chikamoto, Y. (2005) Tobacco control: recent developments in Japan. *American Journal of Health Promotion*, 19(3): 260–265.

AusAID (2007) Australia provides $12 million to combat emerging infectious diseases in our region, www.ausaid.gov.au/media/release.cfm?BC=MediaandID=252_5829_2278_2217_5328 (accessed 22 March 2010).

Ayyar, R. V. V. (2010) India: an emerging donor?, www.norrag.org/issues/article/1332/en/india-an-emerging-donor.html?PHPSESSID=ea018508137f54ef257a1f17bbe581fe (accessed 17 February 2012).

Bajpai, K. (2002) Indian strategic culture, in Chambers, M (ed.), *South Asia in 2020: Future Strategic Balances and Alliances*, pp. 245–304. Carlisle, PA: US Army War College, Strategic Studies Institute.

Barben, D. (2001) The global configuration of the biotechnology regime in comparative perspective, in A. Bamme, G. Getzinger and B. Wieser (eds), *Yearbook of the Institute for Advanced Studies on Science, Technology and Society*, pp. 41–86. Vienna: Profil Verlag.

Barber, S. and Ahsan, A. (2009) The tobacco excise system in Indonesia: hindering effective tobacco control for health. *Journal of Public Health Policy*, 30(2): 208–225.

BAT increases its market share in Indonesia. *Smokers News* 2009; 25 June.

BAT. (2001) *The WHO Framework Convention on Tobacco Control: Update May 2001*. LTDL, Bates 525920523-0528. http://legacy.library.ucsf.edu/tid/fag17a00/pdf

——. (2000) *Information on the Outcome of the WHO second working group meeting 27–29 March 2000*. Geneva, nd, LTDL, Bates 760028629-8635. http://legacy.library.ucsf.edu/tid/mxj45a99/pdf

Benatar, S. R. and Singer, P. A. (2000) A new look at international research ethics. *BMJ* 321(7264): 824–826.

——. and Vaughan, C. L. (2008) Global and local forces shaping the research agenda and the governance of research ethics. *South African Journal of Science*, 104(November/December): 439–442.

Benvenisti, E. and Downs, G. W. (2007) The empire's new clothes: political economy and the fragmentation of international law. *Stanford Law Review*, 60(2): 595–631.

Bhatiasevi, A. and Maneerungsee, W. (2000) HIV/AIDS-compulsory ddi licensing seen as unlikely. *The Bangkok Post*, 2 February.

Biermann, F., Pattberg, P., van Asselt, H. and Zelli, F. (2009) The fragmentation of global governance architectures: a framework for analysis. *Global Environmental Politics*, 9: 14–40.

Boltz, J. (2002) International Tobacco Listserve: FCTC Negotiations updates. Email, 4 April, LTDL, Bates AC5000636469-6471. http://legacy.library.ucsf.edu/tid/fag17a00/pdf

Buse, K., Hein W. and Drager, N. (eds) (2009) *Making sense of global health governance, a policy perspective*. London: Palgrave Macmillan.

——. and Walt, G. (2000) Global public–private partnerships: Part II – what are the health issues for global governance? *Bulletin of the WHO*, 78(5): 699–709.

Butler, D. (2011) Revamp for WHO. *Nature*, doi:10.1038/473430a.

Calder, K. E. (1988) Japanese foreign economic policy formation: explaining the reactive state. *World Politics*, 40(2): 517–541.

Cancer Patients Aid Association (CPAA), Lawyers Collective HIV/AIDS Unit, Delhi Network for Positive People (DNP+), and Médecins Sans Frontières. (2007) *Joint Statement by CPAA, MSF, DNP+ and Lawyers Collective on Novartis Judgment*, 7 August, http://keionline.org/content/view/120/1

Carucci, D. J. and Gottlieb, M. (2008) The future of TDR: the need to adapt to a changing global health environment. *PLoS Neglected Tropical Diseases*, 2(11): e310.

Chan, L., Lee, P. and Chan, G. (March 2008) Rethinking global governance: a China model in the making? *Contemporary Politics*, 14(1):3–19.

Chan, M. (2007) Pandemics: working together for an effective and equitable response. Address to the Pacific Health Summit, Seattle, Washington, 13 June 2007, www.who.int/dg/speeches/2007/20070613_seattle/en/index.html (accessed 4 November 2010).

Charnoz, O. and Severino, J.-M. (2008) From hyper-collective action to global policies. *En Temps Réel*, 36: 1–27.

Chaudhuri, S. (2005) *The WTO and India's pharmaceuticals industry: Patent protection, TRIPS, and developing countries*. New Delhi, New York: Oxford University Press.

Chee, Y. L. (2006) Malaysia: 'government use' route to importing generic medicines. *Third World Resurgence*, 196, www.twnside.org.sg/title2/twr196.htm

Chen, Z. (2008) *Thirty-year health reform and opening up in China* (zhongguo weisheng gaige kaifang 30 nian). Beijing: People's Medical Publishing House.

Cheng, Y., Liu, G. and He, Y. J. (2001) China Tobacco and the WHO FCTC. *Eastern Tobacco News*.

Cheng, Y. H. (2006) Final report on the research of the working group. In STMA, *Countermeasures against the FCTC and approaches to deal with the impact on the tobacco industry in China*, pp. 3–20. Beijing: Economic and Scientific Press.

China Ministry of Foreign Affairs. (2000) *China's Initiation of the Five Principles of Peaceful Co-existence*. Ministry of Foreign Affairs, Beijing, www.fmprc.gov.cn/eng/ziliao/3602/3604/t18053.htm (accessed 12 July 2007).

Chongsuphajaisiddhi, T. and Salazar, N. (1998) Role of the SEAMEO TROPMED network in health human resources development. Southeast Asian Ministers of Education Organization. Tropical Medicine and Public Health. *Southeast Asian Journal of Tropical Medicine and Public Health*, 29(2): 299–310.

Chow, J. (2010) China's billion dollar appetite. *Foreign Policy*, 29 July.

CIDA (2010) Profile project for Asia-Pacific Strategy for Emerging Diseases, I, http://acdi-cida.gc.ca/CIDAWEB/cpo.nsf/vWebProjBySectorSCEn/A1B8E262E239C5FD8525 72A700371141 (accessed 22 March 2010).

Cohen, M., Chen, T., Li, C. L., Chen, A. and Bai, B. (2009) Amendment provides new road map for compulsory licenses. *The China Daily*, 30 November.

Collin, J., Lee, K. and Bissell, K. (2002) The Framework Convention on Tobacco Control: the politics of global health governance. *Third World Quarterly*, 23(2): 265–282.

Commission on Health Research for Development. (1990) *Health research: Essential link to equity in development*. Oxford: Oxford University Press.

Commission on Intellectual Property Rights, Innovation and Public Health (CIPIH). (2006) *Public health, innovation and intellectual property rights*. Geneva: World Health Organization (WHO).

Commission on the Social Determinants of Health. (2008) *Closing the gap in a generation: Health equity through action on the social determinants of health*. Geneva: World Health Organization.

Committee on Economic, Social, and Cultural Rights. (2000) *General comment no. 14: The right to the highest attainable standard of health* (Art. 12 of the Covenant on Economic, Social, and Cultural Rights), 11 August, E/C.12/2000/4. NewYork: UN Economic and Social Council.

Conference of the Parties to the WHO Framework Convention on Tobacco Control. (2006) *First session, Geneva, 6–17 February 2006, Summary Records of Committees, Reports of Committees*. Geneva: World Health Organization.

Cooke, J. G. (2009) China's soft power in Africa, in C. McGiffert (ed.), *Chinese soft power and its implications for the United States: Competition and cooperation in the developing world*, pp. 27–44. Washington, DC: Center for Strategic and International Studies.

Copenhagen Accord. (2009) *UN framework convention on climate change conference of the parties*. FCCC/CP/2009/L.7, 18 December. New York: United Nations.

Correa, C. M. (2002) *Implications of the Doha Declaration on the TRIPS agreement and public health*. WHO/EDM/PAR/2002.3, World Health Organization, EDM Series no. 12. Geneva: World Health Organization.

Costello, A., Abbas, M., Allen, A., Ball, S., Bell, S., Bellamy, R., Friel, S., Groce, N., Johnson, A., Kett, M., Lee, M., Levy, C., Maslin, M., McCoy, D., McGuire, B., Montgomery, H., Napier, D., Pagel, C., Patel, J., de Oliveira, J. A. P., Redclift, N., Rees, H., Rogger, D., Scott, J., Stephenson, J., Twigg, J., Wolff, J. and Patterson, C. (2009) Managing the health affects of climate change. *The Lancet*, 373(9676): 1693–1733.

Cunningham, E. (2011) India boosts ties to Afghanistan with $500m more in aid. *The National*, 13 May, www.thenational.ae/news/world/south-asia/india-boosts-ties-to-afghanistan-with-500m-more-in-aid (accessed 29 Aug 2011).

Daar, A., Abdullah, M. S., Hu, C. L., Whyte, S. R., Hoffman, S. L. and Berger, M. (2006) *Fourth external review of the special programme for research and training in tropical diseases: Towards evolution and growth*. Geneva: WHO.

——. Whyte, S. R., Abdullah, M. S., Hu, C. L., Hoffman, S. L. and Berger, M. (2008) TDR thirty years on: taking stock and envisioning the future for the Special Programme for Research and Training in Tropical Diseases. *PLoS Neglected Tropical Diseases*, 2(11): e314.

Datong Party (2008) The formal establishment of Uganda anti-malaria center aided by China, (zhongguo yuanzhu wuganda kangnue zhongxin zhengshi guaipai, Datong Dangjian), May 20, www.dtdj.gov.cn/dtdj_szyw/2008/0520/article_293.html

Davies, M., Edinger, H., Tay, N. and Naidu, S. (2008) *How China delivers development assistance to Africa. A research prepared for the Department for International Development (DFID)*. Beijing: Centre for Chinese Studies, University of Stellenbosch.

Deere, C. (2008) *The implementation game: The TRIPS agreement and the global politics of intellectual property reform in developing countries*. Oxford: Oxford University Press.

Delamothe, T. and Smith, R. (2004) Open access publishing takes off. *BMJ*, 328 (7430): 1–3.

Dent C. (ed.) (2008) *China, Japan and regional leadership in East Asia.* Cheltenham: Edward Elgar.

Department of Health. (2005) *Research governance framework for health and social care.* London: Department of Health.

Djankov, S., Montalvo, J. G. and Reynal-Querol, M. (2009) Aid with multiple personalities. *Journal of Comparative Economics*, 37(2): 217–229.

Dobson, H. (2005) Global governance, the G7/8 Summit and Japan, in Glenn D. Hook (ed.), *Contested governance in Japan: Sites and issues*, pp. 17–35. London: Routledge Curzon.

Dodgson, R., Lee, K. and Drager, N. (2004) *Global health governance: A conceptual review. Global Health Governance Discussion Paper No. 1.* London: World Health Organisation and Centre for Global Change and Health, London School of Hygiene and Tropical Medicine.

Drahos, P. and Braithwaite, J. (2002) *Information feudalism: Who owns the knowledge economy?* New York: The New Press.

Dreher, A., Nunnenkamp, P. and Thiele, R. (2011) *Are 'new' donors different? Comparing the allocation of bilateral aid between non-DAC and DAC donor countries. World Development*, 39(11): 1950–1968.

Drezner, D. W. (2009) The power and peril of international regime complexity. *Perspectives on Politics*, 7(1): 65–70.

Drifte, R. (1996) *Japan's foreign policy in the 1990s: From economic super-power to what power?* New York: St Martin's Press.

Dubash, N. and Florini, A. (2011) Mapping global energy governance. *Global Policy*, 2(S1): 6–18.

Eberstadt, N. (2006) Growing old the hard way: China, Russia, India. *Policy Review*, No. 136.

Economist, The. (2008) No shelter from the storm: cyclone in Myanmar. *The Economist*, 10 May, 78.

Engelgau, M., Okamoto, K., Kudesia, P., Rajan, V., Rosenhouse, S. and Okamoto, K. (eds) (2011) *Capitalizing on the demographic transition: Tackling noncommunicable diseases in South Asia.* Washington, DC: World Bank.

——. and Dunnill, P. (2007) From scarcity to abundance: pandemic vaccines and other agents for 'have not' countries. *Journal of Public Health Policy*, 28(3): 322–340.

Fidler, D. P. (2005) From international sanitary conventions to global health security: the new International Health Regulations. *Chinese Journal of International Law*, 4(2): 325–392.

——. (2007) Architecture amidst anarchy: global health's quest for governance. *Global Health Governance*, 1(1): 1–17.

——. (2008) Influenza virus samples, international law, and global health diplomacy. *Emerging Infectious Diseases*, 14(1): 88–94.

——. and Gostin, L. (2006) The new international health regulations: an historic development for international law and public health. *Journal of Law, Medicine and Ethics*, 34(1): 85–94.

——. and Gostin, L. (2011) The WHO Pandemic Influenza Preparedness Framework: a milestone in global governance for health. *Journal of the American Medical Association*, 306(2): 200–201.

——. and Ganguly, S. (2010) India and Eastphalia. *Indiana Journal of Global Legal Studies*, 17(1): 147–164.

Fijii, Y. and Price, A. (2000) Debate on global tobacco treaty set to start in Geneva. *Japanese Times*, 9 October, http://search.japantimes.co.jp/cgi-bin/nb20001009a2.html

Fischer-Lescano, A. and Teubner, G. (2006) *Regime-Kollisionen: Zur Fragmentierung des globalen Rechts*. Frankfurt aM: Suhrkamp.

FOCAC. (2006) *FOCAC Beijing Action Plan 2007–2009* (zhongfei hezuo luntan Beijing xingdong jihua), www.focac.org/chn/ltda/bjfhbzjhy/hywj32009/t584788.htm

——. (2009) *FOCAC Sharm el Sheikh action 2010–2012* (zhongfei hezuo luntan Beijing xingdong jihua), www.focac.org/chn/dsjbzjhy/bzhyhywj/t626385.htm

Ford, N., Wilson, D., Bunjumnong, O. and von Schoen Angerer, T. (2004) The role of civil society in protecting public health over commercial interests: lessons from Thailand. *The Lancet*, 363(9408), 560–563, doi:DOI: 10.1016/S0140-6736(04)15545-1, www.sciencedirect.com.ezp-prod1.hul.harvard.edu/science/article/B6T1B-4BP91S1-W/2/4cda28dc20dbda007c550ac8ddb55294

Ford, N., Wilson, D., Chaves, G. C., Lotrowska, M. and Kijtiwatchakul, K. (2007) Sustaining access to antiretroviral therapy in the less-developed world: lessons from Brazil and Thailand. *AIDS*, 21(Suppl. 4): S21–S29.

Forster, P. (2009) *The political economy of avian influenza in Indonesia*. STEPS Working Paper 17. Brighton: STEPS Centre.

Forum on China-Africa Cooperation (2009) *Sharm El Sheikh Action Plan (2010-2012)*, 12 November, www.focac.org/eng/

Frot, E. and Santiso, J. (2010) *Crushed aid: Fragmentation in sectoral aid*, Working Paper No. 284. Paris: OECD.

Führer, H. (1996) *The story of official development assistance: A history of the development assistance committee and the development co-operation directorate in dates, names and figures*. OECD/GD(94)67, www.oecd.org/dataoecd/3/39/1896816.pdf

Funabashi, Y. (2009) Tokyo's trials: can the DPJ change Japan? *Foreign Affairs*, 88(6): 106–117.

Gao, X. (1998) An introduction to administrative protection for pharmaceuticals. *Duke Journal of Comparative and International Law*, 9: 259–262.

Garrett, L. and Fidler, D.P. (2007) Sharing H5N1 viruses to stop a global influenza pandemic. *PLoS Medicine*, 4(11): 1712–1714.

George, J., Sheshadri, R. and Grover, A. (2009) India: intellectual property and access to medicines: developments and civil society initiatives in India, in R. Reis, V. Terto Jr. and M. C. Pimenta (eds), *Intellectual property rights and access to ARV medicines: Civil society resistance in the global south*, pp. 110–136. Rio de Janeiro: Brazilian Interdisciplinary AIDS Association (ABIA).

Gerhardsen, T. I. S. (2007) Drug company reacts to Thai license; government ready to talk. *Intellectual Property Watch (IP Watch)*, 16 February, www.ip-watch.org/weblog/2007/02/16/drug-company-upset-by-newest-thai-license-government-open-to-dialogue/

Ghersi, D. and Pang, T. (2008) En route to international clinical trial transparency. *The Lancet* 372(9649): 1531–1532.

Ginsburg, T. (2010) Eastphalia as the perfection of Westphalia. *Indiana Journal of Global Legal Studies*, 17(1): 27–45.

Glennie, J. (2012) Aid from Brics countries is making a bigger splash. *The Guardian*, 26 March, www.guardian.co.uk/global-development/poverty-matters/2012/mar/26/aid-brics-countries-china-india

Global Fund to Fight HIV/AIDS, Tuberculosis and Malaria, The (2010) *Country pledges*, http://portfolio.theglobalfund.org/en/Home/Index

——. (2011) *Country portfolio*, http://portfolio.theglobalfund.org/en/Country/Index/IDA (accessed 13 February 2012).

Global Health Strategies Initiative (2012) *Shifting paradigm: How the BRICS are reshaping global health and development*. www.ghsinitiatives.org/brics-report

Godlee, F. (2006) An international standard for disclosure of clinical trial information. *BMJ* 332(7550): 1107–1108.

Gomez, E. (2009) The politics of receptivity and resistance: how Brazil, India, China, and Russia strategically use the international health community in response to HIV/AIDS: a theory. *Global Health Governance*, 3(1): 1–29.

Gonzalez Block, M. (2006) The state of international collaboration for health systems research: what do publications tell? *Health Research Policy and Systems*, 4: 7.

Gostin, L. O. (2005) World health law: toward a new conception of global health governance in the 21st century. *Yale Journal of Health Policy, Law and Ethics*, 5: 419.

——. (2008) Meeting basic survival needs of the world's least healthy people: toward a framework convention on global health. *Georgetown Law Journal*, 96: 331–373.

——. (forthcoming 2013) *Global health law: International law, global institutions, and world health*. Cambridge, MA: Harvard University Press.

——. Heywood, M., Ooms, M., Røttingen, J-A. and Chenguang, W. (2010) National and global responsibilities for health (Editorial). *Bulletin of the World Health Organisation*, 88: 719–720, www.who.int/bulletin/volumes/88/10/10-082636.pdf.

——. Friedman, E. A., Oooms, G., Gebauer, T., Gupta, N. Sridhar, D., Chenguang, W., Røttingen, J-A. and Sanders, D. (2011) The joint action and learning initiative: towards a global agreement on national and global responsibilities for health. *PLoS Medicine* 8(5): e1001031; doi:10.1371/journal.pmed.1001031, www.plosmedicine.org/article/info%3Adoi%2F10.1371%2Fjournal.pmed.1001031 (accessed 16 February 2012).

Government bows down to tobacco industry pressures. (2008) *Asian News International*, 3 December.

Government of Canada. (2010) *G8 2010 Muskoka accountability report*. http://g8.gc.ca/wp-content/uploads/2010/06/muskoka_accountability_report.pdf (accessed 30 June 2010).

Government of India (2007) *Ministry of External Affairs annual report*. New Delhi: Ministry of External Affairs.

——. (2009a) *Ministry of Health, Labour, and Welfare: Summary of vital statistics*. New Delhi: Ministry of Health, Labour, and Welfare.

——. (2009b) *Ministry of External Affairs annual report*. New Delhi: Ministry of External Affairs.

——. (2010) *Outcome Budget*. New Delhi: *Ministry of External Affairs.*

——. (2011) *India Technical and Economic Cooperation Programme*. New Delhi: Ministry of External Affairs.

Greenpeace. (2010) *Greenpeace assessment of the Copenhagen Accord*, 7 January, www.greenpeace.org/raw/content/eu-unit/press-centre/reports/greenpeace-assessment-COP15-07-01-10.pdf (accessed 12 March 2010).

Gu, J. and Humphrey, J. (2008) Global governance and developing countries: the implications of the rise of China. *World Development*, 36(2): 274–292.

Gupta, P. (2006) Tobacco control in India. *Indian Journal of Medical Research*, 123: 579–582.

Hackbarth, J. R. (2009) Soft power and smart power in Africa. *Strategic Insights*, 8(1), www.nps.edu/Academics/centers/ccc/publications/OnlineJournal/2008/Dec/hackbarthDec08.html (accessed 12 March 2010).

Hampson, A. W. (1997) Surveillance for pandemic influenza. *Journal of Infectious Diseases*, 176(Suppl 1): S8–13.

Han, L., Koenig-Archibugi, M. and Opsahl, T. (2012) Complex social networks in global health policy: patterns and effects. Paper presented at the International Studies Association Annual Convention, San Diego, CA, 1–4 April 2012.

Hansenclever, A., Mayer, P. and Rittberger, V. (1997) *Theories of international regimes*. Cambridge: Cambridge University Press.

Harinasuta, C. (1972) The programmes and activities of the SEAMEO-TROPMED Project. *Southeast Asian Journal of Tropical Medicine and Public Health*, 23(4): 550–555.

Harman, S. (2012) *Global health governance*. London: Routledge.

HealthBridge. (2007) *Supporting the FCTC process in Indonesia. Final narrative and financial report*. www.healthbridge.ca/assets/images/pdf/Tobacco/HealthBridge%20Indonesia%20TC%20report%2007.pdf

Hechanova, E. R. (2008) Philippines: cheaper medicines act signed into law. *Managing Intellectual Property*, July/August. www.managingip.com/article/1969003/Cheaper-Medicines-Act-signed-into-law.html

Ho, C. S. and Gostin, L. O. (2009) The social face of economic growth: China's health system in transition. *Journal of the American Medical Association*, 301/17: 1809–1811.

Holbrooke, R. and Garrett, L. (2008) Sovereignty that risks global health. *Washington Post*, 8 August, www.washingtonpost.com/wp-yn/content/article/2008/08/08/AR2008080802919.html (accessed 4 April 2012)].

Hook, G. D. and McCormack, G. (2001) *Japan's contested constitution: Documents and analysis*. London: Routledge.

Hook S. W. and Zhang, G. (1998) Japan's aid policy since the cold war: rhetoric and reality. *Asian Survey*, 38: 311–334.

Horvarth, J. S., McKinnon, M. and Roberts, L. (2006) The Australian response: pandemic influenza preparedness. *Medical Journal of Australia*, 185(10): S35–S38.

Howard, L. (1989) The evolution of bilateral and multilateral cooperation for health in developing countries, in M. R. Reich and E. Marui, E. (eds), *International cooperation for health: Problems, prospects, and priorities*, pp. 332–357. Dover: Auburn House Publishing Company.

Huang, M. (2007) The mechanism of Chinese foreign aid: Current situation and trend. *International Economic Cooperation*, 6: 4–11.

Huang, M. and Hu, J. (2009) The formation and development of management system of Chinese foreign aid. *International Economic Cooperation*, 5: 32–39.

Huang, Y. (2010) Pursuing health as foreign policy: the case of China. *Indiana Journal of Global Legal Studies*, 17(1): 105–146.

Hyodo, C. and Katsuma, Y. (2008) *The role and challenges of Japanese NGOs in the global health policymaking process*. Tokyo: Japan Center for International Exchange.

IFENG (2009) Chinese medical team to Africa (zhongguo yuanfei yiliaodui: diandi jilei, jiusifushang), http://phtv.ifeng.com/hotspot/08331/200903/0328_5686_1081660.shtml.

IMS Health. (2010) IMS forecasts global pharmaceutical market growth of 5–8% annually through 2014; maintains expectations of 4–6% growth in 2010. *FiercePharma*, 20 April, press release.

India–Africa Forum Summit. (2008) Africa–India Framework for Cooperation, New Delhi, 8–9 April.

India Brazil South Africa Dialogue Forum (2009) *IBSA agreement on health*, www.ibsa-trilateral.org/index.php?option=com_content&task=view&id=13&Itemid=13 (accessed 13 February 2012).

India Brazil South Africa Dialogue Forum (2011) *IBSA agreement on health*, www.ibsa-trilateral.org/index.php?option=com_content&view=article&id=164&Itemid=92 (accessed 13 February 2012).
Influenza Foundation (Thailand) (2010) http://test.ddc.moph.go.th/objective.html (accessed 20 March 2010).
Information Office of the State Council, People's Republic of China. (2011) *China's foreign aid*. Information Office of the State Council, http://news.xinhuanet.com/english2010/china/2011-04/21/c_13839683.htm (accessed 25 July 2011).
Institute for Health Metrics and Evaluation (2009) *Financing global health report: Tracking* development assistance for health, Seattle, WA: University of Washington. www.healthmetricsandevaluation.org/publications/policy-report/financing-global-health-2009-tracking-development-assistance-health.
——. (2010) *Financing for global health: Development assistance for health*.
Institute of Medicine. (2009) *Sustaining global surveillance and response to emerging zoonotic diseases*. Washington, DC: National Academies Press.
International Commission on Intervention and State Sovereignty. (2001) *The responsibility to protect*. Ottawa: International Development Research Centre.
International Committee of the Red Cross (2004) *ICRC annual report*. Geneva: Switzerland.
——. (2005) *ICRC annual report 2004*. Geneva: Switzerland, www.icrc.org/eng/resources/documents/annual-report/icrc-annual-report-2004.htm
——. (2006) *ICRC annual report*. Geneva: Switzerland, www.icrc.org/eng/resources/documents/annual-report/icrc-annual-report-2005.htm
——. (2007) *ICRC annual report*. Geneva: Switzerland, www.icrc.org/eng/resources/documents/annual-report/icrc-annual-report-2006.htm
——. (2008) *ICRC annual report*. Geneva: Switzerland, www.icrc.org/eng/resources/documents/annual-report/icrc-annual-report-2007.htm
International Finance Facility for Immunisation. (2010) *Donors*. www.iff-immunisation.org/donors.html (accessed 12 March 2010).
International Institute for Population Sciences (IIPS) and ORC Macro. (2006). *National Family Health Survey (NFHS-3)*. Mumbai: IIPS.
International Monetary Fund. (2011) *World economic outlook database*. www.imf.org/external/pubs/ft/weo/2011/ 01/weodata/index.aspx (accessed 25 July 2011).
——. (2011) *IMF data mapper*. www.imf.org/external/datamapper/index.php (accessed 19 February 2012).
International Trade Centre. (2010) *Trade map: Trade statistics for international business development*. www.trademap.org/Index.aspx (accessed 29 August 2010).
Itô, M. (1998) 'Tomouni ikiu chikyu shimin shakai no jitsugen o mezashite: kokusai kyouryoku katsudou ni kakawaru shimin soshiki (NGO) no katsudou' (Aiming towards a global civil society: activities of NGO working in international cooperation), in Yamaoka Yoshinori (ed.), *NPO Kiso Kouza 2 (Lectures on Basic NPO, vol. 2)*, pp. 69–104. Tokyo: Gyousei.
Jakarta Post (2007) RI 'will not share' flu samples, 17 February, www.thejakartapost.com/news/2007/02/17/ri-039will-not-share039-flu-samples.html
——. (2009) Special report: tobacco bill – same old story of another toothless regulation. *Jakarta Post*, 8 May.
Jandoo, T. and Mehrotra, R. (2008) Tobacco control in India: present scenario and challenges ahead. *Asia Pacific Journal of Cancer Prevention*, 9(4): 805–810.
Jentsch, B. and Pilley, C. (2003) Research relationships between the south and the north: Cinderella and the ugly sisters? *Social Science and Medicine*, 57(10): 1957–1967.

Jiang, C. K. (2006) Preamble, advancing research to meet the requirements of decision-making, in STMA, *Countermeasures against the FCTC and approaches to deal with the impact on the tobacco industry in China.* Beijing: Economic and Scientific Press pp. 1–5.

JICA (2010) *JICA annual report 2009*. Tokyo: Japan International Cooperation Agency.

——. (ed.) *JICA Annual Report, various years 1998–2009*. Tokyo: Japan International Cooperation Agency.

Jin, J. Y. (2012) FCTC and China's politics of tobacco control. Paper presented at the fourth GLF Annual Colloquium, Princeton Universty, 15 May.

Jobelius, M. (2007) *New powers for global change and challenges for the international development cooperation: The case of India. FES Briefing Paper 5*. Berlin: Friedrich Ebert Stiftung.

John, S. (2008) *Enforcement of tobacco control policies: Global best practices*. New Delhi: Ministry of Health and Family Welfare.

John, T. J., Dandona, L., Sharma, V. P. and Kakkar, M. (2011) Continuing challenges of infectious diseases in India. *The Lancet*, 377(9761): 252–269.

JTI Weekly News Report (2000) LTDL, Bates No. 530776217-6262. http://legacy.library.ucsf.edu/tid/jhb65a00/pdf

Kamradt-Scott, A. (2009) Disease outbreaks and health governance in the Asia-Pacific: Australia's role in the region. *Australian Journal of International Affairs*, 63(4): 550–570.

——. (2013) The International Health Regulations 2005: a case study in global health diplomacy, in T. E. Novotny and I. Kickbusch (eds) *21st Century Health Diplomacy*. Singapore: World Scientific Publishers.

——. and Rushton, S. (2012) The revised International Health Regulations: socialization, compliance and changing norms of global health security. *Global Change, Peace and Security*, 24(1): 57–70.

Kapczynski, A. (2009) Harmonization and its discontents: a case study of TRIPS implementation in India's pharmaceutical sector. *California Law Review*, 97(1571): 1571–1650.

Karnad, B. (1994) India's weak geopolitics and what to do about it, in B. Karnad (ed.), *Future imperilled: India's security in the 1990s and beyond*, pp. New Delhi: Viking.

Kasai, T and Lee, K. (1997) The changing nature of Japanese health sector aid – from the 1970s into the new millennium. Unpublished manuscript.

Kawai, M., Petri, P. and Sisli-Ciamarra, E. (2009) *Asia in global governance: A case for decentralized institutions*. ADBI Working Paper Series, No. 157. Tokyo: Asian Development Bank.

Kay, A. and Williams, O. D. (eds) (2009) *Global health governance: Crisis, institutions and political economy*. Basingstoke: Palgrave Macmillan.

Kelsall, M. S. (2009) The new ASEAN Intergovernmental Commission on Human Rights: toothless tiger or tentative first step? *Asia Pacific Issues*, 90, September.

Kharas, H. (2009) *Development assistance in the 21st century*. Washington DC: Brookings Institution. www.brookings.edu/~/media/Files/rc/papers/2009/11_development_aid_kharas/11_development_aid_kharas.pdf

Kim, J. (2009) Public feeling for science: the Hwang affair and Hwang supporters. *Public Understanding of Science*, 18(6): 670–686.

Kim, S. W., Fidler, D. P. and Ganguly, S. (2009) Eastphalia rising? Asian influence and the fate of human security. *World Policy Journal*, 26(2): 58.

Kimura, H., Sawada, Y. and Mori, Y. (2012) Aid proliferation and economic growth: A cross-country analysis. *World Development*, 40(1): 1–10.

Kirchanski, S. (1993) Protection of US patent rights in developing countries: US efforts to enforce pharmaceutical patents in Thailand. *Loyola Los Angeles International and Comparative Law Journal*, 16: 569.

Kirton, J. and Mannell, J. (2007) The G8 and global health governance, in A. F. Cooper, J. Kirton and T. Schrecker (eds), *Governing global health*, Aldershot: Ashgate Publishing Company. pp. 115–146.

Knack, S. and Rahman, A. (2007) Donor fragmentation and bureaucratic quality in aid recipients. *Journal of Development Economics*, 83(1): 176–197.

Koenig-Archibugi, M. (2002) Mapping global governance, in D. Held and A. McGrew (eds), *Governing globalization*, pp. 46–69. Cambridge: Polity Press.

—— . (2010) Understanding the global dimensions of policy. *Global Policy*, 1(1): 16–28.

Kohama, H. (1995) Japan's development cooperation and economic development in East Asia, in T. Ito and A. O. Krueger (eds), *Growth theories in light of the East Asian experience*, Chicago, IL: University of Chicago Press. pp. 201–226.

Kondo, M. J. (2009) Japan as the catalyst for improving global public health. *Japan Times*, 12 February.

Krasner, S. D. (1982) Structural causes and regime consequences: regimes as intervening variables. *International Organization*, 36(2): 185–205.

Kunii, O. (2007) Parasitology in Japan: The Okinawa Infectious Diseases Initiative. *Trends in Parasitology*, 23(2): 58–62.

Kuroda, K. (2003) Japan-based non-governmental organizations in pursuit of human security. *Japan Forum*, 15(2): 227–250.

Kurokawa, K., Banno, Y., Hara, S. and Kondo, J. (2009) Italian G8 summit: a critical juncture for global health, *The Lancet*, 373(9663): 526–527.

Lambert, A., Sargent, J. D., Glantz, S. A. and Ling, P. M. (2004) How Philip Morris unlocked the Japanese cigarette market: lessons for global tobacco control. *Tobacco Control*, 13: 379–387.

Lamy, P., Chan, M., and Gurry, F. (2010) *Opening remarks: Creating synergies between intellectual property rights and public health.* Speech made in Geneva: World Trade Organization, World Health Organization, World Intellectual Property Organization. www.wto.org/english/tratop_e/trips_e/techsymp_july10_e/techsymp_july10_e.htm#chan

Lando, H., Borrelli, B., Klein, L., Waverley, L., Stillman, F., Kassel, J. and Warner, K. (2005) The landscape in global tobacco control research: a guide to gaining a foothold. *American Journal of Public Health*, 95(6): 939–945.

Lawrence, S. and Collin, J. (2004) Competing with kreteks: transnational tobacco companies, globalization, and Indonesia. *Tobacco Control*, 13: ii96–103.

Leboeuf, A. (2009) *The global fight against avian influenza*. IFRI Health and Environment Report No. 2. Paris: Institut Français des Relations Internationales.

Lee, K. (2009) Understandings of global health governance: the contested landscape, in A. Kay and O. Williams (eds), *Global health governance, crises, institutions and political economy*, pp. 27–41. London: Palgrave Macmillan.

—— . Chagas L, Novotny T (2010) Brazil and the Framework Convention on Tobacco Control: Global health diplomacy as soft power. *PLoS Medicine*, 7(4): e1–5.

—— . and Fidler, D. P. (2007) Avian and pandemic influenza: progress and problems with global health governance. *Global Public Health*, 2(3): 215–234.

——. and Mills, A. (2000) Strengthening governance for global health research. *BMJ*, 321(7264): 775–776.

——. Sridhar, D. and Patel, M. (2009) Bridging the divide: global governance of trade and health. *The Lancet*, 373: 416–422.

——. Kamradt-Scott, A., Yoon, S. W. and Xu, J. Y. (2012) Asian contributions to three instruments of global health governance. *Global Policy*, 3(3): 348–61.

Lencucha, R., Labonte, R. and Rouse, M. (2010) Beyond idealism and realism: Canadian NGO–government relations during the negotiation of the FCTC. *Journal of Public Health Policy*, 31: 74–87.

Leonard, M. (2008) *What does China think?* London: Fourth Estate.

Lerner, J. (1999) 150 years of patent protection. Unpublished manuscript.

Leroy, J. L., Habicht, J. P., Pelto, G. and Bertozzi, S. M. (2007) Current priorities in health research funding and lack of impact on the number of child deaths per year. *American Journal of Public Health*, 97(2): 219–223.

Levi, M. (2009) *Examining the Copenhagen Accord.* Council on Foreign Relations, 21 December, www.cfr.org/publication/21027/examining_the_copenhagen_accord.html (accessed 12 March 2010). New York: Council on Foreign Relations.

Lewis, M. (2006) *Governance and corruption in public health care systems*. Working Paper No. 78. Washington, DC: Center for Global Development.

Li, J. Y., Li, H. P., Li, L., Li, H., Wang, Z., Yang, K., Bao, Z. Y., Zhuang, D. M., Liu, S. Y., Liu, Y. J., Xing, H. and Shao, Y. M. (2005) Prevalence and evolution of drug-resistant HIV-1 variants in Henan, China. *Cell Research*, 15, 843–849, doi:10.1038/sj.cr.7290356

Li, R. (2009) *A rising China and security in East Asia: Identity construction and security discourse*. London: Routledge.

Li, X. and Wu, J. (2009) Practical experience and challenges of China's aid to Africa (zhongguo duifei yuanzhu de shijian jingyan yu mianlin de tiaozhan). *China Agricultural University Journal of Social Sciences Edition*, 26(4): 45–54.

Limpananont, J., Eksaengsri, A., Kijtiwatchakul, K. and Metheny, N. (2009) Thailand: access to AIDS treatment and intellectual property rights' protection in Thailand, in R. Reis, V. Terto Jr. and M. C. Pimenta (eds), *Intellectual property rights and access to ARV medicines: Civil society resistance in the global south*, pp. 137–163. Rio de Janeiro: Brazilian Interdisciplinary AIDS Association (ABIA).

Lo, C. (2010) Values to be added to an 'Eastphalian' order by the emerging China. *Indiana Journal of Global Legal Studies*, 17(1): 13–25.

Lu, C., Schneider, M. T., Gubbins, P., Leach-Kemon, K., Jamison, D. and Murray, C. J. L. (2010) Public financing of health in developing countries: a cross-national systematic analysis. *Lancet*, 375: 1375–1387.

Lum, T., Fischer, H., Gomez-Granger, J. and Leland, A. (2009) *China's foreign aid activities in Africa, Latin America, and Southeast Asia*. Washington, DC: Congressional Research Service.

Lv, F. (2003) Promoting common development in expanding international economic cooperation. Speech at the Fourth Annual Meeting of China Development Forum, 23 March, http://sanpistudents.blogchina.com/blog/4943174.html

Maasho, A. (2011) India offers $5 billion dollars to Africa, keen to boost ties. *The Globe and Mail* (online), 24 May, www.theglobeandmail.com/report-on-business/international-news/india-offers-5-billion-to-africa-keen-to-boost-ties/article2032463 (accessed 28 July 2011).

Mahal, A. and Yip. W. (2008) The health care systems of China and India: performance and future challenges. *Health Affairs*, 27(4): 921–932.

——. Karan, A. and Engelgau, M. (2010) *The economic implications of non-communicable diseases for India: Health, nutrition, and population.* Discussion paper. Washington, DC: The World Bank, http://siteresources.worldbank.org/HEALTHNUTRITIONAND POPULATION/Resources/281627-1095698140167/EconomicImplicationsofNCD forIndia.pdf

McCoy, D., Chand, S. and Sridhar, D. (2009) Global health funding: how much, where it comes from and where it goes. *Health Policy and Planning*, 24(6): 407–417.

McCurry, J. (2008) G8 meeting disappoints on global health. *The Lancet*, 372(9632): 191–194.

McDorman, T. L. (1992) US-Thailand trade disputes: applying section 301 to cigarettes and intellectual property. *Michigan Journal of International Law*, 14: 90.

McLeod, D. A. (1992) US trade pressure and the developing intellectual property law of Thailand, Malaysia and Indonesia. *University of British Columbia Law Review*, 26(343): 343–374.

Mahbubani, K. and Chesterman, S. (2009) *Asia's role in global governance*. Singapore: Lee Kuan Yew School of Public Policy.

Malone, R. E. (2010) China's chances, China's choices in global tobacco control. *Tobacco Control*, 19(1): 1–2.

Mamudu, H. and Glantz, S. (2009) Civil society and the negotiation of the Framework Convention on Tobacco Control. *Global Public Health*, 4(2): 150–168.

——. Hammond, R. and Glantz, S. (2008) Project Cerberus: tobacco industry strategy to crate an alternative to the Framework Convention on Tobacco Control. *American Journal of Public Health*, 98(9): 1630–42.

March, J. G. (1991) Exploration and exploitation in organizational learning. *Organization Science*, (2)1: 71–87.

Masud, N. and Yontcheva, B. (2005) *Does foreign aid reduce poverty? Empirical evidence from nongovernmental and bilateral aid.* IMF Working Paper Wp/05/100. Washington, DC: International Monetary Fund.

Mathers, C. D. and Loncar, D. (2006) Projections of global mortality and burden of disease from 2002 to 2030. *PLoS Medicine*, 3(11): e442.

Matlin, S. A. and Samuels, G. M. (2009) The Global Health Research and Innovation System (GHRIS). *The Lancet*, 374(9702): 1662–1663.

MDBS (2010) *About us*. www.mbdsoffice.com/aboutus.php (accessed 19 March 2010).

Médecins Sans Frontières (2010) *Untangling the web of antiretroviral price reductions*. http://utw.msfaccess.org/ (accessed 24 August 2010).

Meier, C. and Murthy, C. S. R. (2011) *India's growing involvement in humanitarian assistance*. MGPPi Research Paper No. 13. Berlin: Global Public Policy Institute.

Ministers of Foreign Affairs of Brazil, France, Indonesia, Norway, Senegal, South Africa, and Thailand (2007) Oslo Ministerial Declaration – global health: a pressing foreign policy issue of our time. *The Lancet*, 369: 1373–1378.

Ministry of Public Health (Thailand), and National Health Security Office (Thailand) (2007) *Facts and evidences on the 10 burning issues related to the government use of patents on three patented essential drugs in Thailand: Document to support strengthening of social wisdom on the issue of drug patent.* www.cptech.org/ip/health/c/thailand/thai-cl-white-paper.pdf

Minze, E. D., Tauxe, R. V. and Levine, M. M. (1998) The global resurgence of cholera, in N. Noah and M. O'Mahony (eds), *Communicable disease: Epidemiology and control, 73*, pp. 63–104. Chichester: John Wiley and Sons.

Mishra, P. and Newhouse, D. (2009) Does health aid matter? *Journal of Health Economics*, 28(4): 855–872.

Mitchell, R. B. (2002–2010) *International environmental agreements database project (version 2010.3)*. http://iea.uoregon.edu/ (accessed 15 October 2010).

MOFA, Japan (1987) *Japan's ODA Annual Report 1986*. Tokyo: Association for Promotion of International Cooperation (APIC).

——. (1988) *Japan's ODA Annual Report 1987*. Tokyo: APIC.

——. (1989) *Japan's ODA Annual Report 1988*. Tokyo: APIC.

——. (1992) *Japan's ODA Annual Report 1991*. Tokyo: APIC.

——. (1996) *Japan's ODA Annual Report 1995*. Tokyo: APIC.

——. (2000) Japan's ODA Annual Report 1999. Tokyo: APIC.

——. (2001) *Japan's ODA Annual Report 2000*. Tokyo: APIC.

——. (2001) Japan's ODA White Paper 2001. Tokyo: Ministry of Foreign Affairs, www.mofa.go.jp/policy/oda/white/index.html

——. (2002) Japan's ODA White Paper 2002. Tokyo: Ministry of Foreign Affairs, www.mofa.go.jp/policy/oda/white/index.html

——.(eds) (2003a) *Review of Japan's Official Development Assistance Charter*, www.MOFA.go.jp/policy/oda/reform/review0303.html

——. (2003b) Japan's ODA White Paper 2003. Tokyo: Ministry of Foreign Affairs, www.mofa.go.jp/policy/oda/white/index.html

——. (2007) Japan's ODA White Paper 2007, Japan's International Cooperation. Tokyo: Ministry of Foreign Affairs, www.mofa.go.jp/policy/oda/white/index.html

——. (2008) Japan's ODA White Paper 2008, Japan's International Cooperation. Tokyo: Ministry of Foreign Affairs, www.mofa.go.jp/policy/oda/white/index.html

——. (2009a) Japan's ODA White Paper 2009, Japan's International Cooperation. Tokyo: Ministry of Foreign Affairs, www.mofa.go.jp/policy/oda/white/index.html

——. Japan (eds) (2009b) *The Trust Fund for Human Security: For the 'Human-centered' 21st Century*. Tokyo: Government of Japan, August 2009, www.mofa.go.jp/policy/human_secu/t_fund21.pdf

MOH, the Department of International Cooperation. (2003) Strengthening the implementation of the new strategy to reform the work of health aid to Africa countries: 40 years of the deployment of CMT (jiaqiang shishi xinzhanlue, gaige yuanzhu feizhou yiliao gongzuo: ji zhongguo yuanwai yiliaodui paichu 40 zhounian), *West Asia and Africa*, 5: 15–18.

—— (2009) *International exchange and cooperation in health* (weisheng lingyu de jiaoliu yu hezuo), www.moh.gov.cn/publicfiles/business/cmsresources/mohbgt/. . ./doc3135.doc

Moon, S. (2010) Embedding neoliberalism: global health and the evolution of the global intellectual property regime (1994–2009). Ph.D. dissertation, Harvard University.

Moscow Declaration (2011) First Global Ministerial Conference on Healthy Lifestyles and Noncommunicable Disease Control, Moscow, 28–29 April 2011, www.un.org/en/ga/president/65/issues/moscow_declaration_en.pdf

Muggli, M., Lee, K., Gan, Z., Ebbert, J. and Hurt, R. (2008) Efforts to reprioritise the agenda, in China: British American Tobacco's actions to divert health policy from secondhand smoke to liver disease prevention. *PLoS Medicine*; 5(12): 1729–1736.

NACO (National Aids Control Organization) (2011) *Annual Report 2010–11*, www.nacoonline.org/upload/REPORTS/NACO%20Annual%20Report%202010-11.pdf

National Population and Family Planning Commission of China (2009) *The ceremony of the Chinese donation of medicinal facilities for reproductive health to Uganda was held in Kampala* (zhongguo yuanzhu wuganda shengzhi jiankang yiliao shebei jiaojie yishi zai kanpala juxing), www.npfpc.gov.cn/cn/detail.aspx?articleid=090707091216703828 (accessed 7 July 2009).

Nehru, J. (1961) *India's foreign policy: Selected speeches*. New Delhi: Government of India.

Niu, S. R., Yang, G. H., Chen, Z. M., Wang, J. L., Wang, G. H., He, X. Z., Schoepff, H., Boreham, J., Pan, H.C. and Peto, R. (1998) Emerging tobacco hazards in China: 2. Early mortality results from a prospective study. *BMJ*, 317: 1423–1424.

OECD (1987) *The aid programme of China*. Paris: Organization for Economic Cooperation and Development.

——. *Development co-operation review series, Japan*. Paris: OECD. Various years: 1996, 1999, 2003. www.oecd.org/findDocument/0,2350,en_2649_34603_1_119663_1_1_1,00.html.

——. (2004) *DAC Peer Review: Japan 2003*. Paris: OECD. www.oecd.org/dac/peerreviewsofdacmembers/32285814.pdf

——. (2008) *Debt relief is down: Other ODA rise slightly*, www.oecd.org/document/8/0,3343,en_2649_34447_40381960_1_1_1_1,00.html

OECD (2008) *Scaling up: Aid fragmentation, aid allocation and aid predictability. Report of the 2008 survey of aid allocation policies and indicative forward spending plans*. Paris: Development Assistance Committee. www.oecd.org/dataoecd/37/20/40636926.pdf

Office of the Controller General of Patents, Designs and Trade Marks (2006) *Novartis AG Vs Natco Pharma, 2006, 25 January*. V. Rengasamy, Assistant Controller of Patents and Designs. Mumbai: The Office of the Controller General of Patents, Designs & Trade Marks.

Office of the Preparatory Work for a 30-year History: Exhibition on China's Opening Up (eds) (2008) *Highlights of bilateral economic and trade cooperation* (zhongguo duiwai kaifang 30 zhounian huiguzhan: shuangbian jingmao hezuo dashiji), http://kaifangzhan.mofcom.gov.cn/accessory/dsj_gb.pdf

Ohno, I. (2003) Japan's ODA at a crossroads: striving for a new vision. *Japan Economic Currents*, 31(April): 4–7.

Ollier, P. (2008) Why India's patent battles matter. *Managing Intellectual Property*, 179: 26.

Ooms, G., Decoster, K., Miti, K., Rens, S., Van Leemput, L., Vermeiren, P. and Van Damme, W. (2010) Crowding out: are relations between international health aid and government health funding too complex to be captured in averages only? *Lancet*, 375(9723): 1403–1405.

Orr, R. M. (1990) *The emergence of Japan's foreign aid power*. New York: Columbia University Press.

Oslo Ministerial Declaration. (2007) Oslo Ministerial Declaration – global health: a pressing foreign policy issue of our time. *The Lancet*, 369(9570): 1373–1378.

Park, C. and Menghaney, L. (2010) TRIPS flexibilities: the scope of patentability and oppositions to patents in India, in G. Krikorian and A. Kapczynski (eds), *Access to knowledge in the age of intellectual property*, pp. 415–434. New York: Zone Books.

Patel, N. (2011) India to create a central foreign aid agency. *The Guardian*, 26 July, www.guardian.co.uk/global-development/2011/jul/26/india-foreign-aid-agency (accessed 26 January 2012).

Payne, A.M. (1953) The influenza programme of WHO. *Bulletin of the World Health Organization*, 8(5–6): 755–792.

People's Health Movement (2008) *Global Health Watch 2: An alternative world health report*. London: Zed Books.

Petryna, A. (2005) Ethical variability: drug development and globalizing clinical trials. *American Ethnologist*, 32(2): 183–197.

Philip Morris International (n.d.) *Summary observations*, LTDL, Bates No. 2085283704-3709. http://legacy.library.ucsf.edu/tid/pcm10c00/pdf

Press Information Bureau, Ministry of Commerce and Industry, Government of India. (2005) *Important changes incorporated in the Patents (Amendment) Bill, 2005 as compared to the Patents (Amendment) Bill, 2003*, 23 March, http://pib.nic.in/release/release.asp?relid=8096

Price, A. (2000) Japan tobacco opposes core points of tobacco control accord. *Japan Economic Newswire*, 13 October, http://legacy.library.ucsf.edu/tid/uzn41c00/pdf

Price, G. (2005) *The changing landscape of official humanitarian donorship: The changing landscape of official humanitarian aid. India's official humanitarian aid programme*, HPG background paper. London: Chatham House.

——. (2011) *For the global good: India's developing international role*. London: Chatham House.

Ravishankar, N., Gubbins, P., Cooley, R. J., Leach-Kemon, K., Michaud, C. M., Jamison, D. T. and Murray, C. J. (2009) Financing of global health: tracking development assistance for health from 1990 to 2007. *Lancet*, 373(9681): 2113–2124.

Reddy, S. and Gupta, P. (eds) (2004) *Report on tobacco control in India*. Delhi: Ministry of Health and Family Welfare, Government of India.

——. Arora, M. and Yadav, A. (eds) (2008) *A comparative analysis of WHO Framework Convention on Tobacco Control and the Indian laws regulating tobacco*. Delhi: Ministry of Health and Family Welfare, Government of India and Public Health Foundation of India.

Relax News (2009) Japan, China, S. Korea sign first memorandum on food safety. *The Independent*, www.independent.co.uk/life-style/health-and-families/health-news/japan-china-skorea-sign-first-memorandum-on-food-safety-1826301.html (accessed 23 April 2010).

Revenga, A., Over, M., Masaki, E., Peerapatanapokin, W., Gold, J., Tangcharoensathien, V. and Thanprasertsuk, S. (2006) *The economics of effective AIDS treatment: Evaluating policy options for Thailand*. Washington, DC: The World Bank.

Reynolds, C. (1999) The fourth-largest market in the world. *Tobacco Control*, 8: 89–91.

Rix, A. (1980) *Japan's economic aid: Policy-making and politics*. London: Croom Helm.

——. (1990) *Japan's aid program: A new global agenda*. International Development Issues No. 12, Australian Development Assistance Bureau. Canberra: Australian Government Publishing Service.

——. (1993) *Japan's foreign aid challenge: Policy reform and aid leadership*. London and New York: Routledge.

Rottingen, J. A., Marchiori Buss, P., Davies, S. and Touré, O. (2009) Global-health research architecture – time for mergers? *Lancet*, 373(9659): 193–195.

Rowlands, D. (2008) *Emerging donors in international development assistance: A synthesis report*. Ottawa, International Development Research Centre, Partnership and Business Development Division.

Ruggie, J. G. (2004) Reconstituting the global public domain – issues, actors, and practices. *European Journal of International Relations*, 10(4): 499–531.

Rust, S. M. (1992) US–Thai relations during the 1980s: the issue of intellectual property rights. *US Air Force Academy Journal of Legal Studies*, 3: 161.

Rweyemamu, M., Otim-Nape, W. and Serwadda, D. (2006) *Foresight, infectious diseases: Preparing for the future Africa*. London: Office of Science and Innovation.

S. T. Lee Project on Global Governance Study Group on Global Health Governance. (2009) *Overview and Guidance for Participants of GHG Study Group Workshop, Bellagio, Italy, September*.

Sack, D. A., Brooks, V., Behan, M., Cravioto, A., Kennedy, A., Ijsselmuiden, C. and Sewankambo, N. (2009) Improving international research contracting. *Bulletin of the World Health Organisation* 87(7): 487–487A.

Sagar, R. (2009) What kind of power will India become? *International Affairs*, 85(4): 801–816.

Sahu, S. K. (1998) *Technology transfer, dependence, and self-reliant development in the Third World: The pharmaceutical and machine tool industries in India*. Westport, CT: Praeger.

Sakboon, M. (1999) Bid to help poor fight AIDS virus – drug agency seeks to cut costs. *The Nation (Thailand)*, 13 November, http://lists.essential.org/pharm-policy/msg00306.html

Salter, B., Cooper, M. and Dickens, A. (2006) China and the global stem cell bioeconomy: an emerging political strategy? *Regenerative Medicine*, 1(5): 671–683.

——. Cooper, M., Dickens, A. and Cardo, V. (2007) Stem cell science in India: emerging economies and the politics of globalization. *Regenerative Medicine*, 2(1): 75–89.

Samet, J.M. and Wipfli, H. (2009) Unfinished business in tobacco control. *Journal of the American Medical Association*, 302: 681–682.

Sasuga, K. (2007) Global governance, Japan and the World Bank, in G. Hook and H. Dobson (eds), *Global governance and Japan: The institutional architecture*, pp. 110–125. London: Routledge.

Sato, J., Shiga, H., Kobayashi, T. and Kondoh, H. (2010) *How do 'emerging' donors differ from 'traditional' donors? An institutional analysis of foreign aid in Cambodia*. Working Paper No. 2, March 2010. Tokyo: Japan International Cooperation Agency Research Institute.

Satomura, K., Iwanaga, S., Noami, M., Sakamoto, R., Kusaka, K. and Nakahara, T. (2008) The Framework Convention on Tobacco Control (FCTC) and Japanese anti-tobacco measures. *Tobacco Induced Diseases*, 4(3): 1–3.

Schnirring, L. (2008) Indonesia claims wide support for virus-sharing stance, www.cidrap.umn.edu/cidrap/content/influenza/avianflu/news/may2708 sharing.html (accessed 8 July 2009).

Scoones, I. and Forster, P. (2009) *The international response to highly pathogenic avian influenza: Science, policy and politics*. Brighton: STEPS Centre Working Paper No. 10.

SEARO. (2000) *Regional Committee, 53rd session, provisional agenda, item 16*. New Delhi: World Health Organization.

Seattle Times (2007) Gates Foundation's malaria effort foretells new role for Seattle. *Seattle Times*, 23 September.

Security and Prosperity Partnership of North America (2007) *North American plan for avian and pandemic influenza*. Washington, DC: Security and Prosperity Partnership of North America.

Sedyaningsih, E. R., Isfandari, S., Soendoro, T. and Supari, S. F. (2008) Towards mutual trust, transparency and equity in virus-sharing mechanism: the avian influenza case of Indonesia. *Annals Academy of Medicine*, 37(6): 482–488.

Sell, S. K. (2003) *Private power, public law: The globalization of intellectual property rights*. New York: Cambridge University Press.

Sen, A. (2011) The quality of life: India vs. China. *The New York Review of Books*, 12 May, www.nybooks.com/articles/archives/2011/may/12/quality-life-india-vs-china/?pagination=false (accessed 19 February 2012).

Shearer, J. C., Stack, M. L., Richmond, M. R., Bear, A. P. and Hajjeh, R. A. (2010) Accelerating policy decisions to adopt *Haemophilus Influenzae* Type B vaccine: a global, multivariable analysis. *PLoS Med*, 7(3): e1000249.

Shimkhada, R. and Peabody, J. W. (2003) Tobacco control in India. *Bulletin of the World Health Organization*, 81(1): 48–52.

Silkavute, P. (2008) *Thai APEIR network coordination and collaboration: Countries learning lessons and thinking ahead*. Nonthaburi: APEIR.

Simon, H. A. (1962) The architecture of complexity. *Proceedings of the American Philosophical Society*, 106(6): 467–482.

Smith, T. (2000) *FCTC public hearings and 1st INB session*. JTI, LTDL, 3 November, Bates No. 524408630-8635, http://legacy.library.ucsf.edu/tid/oev03c00/pdf

Smith, R. D. and Mackellar, L. (2007) Global public goods and the global health agenda: problems, priorities and potential. *Global Health*, 3: 9.

Smith, R., Beaglehole, R., Woodward, D. and Drager, N. (eds) (2003) *Global public goods for health: Health economics and public health perspectives*. Oxford: Oxford University Press.

Smokers News. (2009) BAT increases its market share in Indonesia. *Smokers News*, 25 June.

Sridhar, D. (2009) Global health: WHO can lead? *The World Today*, 65(2): 25–26.

——. (2010) Seven challenges in international development assistance for health. *Journal of Law, Medicine and Ethics*, 38(3): 459–469.

——. and Gostin, L.O. (2011) Reforming the World Health Organization. *Journal of the American Medical Association*, 305(15): 1585–1586.

——. Khagram, S. and Pang, T. (2008–2009) Are existing governance structures equipped to deal with today's global health challenges – towards systematic coherence in scaling up. *Global Health Governance*, 2(2): 1–25.

——. and Woods, N. (2010) Are there simple conclusions on how to channel health funding? *The Lancet*, 375(9723): 1326–1328.

Stavins, R. (2009) *What hath Copenhagen wrought? A preliminary assessment of the Copenhagen Accord*. Harvard University Belfer Center for Science and International Affairs, 20 December, http://belfercenter.ksg.harvard.edu/analysis/stavins/?p=464 (accessed 12 March 2010).

Stevenson, M. A. and Cooper, A. F. (2009) Overcoming the constraints of state sovereignty: global health governance in Asia. *Third World Quarterly*, 30(7): 1379–1394.

STMA Working Group. (2006) *Countermeasures against the FCTC and approaches to deal with the impact on the tobacco industry in China*. Beijing: Economic and Scientific Press.

——. (2004) *Research report on the analysis of advantages and disadvantages of impacts on the tobacco economy in China from the fulfillment of obligations under the FCTC*. Beijing: Economic and Scientific Press.

——. Working Group. (2006) Revised suggestions on Chair's text of the Intergovernmental Negotiation Body 4 – second group. In STMA, *Countermeasures against the FCTC and Approaches to Deal with the Impact on the Tobacco Industry in China*, pp. 192–196. Beijing: Economic and Scientific Press.

Strom, S. and Fleischer-Black, M. (2003) Company's vow to donate cancer drug falls short. *The New York Times*, 5 June, www.nytimes.com/2003/06/05/business/05DRUG.html?scp=1andsq=novartis%20strom%20fleischer%20bacandst=cse

Stuenkel, O. (2010) *Responding to global development challenges: Views from Brazil and India*. German Development Institute Discussion Paper. Bonn: German Development Institute.

Swiss Commission for Research Partnership with Developing Countries (1998) *Guidelines for Research in Partnership with Developing Countries*. Bern: KFPE.

Szlezák, N. and Moon, S. (2010) Towards a new set of norms in global pharmaceutical R&D: Changing institutions, changing players and the role of Asia. Working Paper for the S.T. Lee Project on Global Governance. Singapore: Centre on Asia and Globalisation, Study Group on Global Health Governance (GHG).

’t Hoen, E. (2009) *The global politics of pharmaceutical monopoly power: Drug patents, access, innovation, and the application of the WTO Doha Declaration on TRIPS and public health*. Diemen, The Netherlands: AMB Press.

Takemi, K., Jimba, M., Ishii, S., Katsuma, Y. and Nakamura, Y. (2008) Human security approach for global health. *The Lancet*, 372(9632): 13–14.

Tan, Y., Lee, K. and Pang, T. (2012) Global health governance and the rise of Asia. *Global Policy*, 3(3): 324–335.

Tantivess, S., Kessomboon, N. and Laongbua, C. (2008) *Introducing government use of patents on essential medicines in Thailand, 2006–2007: Policy analysis with key lessons learned and recommendations*. Nonthaburi: International Health Policy Program, Ministry of Health.

Thai Health Promotion Foundation. (2010) *About us*, http://en.thaihealth.or.th/about (accessed 20 March 2010).

Thompson, D. (2005) China’s soft power in Africa: from the ‘Beijing Consensus’ to health diplomacy. *China Brief*, 5(21), www.jamestown.org/programs/chinabrief/single/?tx_ttnews%5Btt_news%5D=30973&tx_ttnews%5BbackPid%5D=195&no_cache=1

Thompson, G. (2009) 80 million a day. *ABC News*, 1 January, www.abc.net.au/foreign/content/2009/s2673564.htm

TICAD/UNDP Africa Bureau. (2012) *About TICAD*. www.ticad.net/about.shtml.

Treerutkuarkul, A. (2010) HIV/AIDS drug licence extended. *The Bangkok Post*, 3 August, www.bangkokpost.com/news/health/189154/hiv-aids-drugs-licence-extended

Trust, W. (2005) *Strategic plan 2005–2010: Making a difference*. London: The Wellcome Trust.

Tucker, B. (1999) From arms race to abolition: the evolving norm against biological and chemical warfare, in S. D. Drell, A. D. Sofaer and G. D. Wilson (eds), *The new terror: Facing the threat of biological and chemical weapons*, pp. 205–206. Stanford, CA: Hoover Institution Press.

Tucker, T. J. and Makgoba, M. W. (2008) Public health. Public–private partnerships and scientific imperialism. *Science*, 320(5879): 1016–1017.

Ulrich, A., Waxman, A., de Costa e Silva, L., Bettcher, D., Vesta, G.l. and Sepulveda, C. (2004) Cancer prevention in the political arena: the WHO perspective. *Annals of Oncology*, 15(S4): 249–256.

United Nations. (2006) *Delivering as one: Report of the Secretary-General’s High Level Panel*. New York: United Nations.

——. (2009a) *The Millennium Development Goals report*. New York: United Nations.

——. (2009b). *United Nations Framework Convention on Climate Change. Copenhagen Accord*, FCCC/CP/2009/L.7, 18 December. New York: United Nations.

——. (2010) *Treaty Collection, Status of Treaties*. New York: United Nations, http://treaties.un.org/Pages/ParticipationStatus.aspx

——. (2011) Political declaration of the high-level meeting of the General Assembly on the prevention and control of non-communicable diseases. UNGA 66TH session, Doc. A/RES/66/2 New York, 19 September, www.who.int/nmh/events/un_ncd_summit 2011/political_declaration_en.pdf

UN Secretary-General. (2009) *Global health and foreign policy: strategic opportunities and challenges – note by the Secretary-General*, A/64/365, 23 September. New York: United Nations.

UNAIDS (2005) *The 'Three Ones' in action: Where we are and where we go from here*. Geneva: UNAIDS. http://data.unaids.org/Publications/IRC-pub06/jc935-3onesinaction_en.pdf

United Nations Children's Fund (2000) *UNICEF annual report*. New York: United Nations Children's Fund.

——. (2001) *UNICEF annual report*. New York: United Nations Children's Fund, www.unicef.org/publications/files/pub_ar00_en.pdf

——. (2002) *UNICEF annual report*. New York: United Nations Children's Fund, www.unicef.org/publications/files/Annual_Report_2001.pdf

——. (2003) *UNICEF annual report*. New York: United Nations Children's Fund, www.unicef.org/publications/files/pub_ar02_en.pdf

——. (2004) *UNICEF annual report*. New York: United Nations Children's Fund, www.unicef.org/publications/files/pub_ar03_en.pdf

——. (2005) *UNICEF annual report*. New York: United Nations Children's Fund, www.unicef.org/publications/files/UNICEFAnnualReport2004_eng.pdf

——. (2006) *UNICEF annual report*. New York: United Nations Children's Fund, www.unicef.org/publications/files/pub_ar2005_en.pdf

——. (2007) *UNICEF annual report*. New York: United Nations Children's Fund, www.unicef.org/publications/files/Annual_Report_2006.pdf

——. (2010) *Report on the global AIDS epidemic 2010*. Geneva: UNAIDS.

United Nations Development Program (2011) *Human development index*. http://hdr.undp.org/en/data/trends/ (accessed 25 July 2011).

United Nations Economic and Social Council (2000) E/C.12/2000/4 *General comment no. 4: The right to the highest attainable standard of health*. Committee on Economic, Social and Cultural Rights, Geneva, 25 April–12 May, www.unhchr.ch/tbs/doc.nsf/(symbol)/E.C.12.2000.4.En (accessed 6 August 2012)

United Nations General Assembly (2011) Uniting for universal access: Towards zero new HIV infections, zero discrimination and zero AIDS-related deaths. Report of the Secretary-General, Doc. A/65/797. New York, 28 March, www.unaids.org/en/media/unaids/contentassets/documents/document/2011/A-65-797_English.pdf

UNSIC (2008) *Contributing to One World, One Health: A strategic framework for reducing risks of infectious diseases at the animal–human–ecosystems interface*. New York: A Joint Publication by FAO, OIE, WHO, UNSIC, UNICEF, and the World Bank, UNSIC.

US National Intelligence Council. (2008) *Global trends 2025: A transformed world*. Washington, DC: US National Intelligence Council.

Väyrynen, R. (2001) Sovereignty, globalization and transnational social movements. *International Relations of the Asia-Pacific*, 1: 227–246.

Wagatsuma, T. (1989) Japan's development assistance in health, in M. R. Reich and E. Marui (eds), *International cooperation for health: Problems, prospects, and priorities*, pp. 372–381. Dover: Auburn House Publishing Company.

Waikagul, J. (2006) Southeast Asian tropical medicine and parasitology network. *Parasitology International*, 55(Supplement): S297–S300.

Waldby, C. and Salter, B. (2008) Global governance in human embryonic stem cell science: standardization and bioethics in research and patenting. *Studies in Ethics, Law and Technology*, 2(1): ISSN (Online) 1941-6008, DOI: 10.2202/1941-6008.1031, May 2008.

Wall Street Journal (2009) ASEAN's toothless council. 22 July, http://online.wsj.com/article/SB10001424052970203517304574303592053848748.html (accessed 12 March 2010).

Wan, M. (1995) Spending strategies in world politics: how Japan has used its economic power in the past decade. *International Studies Quarterly*, 39: 85–108.

Wang, N. (2009) Chinese foreign health aid (1963–2003): taking Jiangsu as the center (zhongguo yuanwai yiliaodui yanjiu (1963–2003): yi Jiangsu wei zhongxin). Master's Thesis, College of History Culture, Central China Normal University.

Wang, X., Hu, Y. and Ping, J. (2009) China: multi-sector approaches on improving access to ARVs in China, in R. Reis, V. Terto Jr. and M. C. Pimenta (eds), *Intellectual property rights and access to ARV medicines: Civil society resistance in the global south*, pp. 82–109. Rio de Janeiro: Brazilian Interdisciplinary AIDS Association (ABIA).

Wang, Y. C. H. (2004) The major influence of the FCTC on the tobacco industry in China and consequent suggestions. *Economic Research Reference*, 1857.

Waning, B., Diedrichsen, E. and Moon, S. (2010) A lifeline to treatment: the role of Indian generic manufacturers in supplying antiretroviral medicines to developing countries. *Journal of the International AIDS Society*, 13(35). doi:doi:10.1186/1758-2652-13-35, www.jiasociety.org/content/13/1/35

Ward, H. (2006) International linkages and environmental sustainability: the effectiveness of the regime network. *Journal of Peace Research*, 43: 149–166.

Watal, J. (2001) *Intellectual property rights in the WTO and developing countries*. The Hague: Kluwer Law International.

White House. (2009a) *US–China joint statement*, 17 November. Washington, DC: The White House.

——. (2009b) *Fact sheet: US–India cooperation to protect the health of their people*, 24 November. Washington, DC: The White House.

Williamson, C. R. (2008) Foreign aid and human development: the impact of foreign aid to the health sector. *Southern Economic Journal*, 75: 188–207.

Wilson, D., Cawthorne, P., Ford, N. and Aongsonwang, S. (1999) Global trade and access to medicines: AIDS treatments in Thailand. *The Lancet*, 354(9193): 1893–1895.

Wisartsakul, W. (2004) *Civil society movement to revoke the Thai patent on ddI* (N. Grant Trans.), Bangkok: Médecins Sans Frontières-Belgium.

Wolf, S. (2007) Does aid improve public service delivery? *Weltwirtschaftliches Archiv*, 143(4): 650–672.

Woods, N. (2008) Whose aid? Whose influence? China, emerging donors and the silent revolution in development assistance. *International Affairs*, 84(6): 1205–1221.

World Bank. (n.d.) *The World Bank and Japan: 'Working for a world free of poverty'*, (brochure). Tokyo: World Bank Tokyo Office.

World Health Organization (1983) *International health regulations (1969)*. Third annotated edition. Geneva: World Health Organization.

——. (1995a) *WHA48.13 Communicable diseases prevention and control: New, emerging, and re-emerging infectious diseases*, http://policy.who.int/(accessed 25 November 2006).

——. (1995b) *WHA48.7 Revision and updating of the International Health Regulations*, http://policy.who.int/ (accessed 25 November 2006).

——. (1996) *World Health Report, 1996: Fighting disease, fostering development*. Geneva: World Health Organization.

——. (1999) *WHO International Conference on Tobacco and Health, Kobe, Avoiding the Tobacco Epidemic among Women and Youth*, November 1999, LTDL, Bates No. 321675178-321675248. http://legacy.library.ucsf.edu/tid/yxr53a99/pdf

——. (2000a) *A framework for global outbreak alert and response*. Geneva: World Health Organization.

——. (2000b) *Intergovernmental Negotiating Body on the FCTC, first session, provisional summary record of the fourth meeting, Geneva, 17 October 2000*. http://legacy.library.ucsf.edu/tid/zyb53a99/pdf

——. (2000c) *Intergovernmental negotiating body on the FCTC, first session, provisional summary record of the second meeting, Geneva, 16 October 2000*. http://legacy.library.ucsf.edu/tid/ooc24a99/pdf

——. (2000d) *Intergovernmental Negotiating Body on the FCTC, first session, Geneva, provisional agenda item 8, comments of the fifty-third World Health Assembly on the provisional texts of proposed draft elements of the framework convention on tobacco control (extracts from document WHA53/2000/REC/3, sixth and seventh meetings of Committee A)*, 14 August. http://apps.who.int/gb/fctc/PDF/inb1/e1inb2a1.pdf

——. (2001) *Intergovernmental Negotiating Body on the FCTC, third session, activities since the previous session, progress report, Geneva, 16 October*. http://legacy.library.ucsf.edu/tid/yer80d00/pdf

——. (2002a) *Intergovernmental Negotiating Body on the FCTC, fourth session, activities since the third session, Geneva, 15 March*. http://apps.who.int/gb/fctc/PDF/inb4/einb44a1.pdf

——. (2002b) *Intergovernmental Negotiating Body on the FCTC, fifth session, Geneva, activities since the previous session, regional intersessional meetings on the WHO Framework Convention on Tobacco Control, Doc. A/FCTC/INB5/4 Add.1, 4 October*. http://apps.who.int/gb/fctc/PDF/inb5/einb54a1.pdf

——. (2003a) *Revision of the International Health Regulations: severe acute respiratory syndrome (SARS). Report by the Secretariat. Document: A56/48: 4–5*. Geneva: World Health Organization.

——. (2003b) *Severe acute respiratory syndrome (SARS): Status of the outbreak and lessons for the immediate future, unmasking a new disease*. Geneva: World Health Organization.

——. (2003c) *The World Health Organization Framework Convention on Tobacco Control*. Geneva: World Health Organization.

——. (2004a) *Consultation on the revision of the International Health Regulations (IHR) in the western Pacific region*. Manila: Regional Office for the Western Pacific.

——. (2004b) *International Health Regulations: Report of the first regional consultation of national IHR focal points on the revision of International Health Regulations, New Delhi, India, 13–14 April 2004*. New Delhi: Regional Office for South-East Asia.

——. (2004c) *The Mexico Statement on health research: Knowledge for better health: Strengthening health systems*. Geneva: World Health Organization.

——. (2006) *Conference of the parties to the WHO Framework Convention on Tobacco Control. First session, Geneva, 6–17 February 2006, summary records of committees, reports of committees*. http://apps.who.int/gb/fctc/PDF/cop1/cop1_06_cd_procesverbauxrapportscommissions-en.pdf

——. (2007a) *Conference of the parties to the WHO Framework Convention on Tobacco Control. Second session, Bangkok, 30 June–6 July 2007, summary records of committees, reports of committees*. http://apps.who.int/gb/fctc/PDF/cop2/COP2_07_CDSummaryrecords-en.pdf

——. (2007b) *Everybody's business: Strengthening Health Systems to Improve Health Outcomes. WHO's Framework for Action*. Geneva: World Health Organization.

——. (2007c) *Intergovernmental meeting on pandemic influenza preparedness: Sharing of influenza viruses. List of participants*. Document: A/PIP/IGM/DIV/2_Rev.1. Geneva: World Health Organization.

——. (2007d) *WHA56.28 Revision of the International Health Regulations*, www.who.int/gb/e/index.html (accessed 23 January 2007).

——. (2007e) *The World Health Report 2007: A safer future: global public health security in the 21st century*. Geneva: World Health Organization.

——. (2008a) *Call for applications: candidates for expert roster*, www.searo.who.int/en/Section10_14455.htm (accessed 24 April 2010).

——. (2008b). *Global strategy and plan of action on public health, innovation and intellectual property*. Resolution 61.21, Sixty-first Congress. Geneva: World Health Organization.

——. (2008c) *Intergovernmental negotiating body on a protocol on illicit trade in tobacco products, first session, summary records, Geneva, 11–16 February*. http://apps.who.int/gb/fctc/PDF/it1/FCTC_INB-IT_REC1-en.pdf

——. (2008d) *Report of WHO's Tobacco-Free Initiative on its activities undertaken specifically on the implementation of the WHO Framework Convention on Tobacco Control* (decision FCTC/COP2(10), http://apps.who.int/gb/fctc/PDF/cop3/FCTC_COP3_13-en.pdf

——. (2008e) *The International Health Regulations (2005)*, 2nd edn. Geneva: World Health Organization, 2008.

——. (2009a) *Global health and foreign policy: strategic opportunities and challenges. Background paper for the Secretary-General's report on global health and foreign policy, 11 May*. Geneva: World Health Organization.

——. (2009b) *Human resources: annual report, report by the Secretariat for the sixty-second World Health Assembly, 14 May 2009*. Provisional agenda item 18.2. http://apps.who.int/gb/ebwha/pdf_files/A62/A62_34-en.pdf

——. (2009c) *Protecting health from climate change: Connecting science, policy, and people*. Geneva: World Health Organization.

——. (2009d) *WHO global influenza surveillance network*, www.who.int/csr/disease/influenza/surveillance/en (accessed 7 July 2009).

——. (2010a) China wrestles with tobacco control. An interview with Dr Yang Gonghuan. *Bulletin of the World Health Organization*, 351–352.

——. (2010b) *Global status report on non-communicable diseases*.

——. (2010c) *Implementation of the International Health Regulations (2005): Report by the Director-General*. Document: A63/5, http://apps.who.int/gb/ebwha/pdf_files/WHA63/A63_5-en.pdf (accessed 24 April 2010).

——. (2010d) *International Health Regulations (IHR): Activities*. www.who.int/ihr/activities/en/index.html (accessed 22 April 2010).

——. (2010e) *Scale of Assessments 2010–2011, report by the Director-General for the sixty-third World Health Assembly*, Provisional agenda item 15.4, 16 February. http://apps.who.int/gb/e/e_wha63.html

——. (2010f) *Third Regional Meeting of National IHR Focal Points, Dhaka, Bangladesh, 15–17 February 2010: Draft Recommendations*. www.searo.who.int/LinkFiles/BCT_Draft_Recommendations15feb2010.pdf (accessed 24 April 2010).

——. (2010g) *World Health Report 2010*, www.who.int/whr/2010/en/index.html

——. (2011) *World Health Statistics 2011*. Geneva: Switzerland, www.who.int/gho/publications/world_health_statistics/2011/en/index.html

——. (2012) Global Influenza Surveillance and Response System (GISRS) www.who.int/influenza/gisrs_laboratory/en/index.html (accessed 2 October 2012).

World Intellectual Property Organization. (2010) *A medium term strategic plan for WIPO, 2010–2015: First draft presented to member states by the Director General on May 27, 2010*. Geneva: WIPO. www.wipo.int/export/sites/www/about-wipo/en/pdf/mtsp.pdf

World Trade Organization (2001) *Declaration on the TRIPS Agreement and Public Health*, WT/MIN(01)/DEC/2. Geneva: World Trade Organization.

—— . (2002) Ministerial Declaration on the TRIPS Agreement and Public Health, WT/MIN(01)/DEC/2, 41 I.L.M. 746.

WPRO. (2005) *WPR/RC56.R4: Asia Pacific strategy for emerging diseases. WPRO resolution WPR/RC56.R4*. www.wpro.who.int/rcm/en/archives/rc56/rc_resolutions/wpr_rc56_r04.htm (accessed 22 March 2010).

——. (2010) *Countries reaffirm commitment to health security*. www.wpro.who.int/rcm/en/rc61/press_releases/pr_20101013.htm (accessed 21 October 2010

Xinhuanet. (2007) *WHO urges Indonesia to share live H5N1 virus samples*, www.xinhuanet.com/english/home.htm

Xinhuanet. (2009) Chinese medical team for foreign aid (zhongguo yuanwai yiliaodui, xinhua wang), www.xinhuanet.com/english/home.htm

Yan, W. (2010) Patent conditions amended for drugs. *The China Daily*, 5 February.

Yanagihara, T. and Emig, A. (1991) An overview of Japan's foreign aid, in S. Islam (ed.), *Yen for development: Japanese foreign aid and the politics of burden-sharing*, pp. 37–69. New York: Council on Foreign Relations Press.

Yang, Q. (2009) Health messenger: 41-year history of Zhengjiang medical team to foregin countries (jiankang shizhe: Zhejing yuanwai yiliaodui qingqing feizhou 41 nian, Jinrizaobao). *Today Morning News*, 3 October.

Zacher, M. and Keefe, T. (2008) *The politics of global health governance, United by contagion*. London: Palgrave Macmillan.

Zhang, F., Dou, Z., Ma, Y., Zhao, Y., Liu, Z., Bulterys, M. and Chen, R. Y. (2009) Five-year outcomes of the China national free antiretroviral treatment program. *Annals of Internal Medicine*, 151(4): 241–251. www.annals.org/cgi/content/abstract/151/4/241

Zhao, B. (2006) *Analysis of focal issues in negotiations on the formulation and adoption of the FCTC*. Beijing: State Tobacco Monopoly Administration.

Zhou, H. (2008) Chinese foreign aid and 30 years of opening up (zhongguo duiwai yuanzhu yu gaige kaifang 30 nian, shijie jingji yu zhengzhi). *World Economics and Politics*, 11: 33–43.

Zhou R. (2004) Improve cognition and take measures to effectively reply to the FCTC. *Tobacco Science and Research*, 22.

—— . and Cheng, Y. Z. (2006) List of participants of the working group meeting, in STMA, *Countermeasures against the FCTC and approaches to deal with the impact on the tobacco industry in China*. Beijing: Economic and Scientific Press.

Index

Locators shown in *italics* refer to figures, tables and boxes.